Suckle · Sleep
Thrive

Breastfeeding Success through Understanding
Your Baby's Cues and Unique Temperament

Andrea Herron, RN, MN, CPNP, IBCLC
Lisa Rizzo, BS

Foreword by Phyllis Klaus, LMFT, LMSW
Photography by Lisa Maksoudian

Praeclarus Press, LLC
©2019 Andrea Herron and Lisa Rizzo. All rights reserved.

www.PraeclarusPress.com

Praeclarus Press, LLC
2504 Sweetgum Lane
Amarillo, Texas 79124 USA
806-367-9950
www.PraeclarusPress.com

DISCLAIMER

The information contained in this publication is advisory only and is not intended to replace sound clinical judgment or individualized patient care. The authors disclaim all warranties, whether expressed or implied, including any warranty as the quality, accuracy, safety, or suitability of this information for any particular purpose.

Any advice found in this book is not a substitute for medical advice from your healthcare provider. Some of the names of mothers and babies that appear in the text have been changed to protect their privacy.

ISBN: 978-1-946665-20-1

Cover Design: Ken Tackett
Cover Photo: Lisa Maksoudian
Developmental Editing: Kathleen Kendall-Tackett
Copyediting: Chris Tackett
Layout & Design: Nelly Murariu

To Ruth Wester for
helping babies all over the world.

CONTENTS

Foreword

by Phyllis Klaus, LMFT, LMSW

Every once in a while, a book comes along that can fill a void. This book, *Suckle, Sleep, Thrive*, based on over 40 years of experience, addresses almost every concern that a mother may have as she takes on the role of nourishing and nurturing her baby. The issues facing new parents, both in their development as parents and the baby's enormously busy development in every dimension, is explored.

I'm very impressed with the clarity and the depth in which this book describes the intricacies of what is involved in the newborn's abilities to adjust to the world outside the womb. Therefore, when holding your newborn for the first time and having already become acquainted with the knowledge of what delights await you, these first moments of meeting will have a deeper, richer meaning. Reading this book will apprise you of little actions that you may otherwise miss. It's a puzzle to unravel at times, but it is also a joy just to see how your baby responds through facial expressions, body movements, sounds, and hundreds of little actions that connote the myriad of needs and emotions that the baby is attempting to express.

Having been imbued with the tender art and delight of baby watching by my late husband, Dr. Marshall Klaus, a very kind, sensitive, and aware neonatologist, imagine my delight when I first read *Suckle, Sleep, Thrive* by Pediatric Nurse Andrea Herron and journalist Lisa Rizzo. Herron and Rizzo have taken the art of baby watching, not only to the level of art, but to the level of science and sensitive caretaking.

This book and the incredible descriptions and observations can help parents unlock the mysteries of a baby's needs, emotions, and distinct cues for help and interaction.

I cannot emphasize strongly enough the importance of reading this book before you have a baby and having it nearby after you have a baby. You will find an understanding to almost every action, behavior, response, sound, movement, and distress that your baby shows, and this will prevent a misdiagnosis of your baby's particular activity. This leads to better decisions on how to actually meet the baby's specific needs.

How easy it is to misread the signals the baby is giving and become discouraged or worried that the baby is not getting enough, and stop breastfeeding attempts without fully understanding the situation. There seems to be a disconnect culturally in many situations on how to read what the baby is actually communicating versus what misinterpretation is happening.

Breastfeeding is such a sensitive, personal issue that women, and sometimes caregivers, can too quickly give up. By not understanding how to help a negative situation, caregivers and/or family members may quickly suggest supplementation, which does a major disservice to breastfeeding.

There are sections in this book that describe typical situations, such as traumatic birth or separation from the baby, that may come up, which may convince a new mother to give up breastfeeding. *Suckle, Sleep, Thrive* comes to the rescue by helping the mother recognize what might be interfering and reinfuses the situation with the potential for helpful resolution. The descriptions of other options can often avert a negative situation. Viewing the photos and graphics enhance the information described.

New mothers have an expectation that breastfeeding is natural, easy, and occurs right after birth. But in reality, even for early onset breastfeeding, there are many events that interfere with this natural, human activity. Even for those situations where everything is working ideally, research shows that full-time comfort in breastfeeding can take 10 to 12 weeks to establish. When you understand all the factors that help or hinder breastfeeding, you can be kind to yourself and feel more reassured that the answers will be available.

Phyllis Klaus, LMFT, LMSW is a psychotherapist working with families in the perinatal period for over 40 years. She co-authored *Your Amazing Newborn, Bonding, The Doula Book* and *When Survivors Give Birth*. She is a founder of DONA International and PATTCh (Prevention and Treatment of Traumatic Childbirth).

Preface

by Andrea Herron, RN, MN, CPNP, IBCLC

In the 40 plus years that I've been working with breastfeeding moms, I often notice how mysterious a new baby seems to many parents. They ask, "How do I know when my newborn is hungry? How do I know when my baby is full? How do I know if I have enough milk? What am I doing wrong when he cries? When will we have a schedule?"

Part of the problem mothers have with establishing a successful breastfeeding relationship with their baby are the many rules and schedules they are instructed to follow. They are not shown how to "watch" their baby—to really observe what the infant is telling them through his/her inborn ability to communicate, using natural reflexes and behavioral cues. In general, there seems to be a deficit of common knowledge about what those early cues look and sound like—behaviors that could potentially tell parents exactly what their newborn needs.

Through my past work at the UCLA Marion Davis Pediatric Clinic, I saw that when mothers were more involved with their babies, the children had better life outcomes, were generally healthy, acted out less, and performed better in school. I left UCLA in 1982 with a master's in nursing determined to find a way to help mothers with breastfeeding and infant behavior. Through my graduate studies, I learned how important the breastfeeding relationship is—how it's critical to the long-term physical and mental health of the mother and baby. After graduation, I began a job at the California Public Health Clinic in San Luis Obispo, California and began searching for others who might be interested in promoting breastfeeding. Kathleen Huggins, another clinical nurse specialist, was also interested. Together and with a common purpose, we enrolled in the new UCLA Lactation Consultant Course. In 1983, armed with our crisp new lactation certificates, we set out to change breastfeeding in San Luis Obispo. Little did we know, we were pioneers in the new field of lactation consulting.

At that time, we saw that women who wanted to breastfeed were not succeeding. They lacked correct lactation information and support. Women needed a place to go to get support and resolve breastfeeding problems. The need was so great that Kathleen and I resigned from our jobs and became full-time lactation consultants. We wanted to promote breastfeeding, as well as help mothers and babies individually. One idea was that a book should be written. As we commuted to Los Angeles, we brainstormed and outlined Kathleen's first book, *The Nursing Mother's Companion*. We also developed plans to start a community breastfeeding warmline. Our goal was to educate mothers and physicians, so we could increase breastfeeding rates and start breastfeeding clinics. Kathleen went on to finish the book and I went on to have a baby.

Starting the warmline increased the breastfeeding rates in San Luis Obispo to the highest in California, in the first state survey that was done. Kathleen proceeded to start her hospital breastfeeding clinic. I began the Growing with Baby center located in an old Victorian house in downtown San Luis Obispo. It's been the home of weekly classes and support groups, along with my lactation practice for more than 30 years.

In my day-to-day interaction with breastfeeding mothers, it became apparent how valuable the infant development information I learned and shared over the years was to the beginning parent/infant relationship. Just interpreting infant cues and temperament for the parents seemed to alleviate their stress. Repeatedly, the parents would express that they felt more confident when they understood their baby's communication. The importance of relaying this information was brought home to me when my son was a young baby. My friend and I were sitting and talking while I nursed him. After a while, I could see that his eyes were red, and he was starting to look disorganized. I said to her, "It's time to swaddle him and put him to sleep."

"How do you know that?" she asked. I had to think about it. How did I know this? Because it had been the focus of my training. It's the same response I get from the mothers who come to Growing with Baby. Today's parents are more stressed and isolated than ever before. They need to understand how to watch and learn what their baby is saying. We need another breastfeeding book because there is not a book that addresses normal infant behavior in relation to breastfeeding challenges—real or perceived. Issues, such as mothers restricting their diet, then feeling hungry when their babies are going through normal gassy and fussy stages. When babies aren't understood, their needs may not get met, which can lead to future low self-esteem and all its consequences.

For mothers, there is a preconceived idea that babies should sleep all night and eat on a schedule, reinforced by family, society, media, and hospital instructions. In the hospital, mothers are asked to report each time and the number of minutes their newborn ate. They are told their infant must eat 8 to 10 times for 20 minutes each session. It does not consider different breastmilk storage capacities in mothers, and various infant stomach size, nor the infant's ability to organize—stay awake and alert to feed for long periods. So, it is very confusing to mothers who are looking for instructions after the hospital stay but experiencing a mismatch when it doesn't work with their reality, their anatomy, or their baby.

This book goes beyond traditional breastfeeding books by showing you ways to understand your newborn early-on, during a time that is critical for successfully establishing breastfeeding. It is important that mothers quickly learn this about their baby and understand his way of communicating his needs, so she can figure out how she can tailor her care to any sensitivities the infant might have that affect breastfeeding dynamics and confidence. I hope you can take the first month after birth to really concentrate on yourself and your baby. Watch your newborn closely and try to answer, "what is my baby trying to tell me? What does this baby want?" When your baby is looking around with his mouth open, watch his subtle cues instead of the clock. If it has only been 60 minutes but his little mouth is open and searching, realize that it is okay to feed the baby, despite what your well-meaning family might say. When you bring your baby to the breast, you will learn by his response whether he was hungry or not. This book will teach you each of these cues and behaviors. For example, in the above scenario, the response you might see to confirm hunger is that the baby sucks and swallows vigorously at the breast, then slowly becomes relaxed before coming off and looking at you with a sweet, contented smile.

My wish for all mothers is that they learn their baby's unique communication. By understanding from the start each of your baby's ways of signaling hunger, satiation, fatigue, overstimulation, discomfort, illness, desire to engage, and needing a break, you will be empowered to provide the right response that will nurture a loving and trusting relationship with lifelong benefits. Welcome to the journey of understanding your baby and hopefully, the feeling of, "I know what this baby wants." Soon, your baby will suckle, sleep, and thrive.

Introduction

When you take your newborn into your arms for the first time, you silently promise to love, cherish, and protect him. We all start out with the best intentions and, most often, are innately gifted with maternal intuition. We want to meet our baby's needs for nourishment, safety, and warmth. Long-term, we want good health and happiness for each one of our children. More and more women in America are also wanting to give their babies the gift of breastmilk (CDC, 2016) for the countless lifetime benefits breastfeeding offers, which unfortunately cannot be duplicated by any other life experience.

If it were just mother and baby during this transition to parenthood, breastfeeding would be less complicated. Unfortunately, our current Western society adds many more factors to this happy, healthy breastfeeding equation. Often, it causes interference so profound that it derails our best intentions, clouds our intuition, and may even stop us in our tracks. It's everything from dated hospital practices and smartphones to social commentary and lack of education. The results are damaging. It prevents parents from the simple act of watching and understanding their baby's most subtle behaviors—cues newborns give to signal their needs. When these early signals are missed, the immature newborn's reflexes respond more intensely to internal feelings of hunger, fatigue, or discomfort. When parents miss those behavioral cues, the baby elevates his communication to crying. After this cycle happens repeatedly, the infant becomes tense and may work himself up into a frenzy. The parents struggle to calm him. This uncontrollable crying interferes with taking the breast and his hunger grows deeper. The mother's difficulty getting the baby to take the breast compromises her confidence.

After repeated difficulty and confusing newborn crying spells, the mother begins to believe that there is something wrong with her milk. She gets so far from her ideal vision of what breastfeeding would be like that she puts her most pressing wish for her baby aside and decides to stop breastfeeding. She suffers guilt and sadness (Palmér et al., 2012). Unfortunately, this scenario is all too common.

In fact, more than 80% of women who give birth in American medical centers start out bringing their baby to the breast, but nearly half give up breastfeeding exclusively within the first 3 months of their infant's life, according the nation's Breastfeeding Report Card (CDC, 2016). By their baby's 6-month mark, only about 22% offer breastmilk alone (CDC, 2016), despite the American Academy of Pediatrics (AAP) and the World Health Organization (WHO) that recommend babies receive human milk exclusively for their first 6 months of life (AAP, 2012; WHO, 2016).

These statistics beg the question: If most new moms in America choose to breastfeed, why are so many ceasing soon after? A striking disparity shows ending breastfeeding is vastly due to difficulties rather than maternal choice (Dennis, 2002). In developing the contents for this book, we analyzed a body of research about women who discontinue breastfeeding during their first 3 months postpartum. We wanted to really understand the root of the problem—what factors influenced mothers to give up breastfeeding earlier than planned and how we can help those determined to succeed. Undoubtably, Andrea Herron was qualified to take on this task with her 40 years of experience as a pediatric nurse practitioner (one of the first nationally certified in the U.S.) and thousands of mother/baby breastfeeding success stories behind her through her private lactation practice, Growing with Baby in San Luis Obispo, California. By partnering with investigative journalist Lisa Rizzo, surely, we could find answers and determine the best way to help. The research unveiled an information gap echoed over and over in scientists' conclusions in a field that Andrea specialized in.

PROBLEMS MISDIAGNOSED

Surprisingly, overwhelming research showed that there was a correlation between breastfeeding problems and a lack of under-standing of early infant development—specific to the breastfed baby. Furthermore, the dynamics of normal breastfeeding interaction, including the ways and frequency breastfed babies signal their needs was generally misunderstood by new parents and the older generations who advised them based on their knowledge of bottle-feeding norms. Consequently, many mothers misinterpret normal newborn behaviors for problems and subsequently, stop breastfeeding unnecessarily (Gatti, 2008).

For example, in study after study, one of the top reasons mothers cited for quitting was not their free will and desire, or their choice, but the misbelief that they did not make enough milk to meet their baby's demand. The common response was, "breastmilk alone did not satisfy my baby" (Li et al., 2008). What's especially concerning is that mothers are blaming the quantity and quality of their milk, but few researchers, clinicians, and breastfeeding women evaluate the actual milk supply as a true indication of a problem, according to an integrative review of research conducted by Lisa Gatti, RN, MSN, in her study published in the *Journal of Nursing Scholarship*. In fact, "verification of actual milk supply is extremely rare," she writes.

Instead, moms are concluding that their milk supply is inadequate based on their infant's "satisfaction" cues. Normal challenging behaviors like fussiness and frequent "hunger" signaling during the first 3 months of infancy mimic problems and confuse parents. American culture dictates that all newborn babies do is "eat, sleep, and poop." Parents are often surprised to learn that reality is quite different, and much time is spent settling their baby to sleep. "Many women perceive crying, fussiness, and wakefulness as signs that their infant is not receiving enough milk," Gatti writes. "While these signs might be part of an infant's feeding cues, they can also be normal infant behavior, and might vary as infant temperaments vary."

When parents offer formula and the baby empties the bottle, they are sure hunger is not the cause of their baby's fussiness. But because lactating women can't see the amount of milk in their breasts, they may not be confident that they have enough for their baby. In addition, most parents haven't studied infant development, and thus, lack the knowledge to understand how babies communicate their wants and needs. This can leave parents scrambling to keep their newborn calm and nourished. A baby whose signals are being misunderstood might even struggle to put on weight. Repeatedly, this interaction causes mothers to become particularly stressed about breastfeeding and, as a result, they begin to misdiagnosis problems, including milk-supply issues, before their body has a chance to activate a full milk supply, which takes several weeks.

IT'S COMPLICATED

So, if it takes time to build a milk supply, why are mothers quick to reach for the bottle? Breastfeeding has become more complicated than it should be, thanks to a common knowledge deficit of breastfeeding norms and breastfed-baby behaviors following half a century where parents primarily bottle-fed formula. In addition, mothers face increasing interference, socially and medically, which inhibit normal biological processes and lead to challenges. Science concurs: most mothers cope with problems, especially in the early stages of infancy (Binns & Scott, 2002). While breastfeeding success is entirely possible in the face of problems, it just takes more work and support to overcome.

A contributing factor to early weaning, scientists say, is that many mothers are blindsided when problems arise because their expectations are unrealistic, often due to the lack of public education on the feeding method and the idea that natural is synonymous with "easy." Sometimes breastfeeding advocates paint a picture that's too rosy because they want to encourage as many pregnant women as possible to choose breastfeeding with their "Breast is Best" rhetoric. Some publications go as far as to promise "stress-free," "pain-free" breastfeeding (Rapley & Murkett, 2012). With all due respect, that vocabulary just doesn't fit-in with the adjustment to parenthood period—surely one of the most demanding times of life. Even when breastfeeding is convenient and easy—an opportunity to rest, cuddle, and bond—taking care of a newborn is still new and tiring. Not understanding that working through problems is a part of the normal experience leads many mothers to stop breastfeeding soon after their baby is born (Mozingo et al., 2000).

The Surgeon General's Call to Action to Support Breastfeeding echoes this American dilemma.

Not surprisingly, some women expect breastfeeding to be easy, but then find themselves faced with challenges. The incongruity between expectations about breastfeeding and the reality of the mother's early experiences with breastfeeding her infant has been identified as a key reason that many mothers stop breastfeeding within the first 2 weeks postpartum (Office of the Surgeon General, 2011).

It is no mystery why, by-and-large, mothers are supplementing with bottles of formula early on, or calling it quits before receiving an accurate diagnosis, whether it be insufficient milk supply, dairy allergies, or some other problem. In today's economic climate, where doctors must see so many patients a day to keep their practice going, they don't typically have the time or the training to solve these breastfeeding problems. For an exhausted mother, the sound of her inconsolable child makes her desperate for a quick fix. Instead, a breastfeeding mother must turn to her intuition regularly for sound parenting choices—and justly so. She surely knows her body better than anyone else. But then, why are so many of us getting it wrong, targeting lack of milk as the problem? One answer: the unpredictability of future breastfeeding success with even the best intentions is unsettling for women. Mothers are quick to blame themselves and take on unnecessary guilt.

Many pregnant women worry about whether they will be able to breastfeed or produce enough milk. In an Australian study, anxiety over the sufficiency of a mother's breastmilk supply was the most serious early problem in that it often resulted in the actual cessation of breastfeeding (Binns & Scott, 2002). Marketers know this truth, hence why they distribute free bottles, pacifiers, and formula to expectant parents. Stress makes the free can of formula sitting on her shelf even more tempting. A mother who does not feel the support of her partner, the pediatrician, and family to continue breastfeeding is more likely to trade the breast for the bottle.

BREASTFED BABIES MISUNDERSTOOD

When breastfeeding mothers compare their baby to their formula-feeding friend's baby, they sometimes find that the bottle-feeding infant has longer intervals between meals and longer stretches of sleep at night. Scientific research into how mothers perceive their baby's temperament shows astounding differences. Mothers who breastfeed commonly perceive that other people's formula-fed babies are more content while they see their baby's temperament as challenging (de Lauzon-Guillain et al., 2012). The Cambridge Baby Growth Study also found evidence that suggests some mothers believe the main cause of infant distress is hunger. For parents who don't understand normal newborn behaviors and the dynamics of breastfeeding, the frequent signaling is interpreted as difficult. Through the study, it became apparent to researchers that breastfed babies require a unique understanding for continued breastfeeding success.

In their first 3 months of life, breastfed babies must signal more to their parents to alert their hunger, take longer to eat, and feed more often, the study found (de Lauzon-Guillain et al., 2012). Because of the natural dynamics of breastfeeding, they control their intake and learn to signal when their blood sugar level drops or they feel hungry. They learn to ask for what they need instead of waiting passively, which long-term, makes them more confident and assertive. This active interaction is commonly misunderstood as more demanding and difficult because it does not fit in with our current cultural expectations of infant behavior that originated from bottle-feeding norms. Also, a baby in control of how much he eats, and when, conflicts with the Western idea that the parents should be in charge of the routine.

"Humans often perceive infant crying as stress, but for infants, irritability is a normal component of signaling to parents," the Cambridge authors wrote.

Healthy babies are born programed to speak-up. They cue their mother to give them the fuel they need to grow and thrive. Bottle-fed babies are tending to be overfed with a food that is not digested as quickly. If the bottle-fed baby feels hungry sooner than the mother expects based on the amount of formula the child last consumed, she may ignore that signal thinking; *you can't be hungry. I just fed you 3 ounces.* She might misinterpret the cue and hold off on feeding until the schedule dictates. When the mother fails to reciprocate the baby's "off-schedule" hunger cue, the infant essentially shuts-down. Over time, the baby learns to stop signaling as often. Basically, by ignoring a behavior, you extinguish it. From the looks of it, the baby appears less demanding and more content. But long-term, it can impact the baby's ability to communicate personal needs.

Except for this report, there has been little discussion about the role infant behavior has on breastfeeding duration (de Lauzon-Guillain et al., 2012). The Cambridge researchers also identified an information gap in public knowledge, which they concluded was partly responsible for the common premature cessation of breastfeeding. They said that even though their results are profound, they do not intend for it to discourage the choice to breastfeed. On the contrary, they recommend parents increase their awareness of the behavioral dynamics of breastfeeding, gain a better expectation of normal infant temperament, and find support to cope with difficult infant phases, so that mothers can prevent the misdiagnosis of problems that might otherwise lead to premature weaning.

In an ideal world, we would also see researcher Gatti's recommendation come to fruition—one that would fill the information gap and improve breastfeeding outcomes. "Obstetric and pediatric providers should therefore explicitly discuss information about normal newborn behaviors, appropriate feeding cues, differences in infant temperament, and proper ways to assess infant intake," she writes (Gatti, 2008). Unfortunately, this isn't the status quo.

THE SOLUTION: BABY WATCHING

This book has been developed in direct response to numerous researchers' calls to action. Like the scientists, we believe you can increase your odds of breastfeeding success by truly understanding YOUR breastfed baby and following evidence-based guidelines that support lactation. Not only will *Suckle, Sleep, Thrive* teach you how to establish breastfeeding, but how to reach your breastfeeding goals. We'll walk you through common challenges that arise during the first 10-week learning curve that cause many mothers to give up, including confusing newborn behaviors, breast-attachment issues, and perceived insufficient milk supply.

Pediatric Nurse Andrea Herron teaches an infant-led parenting approach called Baby Watching, designed to help parents understand their newborn's individual cues and temperament. Unlike many other books that instruct parents to listen to their baby's cues, this book describes, in-depth, what subtle behaviors babies do to communicate each of their needs. It offers a sound maternal response for each one and suggestions on how to rebound when cues are missed, and the newborn is stressed, so you can calm your baby, meet his needs, and breastfeed effectively.

During 40+ years of working with babies and their families, Andrea developed best practices for supporting newborn development by adopting the findings of researchers and groundbreaking child psychologists, while cataloging the knowledge from her own clinical lactation experiences. What she established were successful methods to help parents identify their baby's individual temperament and needs that impact feeding, calming, sleep, and activity. Through breastfeeding support groups, talks, and consults, Andrea has taught thousands of mothers how to use this knowledge to help them respond correctly to their baby's behaviors and cues.

WHY IT'S IMPORTANT

In the first weeks of life while the infant is fragile and developing so rapidly, the baby's needs take precedence. Parents practicing Baby Watching pick up and hold their newborn often and try to respond appropriately to his early need cues before he begins to cry because crying interferes with breastfeeding. When you regularly attend to your baby with a prompt and correct response, you create a secure attachment that tells him he is loved and important. Research shows that babies who are regularly left to cry, rather than those who receive a response, are less likely to develop a secure attachment relationship with their mother (Leach, 2010). Stress as a result of an insecure attachment to the mother is also likely to damage a baby's capacity to learn.

THE BENEFITS

Baby Watching is bound to encourage strong attachment in the mother-infant relationship and healthy physical-emotional development in the baby. Through Baby Watching, you will answer:

> » What should I expect for my baby's patterns for eating, sleeping, crying, and growing?

> » What is my newborn trying to tell me and how can I best meet these needs?

> » What are my baby's unique characteristics and sensitivities that affect nursing, sleep, calming, and our interaction? What can I do to tailor my care to meet these unique needs?

HOW TO USE THIS BOOK

In the most ideal scenario, you would read this book during your pregnancy. When your nesting instinct kicks in and you feel the need to educate yourself and prepare, this is the best time to start learning about babyrearing, the intuitive way. You can get the most out of this book if you read the first three parts before your baby arrives. Read on, and you will further your opportunities to prevent pitfalls that have challenged countless mothers. Main topics include establishing breastfeeding, returning home and getting to know your baby, and overcoming common challenges that arise while working through the learning curve. When you are pondering your baby's behaviors and beginning to blame your body or your choices, thumb through this trusted guide. As you read the compelling stories of real mothers and babies, you will be assured that you are not alone in this difficult yet wonderful journey. You will find answers, gain confidence in your mothering skills, and together, your family and that growing baby will begin to thrive. Soon, you will feel proud of your ability to grow another person with your body and build a predictable rhythm that you can both count on.

AUTHORS' NOTE

You may notice the use of "he" throughout the book, referring to all babies. Although, we cherish female babies as much as males, the pronoun has been selected for clarity and ease in being able to often and simply refer to the mother as "she" without confusion.

· ·

PART I

A Warm Welcome to the World: Beginning the Breastfeeding Bond

· ·

. . . .

CHAPTER ONE

From Belly to Breast: Establishing Breastfeeding in the Hospital

Chapter Goal: Ease your newborn's transition to life outside the womb and establish breastfeeding using a biologic approach.

FROM BELLY TO BREAST

For many women, childbirth is the most difficult physical challenge of their life to date. Our culture glamorizes having a baby, romanticizing the whole neonatal experience, and often leaving us unprepared for this reality. If you feel overwhelmed by your birth experience and the thought that you suddenly have to be a pro at breastfeeding, put the worries aside and turn your focus to enjoying the precious miracle you created. Breastfeeding is a skill that you will learn together through time and practice. The first step turns out to be the most important and is also the easiest. A few early decisions like taking time for skin-to-skin bonding, and staying together can build your breastfeeding foundation and give you the peaceful and safe start you all deserve.

FIRST THINGS FIRST: VITAL TASKS

Before your newborn can begin to breastfeed, interact, or love, he has a major transition to go through. He must first regulate changes to his central nervous system after leaving the protective uterus. Immediately after birth, he must adapt from dependency upon your body, and all that it provides through the placenta and womb, to the independent functions of his heart, lungs, and nervous system (Hillman et al., 2012; March of Dimes, 2003). His body that was positioned in a tight fetal ball is now open and needs to be controlled to help him contain his body's movements and startles. Before, you kept him warm. Now, he must begin regulating his own body temperature.

At first, he will feel all-out-of-sorts and unsettled after the shock of being born. He can now feel sensations like cold and roughness, see lights that are too bright, hear sounds that are startling, and, worst of all, he can experience hunger. Pre-birth, his environment met his every need. Now, rather than automatically getting nourishment from the placenta, he will have to work for it, suckling often. Your newborn must learn to eat, breathe, and excrete on his own, and sometimes all at once. He will need help falling asleep and reaching a state of calm. First and foremost, he needs the warmth and comfort of his mother's body during this period of adaptation. The secret to helping your baby transition to the outside world is making life, much like the way things were in the womb, where he did not feel cold, dirty, or overstimulated. Your movements rocked him to sleep, and he always felt safe and snug within the limits inside your body. Breastfeeding and skin-to-skin contact will give you both a sort of closeness, like in the womb, when you two become one again.

SKIN-TO-SKIN BONDING

As soon as possible after birth, lean back and have your unwrapped, undressed baby placed on your bare chest. Turn his head to the side so that the mouth and nose are unobstructed. Soak in the moments and allow your little one to lead the way. To your surprise, he might gaze into your eyes and even search for the nipple. Together, you will most likely find a natural and comfortable nursing position. The American Academy of Pediatrics (AAP) recommends that mothers and newborns are kept like this, chest-to-chest, until the completion of the first feed (Gartner et al., 2005). Following a thorough standardized assessment, well-babies without risk factors are candidates for skin-to-skin care.

Safety During Skin-to-Skin Care

The AAP recommends skin-to-skin time be supervised in the delivery environment by a healthcare professional who can continuously monitor the baby's breathing, color, and muscle tone (Feldman-Winter et al., 2016). This is to prevent an episode of sudden unexpected postnatal collapse, a rare incident where a well-appearing, full-term newborn with Apgar scores of eight or more, suddenly stops breathing. This can typically occur during skin-to-skin care within the first 2 hours of life but can happen up to 7 days after delivery, thus regular monitoring is recommended (Feldman-Winter et al. 2016).

During your hospital stay, and while rooming-in with your baby, if you don't feel alert enough to stay awake during skin-to-skin time or breastfeeding, ask an alert support person to monitor you. If you are too tired or medicated to take care of your baby, put him in his cradle and tell the staff. If you are recovering from cesarean surgery, have someone help you lift the baby from the bassinet to your arms and back as needed. Too many women strain themselves post-surgery, trying to awkwardly lean and pick up their baby while confined to bed.

Researchers have observed that healthy full-term newborns go through nine phases beginning immediately after birth when left skin-to-skin with their mothers (Widström et al., 2011). **Phase 1**- the first cry, which expands the lungs and fills them with air; **Phase 2** - several minutes of rest; **Phase 3** - an awakening when the newborn starts to move his head and shoulders; **Phase 4** - activity when he begins to search for the breast with his mouth; **Phase 5** - another period of rest; **Phase 6** - sometime between 50 and 90 minutes after birth, a healthy-term baby held skin-to-skin might spontaneously crawl to the breast and search for the nipple (Morrison, 2006); **Phase 7** - time getting familiar with the mother's breast, licking the areola, and rubbing the nipple; **Phase 8** - suckling which, unfortunately, may be delayed after a medicated birth; **Phase 9** - sleep for about 90 to 120 minutes.

Researchers believe that when this natural process is allowed to happen peacefully through skin-to-skin time with the mother, known as Kangaroo Care, it supports the newborn's ability to self-regulate (transition into an alert state) and get himself organized to breastfeed (Widström et al., 2011). On the contrary, routine hospital care often interferes with Mother Nature's intentions. In some hospitals, newborns go from womb to warming unit for assessments, treatments, and swaddling before meeting their mother (Widström et al., 2011). After a 5-to-10-minute visit in her arms, they are typically transported to a nursery for newborn care.

The mother also has responses that are physical and hormonal in nature from bare-bonding soon after birth. Her infant's touch enhances her levels of oxytocin (Matthiesen et al., 2001). Oxytocin is the hormone responsible for uterine contractions (decreasing bleeding) and milk ejection. Researchers found that the mothers who got to experience Kangaroo Care had less breast engorgement, and overall greater maternal self-confidence, which equated to more breastfeeding success (Morrison, 2006). Among all the biochemical and physiologic benefits, this immediate togetherness, most importantly, increases infant survival by helping transition the baby to the outside world. Skin-to-skin contact is a proven method of stabilizing the baby's body temperature while reducing startles and the stress of the birth experience (Moore et al., 2007). As the baby calms on his mother's chest, he begins to relax and breathe more deeply, which facilitates his task of learning to regulate inhaling, exhaling, and processing oxygen through his lungs after relying on an umbilical cord.

In the most ideal scenario (a healthy newborn and complication-free vaginal birth), your baby would not be separated from you before the first feed (Righard & Alade, 1990). Newborns who are separated from their mothers for long periods after birth begin to show stress responses like crying, which can cause low blood sugar and temperature instability (they get colder), which then leads to breastfeeding problems (Moore et al., 2007). For these reasons alone, it is vital that your newborn baby has unlimited access to you. Since mother/baby vital signs are taken frequently and immediately after birth, request to keep your infant on your body as much as possible during these routine checks.

Boarding Environment: Room Together

To ease the newborn's transition, it helps to keep your baby's heart as close to yours as often as possible, especially in the first few hours after birth. Sharing a room with your newborn, rather than sending him to a nursery, is one way you can achieve this goal. Numerous recent studies support the modern practice of mothers keeping their babies in their hospital room because it has been shown to reduce newborn health complications, decrease the rate of sudden infant death syndrome (SIDS), improve mother-infant bonding, and increase how frequent a mother breastfeeds (Moore et al., 2007).

In some hospitals, the routine practice of mother/infant separation hijacks many early learning opportunities, which may interfere with breastfeeding. Separation in the hospital can reduce the mother's milk supply and discourage on-cue feeding, which is essential for building the foundation for a successful nursing experience in general (Moore et al., 2007).

A Change in Care

Did you ever hear stories about how your grandfather waited in the father's room and didn't get to see the baby until after he was in the nursery? How your grandmother had a general anesthesia and didn't see the baby for 24 hours? We take for granted that our infants remain near us and stay close to their family unit from the moment they are born. It wasn't always that way. Thanks to the observations and research of Dr. Marshall Klaus and his colleague Dr. John Kennel in the early 1970s, maternity practices changed. Their book, *Maternal-Infant Bonding* released in 1976, emphasized that early contact between mother and baby enhanced their connection and was a critical component of long-term attachment. Klaus and Kennel's findings were the beginnings and stimulus of the family-centered care one now receives during a hospital birth today. After many years of continuing research and many other valuable contributions to the promotion of humanizing maternal care, Dr. Klaus passed away in 2017 at the age of 90.

FREEDOM FOR THE FIRST FEED

Breastfeeding within the first hour after birth is correlated with infant vitality, future milk intake, and breastfeeding success (Mohrbacher, 2010). If you miss this window, it is not detrimental (see Problem Prevention Tip box). We have great science that shows this time is helpful for breastfeeding, but there is a grace period. Many mothers don't get to bring their baby to the breast right away and go on to breastfeed for as long as they wish.

Problem Prevention Tip for
Separated Mothers and Babies

If you have risk factors for insufficient milk supply (listed on page 352) and circumstances that cause you to miss the first hour or more skin-to-skin with your newborn, ask for assistance to start expressing your milk. If you are being recovered separately from your baby after cesarean, Dr. Jane Morton with Stanford University School of Medicine recommends you reduce the impact of separation by hand expressing your colostrum and having it transferred to your baby for spoon-feeding (Morton, 2016). Request that your partner have access to you in the recovery room to retrieve the milk in a vile to spoon or dropper feed the baby.

Good science shows that the more colostrum expressed during the first hour, the more you will have later, and the sooner your milk will arrive (Parker et al., 2012). Even if the colostrum goes to waste, expression will activate your milk production, signaling your body to produce more. When you do set out to nurse for the first time, your breasts will be fuller, making it easier for your newborn to get milk (see hand-expression).

In the beginning, try to relax and get acquainted with the baby. Ease the pressure of the first feed by not getting caught up in all the technicalities of breastfeeding. Try to work out breastfeeding by doing what feels natural. In a clinical setting, there tends to be many people giving various instructions to obtain the perfect breastfeeding hold. The instructions may involve more steps than you can keep in your brain. The truth is that the baby is in charge of taking the breast and is innately driven to seek it. You are in charge of presenting the breast in a way that accommodates the baby's natural reflexes. If you let your newborn lead, you can see what he wants to do rather than having to think about all the rules. Then, you will be able to observe how you can help guide or support him. With this method, mothers and babies are often able to find a way to "dance" together and get that first feed going correctly.

First Milk and Infant Stomach Capacity

Although your milk supply may take another 72 hours or so to come in, your breasts can offer colostrum—pure nutrition that is loaded with easy to digest carbohydrates, protein, and antibodies. You may feel like you do not have much colostrum to offer your newborn. Worries aside, this early milk is more about quality than quantity. Although low in volume, it is the best possible food for your infant who can only handle very small amounts at a time. A day-old baby has a stomach capacity about the size of a marble. It can only contain about 5 to 7 milliliters and the stomach walls can't stretch yet to make room for more. By day three, the newborn stomach is larger and can hold about 3/4 of an ounce to a full ounce. A week-old baby fills up with 1.5 to 2 ounces. The low volume gives the baby an opportunity to learn how to coordinate the breastfeeding rhythm—suck, swallow, breathe—without choking. This is practice time.

Babies fresh from the womb are wide awake. They have inborn survival reflexes that make them capable of climbing up the mother's abdomen to find the breast (Klaus & Klaus, 2000; Righard & Alade, 1990; Varendi et al., 2002,). When they feel pressure on their feet, they push. This, combined with the reflexive movements of the arms, mimics crawling. As he moves, the baby's hands, still moist with amniotic fluid, which he is accustomed to swallowing, brushes the mother's body, enticing him to follow with his mouth. He moves his face from side-to-side with the mouth open in what is called rooting—a breast-seeking behavior. When he sees the dark target of the breast, the areola, his eyes brighten, and he pushes his head up. The baby's strong sense of smell draws him onward. Then, he may brush his little hand across the nipple, causing it to become erect and, perhaps, even leak colostrum. He begins to peck and bob his head. When his chin hits the breast first, it makes the newborn's mouth open wide and his tongue come forward. Then, he may try to take the nipple into his mouth and suckle. Your smart little baby can even use his hands to push the breast, bringing the nipple closer to his mouth.

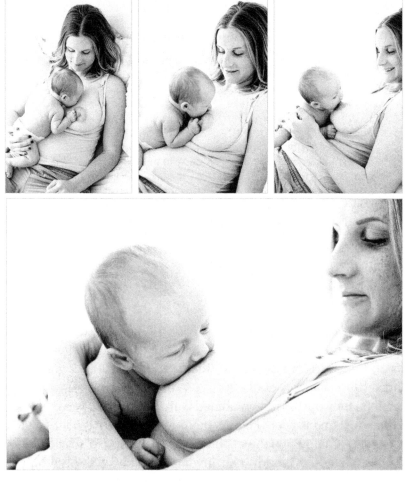

When placed tummy to tummy with her mother and with little help, this newborn used her reflexes to find the breast, scoop it into her mouth, and begin nursing. The mother lit up with confidence seeing how capable her little baby was.

Learning After the First Feed

An important skill that will help you succeed at breastfeeding is understanding your baby's feeding cues and reflexes, including how they relate to the timing of offering your breast. It reflects your infant's particular style of "baby talk," which signals that he is ready to eat. For one, notice the newborn's readiness to find the nipple. Babies open their mouth wide and reach with their little tongue. They sometimes turn their head side-to-side. They might bring their fists to their mouth and suck. Offer your breast when you observe these behaviors.

Leaning-Back Position

In the hospital and while you are getting used to breastfeeding, a semi-reclined position will help your baby take the breast and make you both more comfortable.

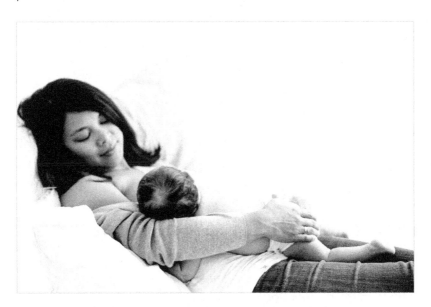

When the mother leans back, the baby lies above her breast rather than underneath. This position, which promotes infant-led feeding, has many advantages, such as preventing nipple injury and limiting choking at the breast.

Modern Breastfeeding Developments

In the last decade, two practitioners used scientific findings to change modern day breastfeeding education and practices. Dr. Suzanne Colson, RM, PhD, coined Biological Nurturing and Laid-Back Breastfeeding to describe using semi-reclined breast-feeding postures that stimulate and support innate feeding reflexes. She and colleagues found that natural breastfeeding reflexes are triggered when the newborn lies abdomen down rather than in a back-down posture (Colson et al., 2008). The researchers further discovered that breastfeeding is innate for mother and child. We can also credit Dr. Christina Smillie, MD, FAAP, IBCLC, FABM, for developing baby-led breastfeeding, which guides mothers to follow their baby's cues in attaching to the breast and much more.

Lean back in a semi-reclined position, as if resting on a couch while watching TV. Your body and head should feel supported so that you can tilt your head down without strain. Then, position the baby (dressed in a diaper) on top of your body with your torsos facing, belly to belly. Make sure that your newborn's entire body is touching yours. His feet need to be supported by your body. This full body contact and support stimulates the baby's inborn reflexes, allowing him to find the breast and take it into his mouth. Allow the baby to lead freely, rather than restraining him into a position. The baby may stop and suck his hand, so be patient. He may just need a moment to settle.

It Takes Two: Helpful Hints to Get You Started

While healthy babies are born with natural reflexes to breastfeed, they need their mother's assistance until they develop muscle strength in their upper body. Learning how to offer your breast in a way that your baby can easily and comfortably take is an important skill that will help you successfully breastfeed. The baby milking the breast correctly is the key to stimulating an adequate milk supply and keeping the baby well-fed and content.

In the laid-back position, as the infant crawls to take the breast, you can support him by keeping your arms close to cradle him, so when he moves towards the breast, his movements don't make him fall over towards your armpit. For example, if the baby is aiming for the right breast, use the right arm. The baby's body should be free to move. If his arms and legs are trapped in a swaddle, he won't be able to help himself. When he pushes up with his hands, recognize that he is not fighting you at the breast, but rather, using his reflexes to move.

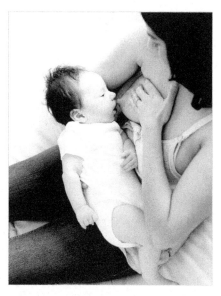

A mother helps her baby take the breast by making a small adjustment with her left hand just before she pulls her baby close to her body.

As you observe your infant's movements and see what he wants to do naturally, you can help direct him to the nipple or notice when he wants to find it himself. Ask yourself, "what is my baby like? Does he need more help latching on? If I help, does that agitate him?" Check to see if you need to assist by shaping the nipple. Sometimes it just takes pressing above the areola with one finger or pressing right below the areola with the index finger to create a soft round bulge that the baby's tongue can feel.

What the Baby is Trying to Do

When the baby's chin brushes the areola, his reflexes cause him to open his mouth and bring his tongue out past his lower lip to scoop the areola in with his tongue. He then draws it deep into his mouth along with the nipple. Very strong and consistent pressure keeps the mother's breast in the baby's mouth (Geddes et al., 2008). While holding the nipple deep in his mouth, the tip of his tongue is over the gum, while the lower lip folds down on his chin. He then lowers his jaw while keeping the tongue in place, which increases vacuum, allowing the milk to flow into his mouth. Then, he raises the jaw with the tongue as a unit to stop the milk flow while swallowing. The mother's nipple elongates when the tongue is up and shortens slightly when it is down.

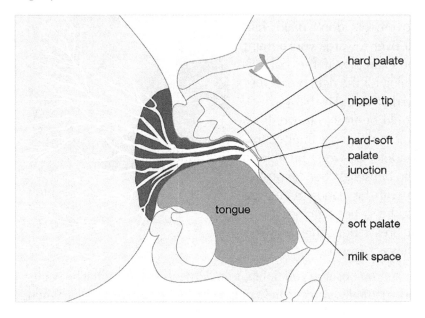

ILLUSTRATION 1.1 Infant Sucking and Milk Removal. Source: ©Medela 2018. Used with Permission.

In order for the baby to nurse without hurting the mom, his body must be well supported and pressed against her body. He must have his tongue and jaw deep on the breast because it is primarily the tongue and lower jaw that work in unison to milk the breast. When the baby is correctly positioned, you will see the top part of the areola near the baby's upper lip. His nose will be slightly off the breast. His upper lip will be long, thin, and not tucked under. The upper and bottom lips will be stretched and not touching each other. The lower lip will be curled down on the chin, and you may see the tongue on top of it. The baby's chin will be plastered against the breast and areola, which will be deep in his mouth. You will see much less of the bottom of the areola than the top.

The milk is in the breast—not the nipple. The pressure of the baby's chin on the lower breast massages and stimulates milk flow. The mother must support her breast in a way that does not interfere with what the baby needs to do. Breastfeeding success happens when the newborn is fully awake and ready to nurse. Once the baby is on the breast, you will know he is doing well if you feel a strong pull and not a pinch, and you hear intermittent sucks and swallows with concurrent cramping in your uterus.

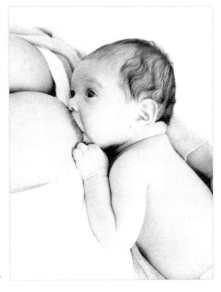

This mother and baby illustrate a perfect attachment using laid-back breastfeeding. Note, there is less areola visible on the bottom than on the top. The infant begins wide awake and ready to complete a feed.

After a good feeding, the baby will relax. He might come off the breast, turn his head sideways, and lay his cheek on the breast. If he seems relaxed and finished, you'll want to move the baby to the chest area underneath your chin, close enough to kiss the top of his head. Turn his head to the side. This will prevent your newborn from sinking his nose into the soft tissue of the breast, which could interfere with his breathing (see Safety During Skin-to-Skin Care Box). If the infant is healthy and normal, he does not have to eat a lot at this moment. This is no time for pressure—it's about exploration and learning. The more you observe and support, the more you will figure it out together and learn to breastfeed without rules. This is the whole idea of biologic nursing—familiarity and practice.

CHECK-LIST

Verify that your baby is on the breast correctly.

[_] He has the nipple and a large part of the areola (more of the bottom than the top) deep in his mouth.

[_] His nose is slightly off the breast.

[_] His chin is pressing against the breast.

[_] His upper lip is long and thin but not tucked under.

[_] His lower lip is folded down on his chin.

[_] His lips are stretched and not touching each other.

[_] The cheeks are full and without dimples.

[_] You feel a strong pull.

[_] If there is any discomfort, it passes within 10 to 30 seconds.

[_] After the baby lets go of the breast, the nipple appears elongated and round without creases, blanching, injury, or unusual shape.

BREASTFEEDING STEP-BY-STEP

Once hunger sets in, you might find a need to get down to business with some technical help. Even seasoned moms who nursed children well into toddlerhood have to start over with each newborn. Patience pays off. Once babies are a few months old, they simply need to be brought near a bare breast, and then they just help themselves. This step-by-step guide will give you some valuable tips—a recipe for success. You'll start by nixing cookie-cutter holds and getting comfy. Then, lean back and bring the baby to your body. You'll see if the breast needs support, then promote a deep latch-on. Finally, conduct a checklist to confirm the baby is on the breast correctly, transferring milk, and making breastfeeding comfortable for you.

ACTION PLAN

Recipe for Success
(1) Nix cookie-cutter holds & get comfy
(2) Lean back & bring the baby to your body
(3) See if the breast needs support
(4) Promote a deep latch-on
(5) Conduct a mental check-list

1. Nix Cookie-Cutter Holds & Get Comfy

Since mothers and babies come in many shapes and sizes, there is not one magic way to sit and hold a baby that is right for everyone. Any position that is comfortable is likely correct if the baby is content after feeding. This text emphasizes the laid-back nursing style, developed by Dr. Suzanne Colson (see box on page 12). It is a biologic approach that uses gravity and promotes the newborn's innate reflexes to self-attach while preventing neck and back strain in the mother. Mothers and babies often do best in this nursing style. When the milk begins to flow, the baby will have more control in this position and will choke less.

When the baby is positioned in a way that he must move against gravity like when the mother is seated upright, it causes him to startle and make uncoordinated arm and leg movements, frustrating them both. Mothers complain that their baby is fighting at the breast. A semi-recline or "hammock position" is more efficient and comfortable (Douglas & Keogh, 2017). If you prefer an upright position, or your baby is struggling to find the breast, you can use pillows and cushions to provide more support and assistance. While upright positions often interfere with the newborn's inborn reflexes, there are times when they are more comfortable for the mother, including circumstances where the baby needs more direction and support.

2. Lean Back and Bring Your Baby to Your Body

To get started, lean way back and place your lightly-dressed newborn on your bare skin with his hips against your lower stomach. The baby's feet will rest on your opposite thigh (feet support helps trigger the baby's feeding reflexes). His chin and chest should face the breast at the level of the nipple, where the breast falls naturally. You can get into a comfortable semi-upright position from many starting points. For example, you can cradle your baby by either using the same arm as the offered breast or the opposite arm, if that gets him in a better position for your breast. This is often referred to as a cross-cradle hold. When using the opposite arm, support your baby's shoulders, back, and buttocks with the hand and forearm of your right arm if you intend to offer the left breast, and vice versa. Hold his neck and shoulders so his chin is pointed toward your breast. The baby's whole body and head should be turned toward your body. Take care to keep your fingers away from the baby's head and upper cheeks/ temples, to not inhibit his jaw movement. Let his arms hug the breast. Holding your infant this way across your body can give you more control over his head and neck.

With your free hand, hold your breast in a way that you can tilt the nipple toward the baby's upper lip. Your hand may make a U or C-shape. Press a little bit more firmly with your thumb on top of the breast to tilt the nipple. Take care that your bottom fingers are not in his chin space. Bring the baby to the breast with the chin leading toward the inner areola. The baby's upper lip should be close to the nipple.

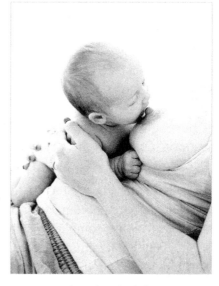

You can see that when the baby is in charge of taking the breast, her chin hits first allowing the lower jaw and tongue to scoop up a good amount of breast tissue into her mouth, promoting a comfortable latch and effective feed.

Let his chin touch first, which will stimulate his reflex to bring his tongue out to scoop the areola into his mouth with his lower jaw. After he takes part of the areola, relax your hand and let the nipple roll in last. Tuck your baby's body close and relax.

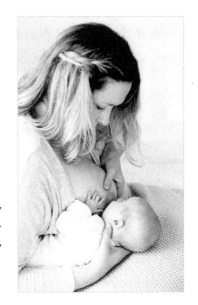

To promote good attachment, try not to push the head into the breast, or he will be inclined to push away. It can lead to attachment problems, fussy feeding behaviors, and breast refusal (Noble & Bovey, 2016). It also interferes with breathing and three essential feeding reflexes: the rooting reflex, the gape reflex (opening the mouth wide), and tongue-extrusion reflex (sticking the tongue forward to grab the breast) (Noble & Bovey, 2016).

Notice how the mother's hand is supporting the baby's head at the base of the skull and not against the back of the head, which would otherwise cause the baby to pull on the nipple.

A baby with a deep hold of the breast with a comfortably seated mother will be able to drink adequate amounts of milk without causing nipple pain. Do a check; your forearm should support the middle of the baby's back with the palm of your hand below the base of his head, thumb behind one ear, and index finger behind the other. Or, the baby is cradled with his head free and his body closely pressed against you. The rule of thumb is to hold the baby so that his body is facing the breast with the chin pointing toward it, while his nose or upper lip (depending on your nipple type) lines up with the nipple. It is important that you feel comfortable and the baby is well supported and secure while able to easily reach your breast.

3. See if the Breast Needs Support

Breasts and nipples come in many sizes and combinations. For example, one woman may have large breasts and small nipples/areolae. Another woman might have very small breasts with large nipples. Some have nipples that point up, others point down, and many point to the side. Based on your anatomy, how big or small, soft or firm your breasts are, you will need to help your baby take the breast with a deep mouthful to adequately transfer milk. Remember, it's the mother's job to present the breast, and it's the baby's job to take it. You don't put it in the infant's mouth like you would a bottle. The way you offer it will depend on the unique shape and size of your breasts, nipples, and areola.

Relaxed Breasts

If the breast is relaxed with lax tissue and nipples pointing downward, bring it up to the baby. Some women need to pinch way behind the areola, pulling back toward the chest in a way that makes the nipple stick out. If your breast is low, it may be necessary to lift it with your free hand.

Large, Heavy, or Lax-Skin Breasts

Women with larger, heavier breasts may need to support them to help the baby. If this describes your anatomy, place your index finger of your free hand at the base of your breast by your ribs, with the thumb on top. Lift up with your index finger while gently pushing down with your thumb. Make sure that your hand is away from the areola. Also, keep your fingers away from the baby's face because it can impede suckling. If necessary, move them back towards your ribs. If the breast is really large, you may need to make a pinch from the side, close to the areola, but you don't have to hold the breast (see scissors hold on page 288). If the areola feels hard and full, it may be a result of excess IV fluids given during labor. Leaning back and doing reverse-pressure softening will help (see areolar edema/engorgement). Position the baby at the natural level of your nipple.

You may have to "sandwich" your breast if it is large and/or the skin is lax. When you do that, you want to make the area smaller in the direction the baby opens his mouth. That generally happens when you have your thumb by the baby's nose and the index finger by his chin. Use your fingers to gently lift the area of your breast that would lie on the baby's chin. The weight of the breast is resistance against movement of the jaw. It can be very tiring. When you lift that weight off his chin and gently press the breast to stimulate milk flow with your fingers, it alerts the baby, then he can continue feeding without tiring. If you are laying back, gravity will do it for you. While sitting more

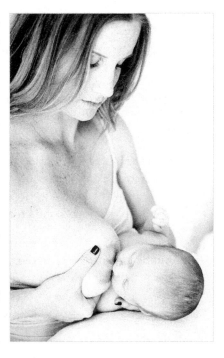

A mother supports her breast by making a breast "sandwich." This wide pinch helps the baby get a deep grab of the nipple and areola, especially when the breasts are large, full, or hanging.

upright, you may need to support the breast throughout the entire feed until the two of you become comfortable nursing together.

Small, Firm Breasts

If you have small, firm breasts, it may not be necessary to support them. However, if the nipples point upward, take care not to press above the areola because it may push the nipple further up and lead it to rub on the baby's palate (top of the mouth)—a move sure to cause sore nipples. The following chart will offer you some hints to help you present your breast, no matter what size or shape, so your baby can get a full feed without causing you discomfort.

TABLE 1.1: Aid for Your Anatomy.

BREAST TYPE	MINDFUL TIP
Large	Rather than lift the breast, bring the baby to the natural level of the nipple while sandwiching the areola.
Small Breast Long Torso	You may need to elevate the baby with a thick, firm pillow (such as The Breast Friend Pillow). Take care to keep your hands out of the baby's way. You may not need to sandwich the breast.
Athletic	Small, firm breasts with nipples that point up may result in the nipple rubbing on the roof of the baby's mouth (palate). Slight pressure under the areola will prevent this.
Relaxed	For breasts with lax skin and nipples that point downward, wear a supportive bra. Roll a small cloth diaper and place it under the breast to prop it up. Be sure that any lax skin does not block air to the baby's nose.
Firm	A hard, firm breast may be engorged. See reverse pressure softening. Sandwich the breast as much as possible with your fingers out of the way to make it easier for the baby to get enough breast into his mouth.

4. Promote A Deep Latch On

Babies have natural reflexes that allow them to take a deep hold of the breast. We just need to offer the breast in a way that takes advantage of the reflexes. The milk ducts are in the areola area behind the nipple and are superficial (not deep in the breast). For the baby to milk the breast, he must have more than the nipple in his mouth. If the grasp is shallow, the gums will pinch behind the nipple, putting too much pressure on the ducts and blocking the release of milk, causing nipple trauma while the baby doesn't get enough to eat.

If you are sitting up, keep his nose level with your nipple and allow his chin to gently brush the breast. Make sure his lower lip is well below the nipple. When you feel him take the nipple, use the arm holding the baby's body to tuck him close. Make sure you are, in fact, pulling the baby's body close, rather than pushing his head into your breast or lowering the breast to him. If leaning back, let the baby take the breast, making sure you are holding him in a way that allows clear access to the inner aspect of the nipple and areola. If you are holding the base of the baby's head, you will feel the head push back. It will signal you to pull the baby's body closer.

Make sure the baby is latched on correctly so that he does not injure the nipple. For a proper latch, his mouth should be wide open with the nipple and a good amount of areola inside the mouth (more of the bottom of the areola than the top). As previously mentioned, the lower lip should be curled down on the chin while the upper lip is untucked. If you do not see this and you feel pain, immediately place a clean finger in the corner of his mouth, gently pull to the side, and push down on the bottom gum to break the suction. Release the breast from the baby's hold, then start again. If you try to pull away prior to breaking the suction, you could hurt yourself.

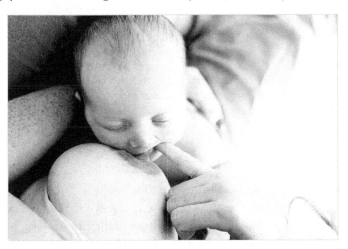

If your baby's latch does not feel right, remove the breast by inserting a clean finger into the corner of the mouth, then gently pull to break suction while pressing down on the lower gum. Pulling the breast out without breaking suction can injure the nipple.

A common initial concern, particularly for the large-breasted woman, is how well the baby can breathe. Newborn babies breathe through their nose. If the nose appears buried in the breast, lean way back so he can push off. Also, pull his hips as close to you as possible. This will make his head go back slightly, freeing his nose and allowing the chin to move deeper into the breast. If the breast is hard and engorged, and pressing the hips forward does not free the nose, you may need to gently press the breast away from his nose with four fingers. Take care not to press too hard because this pressure could cause a plugged duct. Avoid making a dent in the tissue above his nose while breastfeeding because it tilts the nipple up, causing nipple trauma.

Nipple Care

After completing a feed, you can help keep your nipples healthy and reduce soreness by allowing the breasts to air-dry. Some women develop dry, flaky skin around their nipples. Use a gentle odorless soap on your breasts during your normal bathing routine. You will need a nursing bra that allows for one cup size of growth and space for breast pads. You should be able to easily undo the cup with one hand. Wear an all-cotton bra with no under-wires or plastic liners. It will help prevent plugged ducts. Breast pads should be changed regularly and monitored for dryness. Any nipple shields should be washed with hot soapy water after each feed. These devices are susceptible to fungal infections that can affect the baby's mouth and your nipples/areola.

5. Conduct a Checklist

Once your baby is latched on and eating well, sit back and relax while holding his body close. Make sure you feel a strong pull. Most importantly, check that the infant swallows at the breast, which you can tell by gulping and repeated "ka, ka, ka" sounds. As he fills up and really begins to relax, he will do little flutter sucks, and then either pull himself off the breast or fall asleep attached to the nipple. Let him feed until he lets go or falls asleep. You'll know he took in milk if you heard his swallows and loud gulps and after the breast softened. If a few minutes later, he is searching again for the nipple by opening his mouth and bobbing his head around, he is hungry for more. Try to help the baby produce a burp. If after burping, he is still searching, offer the other breast. If the baby is content for at least 60 to 90 minutes afterward and filled his diaper, you know breastfeeding is off to a good start.

CHECK-LIST

You can rest assured the feeding is going well when...
(Herron & Weber, 1998):

[_] The baby has the nipple and a large part of the areola (more of the bottom than the top) deep in his mouth.

[_] You feel a strong pull, not pain after the initial 10 to 30 seconds.

[_] He sucks, then swallows with a regular rhythm.

[_] When you listen closely, you hear "ka, ka, ka" sounds and no loud clicks or slurps.

[_] You see your baby's little body relax as he becomes full.

[_] He is content for 60 to 90 minutes after a complete feeding.

OTHER HELPFUL HOLDS

Breastfeeding mothers use various nursing holds throughout the day to adjust for convenience and comfort. This section describes several other nursing positions.

Lying Down

If recovering from a cesarean, you will not be able to sit up all the way for your first feeds due to potential adverse side-effects recovering from surgery, such as a spinal headache. Nursing while lying on your side will afford you more comfort during breastfeeding until you can sit up. Later, you may find this position to be more restful.

1. Carefully pull yourself onto your side using the hospital bed railing. A pillow pressed against your lower abdomen can help splint your incision.

2. Place your head on a pillow, tucked between your shoulder and bottom ear. The lower arm should extend upward to allow room for your baby to snuggle into your body, and for your breast to relax flat onto the bed. If you skip this step, your arm could get in the way, and you might not be able to lower your breast enough.

3. For comfort, place a pillow between your knees and wedge another behind your lower back.

4. Turn your baby onto his side, bellies facing. Prop a rolled receiving blanket behind his back to keep him in position. Place his body so he is looking up at the breast.

5. With your upper arm, place your hand on his upper back and slide him towards your body so that he rests under your breast. The nipple should face the center of his upper lip.

6. You can adjust the breast's position by rotating your hips. To move the breast up from the bed, rotate the bottom hip up. If the breast is too far above the baby's face, turn the bottom hip away from the baby.

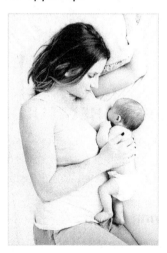

7. Tilt your nipple up by pressing on the breast slightly above the nipple or sandwich the breast while leaning toward the baby. Move closer when he opens up.

8. If the baby buries his nose into the breast during the feed, pull his hips closer or use the flats of your fingers to gently press the top of your breast away from his nose.

The side-lying nursing position is optimal for night feedings and for mothers recovering from cesarean.

Pain Management

Many mothers who experience natural childbirth have the great benefit of mobility and are able to get up, move around, and care for their baby without depending on others to assist them. If you had a vaginal birth without major complications except for an episiotomy, you may be able to tolerate after birth discomfort without the use of narcotic medications. Severe pain after vaginal birth may be a symptom of an underlying medical condition, which can require further treatment.

If you have a cesarean, once the anesthesia drugs wear off, some mothers are overwhelmed by pain and chills that puts them into a state of immobility and shock. Realize that cesarean section is an abdominal surgery. Most surgeries require a patient to rest and recover. It will be hard for you to be responsible for around-the-clock care of a baby. Be kind to yourself and take the medication needed to keep acute pain at bay during the first 48 hours. Before your milk supply arrives, very little medication is passed through your milk because colostrum is transferred in very small amounts. Thereafter, you may be able to get ample pain relief from a non-opioid medication. Research shows that taking opioids for more than 3 days increases risk of dependency (Shah et al., 2017). Return any leftover prescriptions to your local pharmacy so they don't fall into the wrong hands or become misused.

The Football Hold or Clutch Hold

A nursing position known as the "football" hold or clutch hold is also useful for mothers who need to protect a cesarean incision. It can help those who need more control, such as a petite mother with a large baby and/or large breasts, mothers dealing with infant breast-taking difficulties, and babies smaller than 7 pounds. A football hold is not recommended for babies who were breech presentation. It is beneficial for the tense infant that tends to arch.

1. Sit up and place a pillow at your side. Half of the pillow should be behind you.

2. Place the infant on the pillow. He can be held in a sitting position in front of you, or he can rest on his side with the knees toward your armpit. You'll need to hold the baby with the arm that is on the same side as the breast you plan to feed with. Roll your shoulder down, tucking the baby into your side with your elbow back, like you would hold a football. Look down. If his hips are away from your body, pull him closer.

3. Line up the baby's chin to the side of the areola so that his upper lip is near the nipple.

4. With your other hand, hold the breast with your forefingers underneath the areola and the thumb on top. Use your thumb to tilt the nipple up. Bring the baby to the breast and let his chin brush against the underside of the breast. When you feel him start to take the breast, draw him closer, pressing with your forearm so that his chin touches first. If you are small-breasted, you do not need to hold your breast, but it may help to press gently on top of the breast to tilt the nipple up toward his upper lip.

5. As you feel the baby's tongue grasp the areola, use your forearm to put pressure between the shoulder blades, pulling the baby snugly to your body. Keep the nipple towards the upper lip, letting it roll into his mouth last.

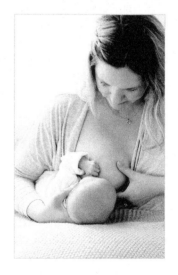

6. After the infant starts nursing, if his weight is not well supported when you tire, pulling may occur and cause nipple soreness. So, once the baby gets into a suckling rhythm, large-breasted women can support the breast by tucking a small, rolled burp or washcloth under the breast. To relieve pressure on your wrist,

The football hold helps mothers avoid putting the weight of the baby near their cesarean wound. Make sure you tuck the baby's body into your side with your elbow and keep your free hand out of the baby's way of taking the breast.

roll another burp cloth under the baby's neck, right below the curve of the head.

7.   Lean back and get comfortable.

The Front Hold

The front hold is an easy position to get into, but mothers should take care that it does not cause back and neck strain, or pulling, which can result in nipple soreness and/or trauma.

1.   Start by leaning back.

2.   Cradle the baby in front of your body where your breast lies naturally. The infant's belly should face and rest against your belly. His chin should be close to the inner aspect of the breast that you are offering. This may be challenging to achieve in this position.

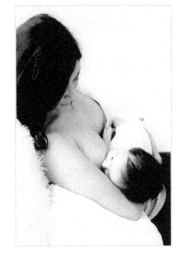

3.   Support the baby's back with the same arm of the breast that you are offering. His back and shoulders should rest on the crook of your elbow.

The front hold is a common position mothers take when out and about, away from the comfort of home.

4.   Bring him to the breast while supporting your breast with the opposite hand. Make sure your fingers are out of the inner aspect of the areola, or the baby will just take the nipple. Use your thumb to tilt the nipple towards his upper lip.

5.   When you feel the baby take the nipple, pull his bottom close with your hand.

BREASTFEEDING MULTIPLES

Nursing twins is challenging, and the learning period may be prolonged if the babies are born early. In the beginning, you may need to pump primarily to establish a copious milk supply before they can nurse (see exclusive pumping). Unfortunately, even once they begin to breastfeed, you may still need to pump and empty the breasts to maintain the milk supply until they can do it on their own, typically after they each reach a weight of 7 pounds.

Feeding Plan

During the learning period, many mothers find it easier to nurse one baby at a time until they are comfortable, and breastfeeding is less challenging. To get through a 24-hour day and make time for the mother to take care of her physical needs, it saves time to get twins on the same feeding and sleeping schedule. Premature twins can be very sleepy and must be woken up to feed every 2 to 3 hours around the clock.

While learning, you can let one nurse until he is sleepy. Burp and lay him down. Nurse the other until he is sleepy. Burp and lay him down. Encourage the first baby to nurse again after resting and repeat for the second. Mothers of twins often find it practical to nurse one baby while bottle-feeding the other with assistance, until the babies nurse more efficiently (see paced bottle-feeding on page 246). If bottle-feeding proves to cause a change in your breastfeeding, try cup-feeding or finger-feeding instead (see Chapter 11).

Nursing Twins Together

Once the twins are nursing well, it will save you time if you learn to feed both babies together. In the beginning, holding both in the football position seems to be the easiest. Laying back with both babies vertical on top of your body (bellies to belly) is another helpful position. Props are essential early on. A nursing pillow designed for twins is highly recommended. The following is a step-by-step guide to logistically get the twins breastfeeding simultaneously:

1. When you set out to feed your babies, position yourself in a safe place with lots of room.

2. Have your nursing pillow in place. Make sure it fits your body so that there are no gaps. Elevate the sides of the nursing pillow with props (rolled receiving blankets or burp cloths) so that the twins tilt toward you to prevent the babies from rolling off the edge.

3. Before placing the twins on the pillow, set them on either side of you.

4. Start with the baby that has an easier time taking the breast. Bring him to the breast with the football hold. Once he starts nursing, turn to your props to free up your hands so you can get the second baby on the breast. Tuck a rolled up receiving blanket under the first baby's neck so you can remove your wrist and hand. If necessary, tuck another blanket behind the nursing baby's back to keep him from rolling away. If your breasts are heavy, prop a rolled-up washcloth under the breast to help support it.

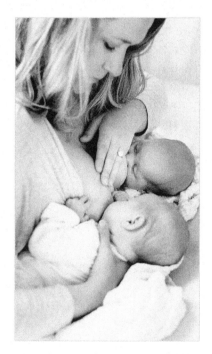

5. Now you are ready for the sibling. Bring the baby to your breast with a football hold on the other side. If the first is nursing correctly, he'll be able to keep the breast in his mouth while you position the sibling.

This mother is able to nurse both her babies at once, using a pillow designed for twins and the football hold. She helps one baby on at a time.

6. Repeat attachment and propping method for the sibling.

7. Once they are nursing together, lean back and take pride in your glorious accomplishment.

8. If they become sleepy, use your hands to gently press on the breasts to help release more milk. You may notice that when one baby stimulates a let-down, the other suddenly starts gulping with big eyes. This chain reaction of dual nursing stimulates the milk production overall and helps a skilled baby get more milk—an added benefit of tandem nursing.

Miscellaneous Tips for Twins

If one baby is larger than the other, and you have one breast that produces more milk than the other, start the larger baby on that breast. If one baby has a harder time with the flow, put the baby on the breast that is easier for him. Pump after or let the more vigorous baby finish the fuller breast if that is the breast the smaller baby prefers.

CHAPTER TWO

Learning the ABCs of Lactation

Chapter Goal: Learn how to bring in an abundant milk supply. Understand what you need to do to keep the milk flowing and ensure long-term success.

MILK-MINDED

Today, most health professionals agree that breastfeeding is the best start any infant can have. The American Academy of Pediatrics recommends that babies be exclusively breastfed for the first 6 months of life (AAP, 2012). Once complementary solids are introduced, the baby should be breastfed for the remainder of the first year, and after that, if it is mutually beneficial for the mother and child. The World Health Organization agrees; exclusive breastfeeding for 6 months is the optimal way to feed infants. After that, they should receive complementary foods with continued breastfeeding for up to 2 years of age or beyond (WHO, 2016).

If you give your baby unlimited access, letting him nurse at least 8 to 12 times in 24 hours, your body will likely make as much milk as the baby needs. Knowing a little bit about how your breasts make milk will help you understand the tremendous physiological changes your body is undergoing during lactation. This chapter will not only teach you how to build your milk supply but how to sustain it. You'll learn how protecting your milk supply and your infant's early experiences will benefit him in many wonderful ways.

Through successful breastfeeding, rest assured, your baby will get what he needs to reach his genetic potential and have optimal health.

ABOUT BREASTMILK

The best food for your newborn is the food your body provides. With few exceptions, breastmilk is made up of all the essential nutrients and protective agents the young infant needs. It is composed of proteins, immunoglobulins, nonprotein nitrogen, enzymes, hormones, growth factors, carbohydrates, and oligosaccharides (Gidrewicz & Fenton, 2014; Lawrence & Lawrence, 2011). There are also minerals, electrolytes, trace elements, vitamins, and water (Kent, 2007). To date, scientists have identified hundreds of ingredients in breastmilk (whereas formula has a few dozen). So far, no synthetic duplicate exists.

Breastmilk is easily digestible, processed relatively quickly from the baby's stomach compared to formula. Digestive enzymes and lipase found in milk help the infant break down the fats for easier absorption. Among the oligosaccharides are potent sugars that can stay alive in the baby's stomach acid. They serve to feed friendly bacteria in the gut, promoting the growth of bifidobacteria (a prebiotic), which helps build a lining that protects the baby from many diseases and harmful germs (Wall et al., 2009). While all mammals produce milk that has some of these qualities, human milk is species specific and contains the exact amount that a human infant needs to grow and thrive. Through your milk, you will pass on anti-infective properties specifically for your baby and tailor-made to protect against germs in your unique environment.

Evolving Nutrition

The beauty of breastmilk is that it is dynamic, changing as it builds. It evolves throughout a feeding, the day, and your breastfeeding experience. For example, the ratio of the fats and proteins changes as the milk matures (Gidrewicz & Fenton, 2014).

First Milk - Colostrum

During the first few days of breastfeeding, milk comes in the form of colostrum. First feeds transfer anywhere from 2 ml to 20 ml (30 ml equals one ounce)—just the right size for your newborn baby's tiny stomach (Walker, 2014). Colostrum is high in protein for the fragile newborn. This early milk has a laxative effect to help clear his intestinal tract of meconium (stool), helping to prevent jaundice (Lawrence & Lawrence, 2011). Colostrum is rich with protective immunoglobulins that coat the newborn's intestine with healthy bacteria (Wall et al., 2009). This seals the baby's gastrointestinal tract, which helps protect against allergies. It is rich with protective white cells that can fight many disease-causing bacteria and viruses. This first milk essentially works like a first immunization.

Colostrum can have an orange cast, yellow tone, be reddish, blue, or even greenish. It gets its bright color from high levels of beta-Carotene, which is a powerful antioxidant (Walker, 2014). It can also have different consistencies (thin or thick and oily), depending on the volume the mother produces. Colostrum is a multipurpose superfood. For one, if your baby has any pain associated with birth trauma or injury, the colostrum may provide pain relief because following a drug-free vaginal delivery, a mother's colostrum is loaded with pain relieving beta-endorphins, which remain elevated for at least 10 days after birth (Zanardo et al., 2001).

Copious Milk Production - Lactogenesis II

With the onset of copious milk production that occurs between 24 and 102 hours after birth, known as Lactogenesis II (milk coming in), there is an increase in the fat and protein content, and concentration of minerals and sugars (Kent, 2007). After day 5, the concentrations remain the same for about a month. As your milk increases, it will become a thinner-looking liquid that has a yellowish tint. This is called transitional milk. Around day 7 to 10, the milk will change to a bluish-white, thin liquid. This is called mature milk. Sometimes the food you eat changes the color of your milk. By 6 weeks, the protein content of mature milk is half that of colostrum (Gidrewicz & Fenton, 2014).

Milk-Intake Changes

The volume of milk your infant takes will change throughout breast-feeding. On the first day, a baby may nurse 3 to 8 times and have an intake of 7 to 123 ml (a teaspoon to 4 oz) of colostrum (Kent, 2007). On the second day and onward, babies generally nurse 5 to 10 times, with an intake that varies from 395 to 868 ml (13 to 29 oz) a day (Kent, 2007). By one month of age, milk intake ranges from 750 to 800 ml (25 to 27 oz) per day (Kent, 2007). Remarkably, this production will be stable for the baby's first 6 months (Kent, 2007).

Not all babies take the same amount. Mothers can have anywhere from 3 to 17 let-downs during a breastfeed, which is when the milk flow increases with a surge of oxytocin hormone, often causing the milk to spray (Kent et al., 2008). Your baby will stay on the breast as long as he needs for his satisfaction and individual growth needs. Hence, there is a milk volume intake variation of 440 to 1,220 ml (14.6 to 40 oz) per day (Kent, 2007).

Long-term Benefits

Breastmilk is the single most beneficial preventative medicine known to man. Through breastfeeding, you will help your baby grow normally and be healthier. It's not only breastmilk, but the act of breastfeeding that will help protect your newborn from illness. This protective advantage continues as long as you breastfeed. Six months of exclusive breastfeeding before introducing complementary food can set the stage for a myriad of benefits. Some are lifelong.

Exclusively breastfed babies are proving to have significantly better health outcomes than formula-fed infants during the first year of life where incidents of numerous infections that require medical care or hospitalization are less (AAP, 2012). Growing evidence credits breastfeeding for reducing the risk of several serious diseases that would otherwise shorten life or affect the quality of it. An analysis of nearly 10,000 studies, reviews, and abstracts found a history of breastfeeding was associated with a reduction in the risk of acute otitis media (ear infection), gastroenteritis (diarrhea), necrotizing enterocolitis (serious intestinal illness where cells die), colds, severe lower respiratory tract infections (bronchiolitis, pneumonia), atopic dermatitis (skin rash), sudden infant death syndrome (SIDS), and long-term, childhood asthma, obesity, type 1 and 2 diabetes, and childhood leukemia (Ip et al., 2007).

For mothers, a history of lactation is associated with a reduced risk of type 2 diabetes, and breast and ovarian cancers (Ip et al., 2007). A study looking at postmenopausal women found that those with a cumulative lactation history of 12 to 24 months had significantly fewer cases of hypertension, hyperlipidemia, heart disease, and diabetes (Schwarz et al., 2009). Breastfeeding mothers also have a lower risk of suffering from postpartum depression compared to women who stop breastfeeding early or choose to bottle-feed from the start (Ip et al., 2007).

The Infant Microbiome

Now more than ever, we are aware that we are what we eat. That certainly includes what the newborn baby eats. In the last decade, scientists discovered that the human body is made up of more microbial cells, including yeasts and bacteria, than human cells. We accumulate microbial cells from our environment and the things we eat and drink, beginning with our experience in the womb, through the birth canal, breastfeeding, and beyond.

The microbiome is the collection of bacteria, viruses, fungi, and other types of cells that live in our body. We have bacteria that are friendly and bacteria that are unfriendly in all of our organ systems. When the bacteria are in balance, we are healthy, and this is called symbiosis. When the bacteria are out of balance, then we have dysbiosis, or illness. Bacterial cells outnumber the human cells in the body by an estimated factor of 10, with 100 trillion microbes living in the gastrointestinal system alone (Embleton et al., 2015). The majority, 80%, of all antibody-producing B cells are in the gut (Benckert et al., 2011). Thanks to the ongoing government-funded Human Genome and Microbiome Projects, a vaginal delivery and breastfeeding have been proven to be the first and most beneficial ways to quick-start a healthy microbiome, a method critical for a lifetime of disease prevention and immune system support.

So, what can you do? If you wind up having a C-section, consider vaginal seeding, which is when sterile gauze is dipped in saline then inserted vaginally. After delivery, the gauze is wiped on the baby's skin to seed the newborn's microbiome with bacteria from the mother's birth canal. Her colostrum then finishes the process. Other tips include making sure your newborn is placed on your chest immediately after birth and breastfeeding as soon as possible. Ask to delay the first bath. Between you and the baby's father, keep your newborn skin-to-skin as much as possible. Ask to have the frequent infant vital checks conducted when the baby is on your body. To support a healthy microbiome, some experts even recommend using your own blankets, bedding, and first newborn clothes from home (Simkin, 2015).

ACTION PLAN

Build & Protect Your Baby's Microbiome
(1) Try to have a natural childbirth
(2) Take baby from womb to chest
(3) Delay the first bath
(4) Breastfeed soon after birth
(5) Keep baby skin to skin with mother and/or father
(6) Consider vaginal seeding after C-section
(7) Use clothing and linen from home
(8) Prevent separation

HOW THE BODY PREPARES FOR LACTATION

Pregnancy hormones prepare the breasts for lactation. During pregnancy, blood flow to the breasts just about doubles in volume (Geddes, 2007), making the veins visible and the skin appear thinner. Breast tissue and alveolar growth, combined with a branching of the ductal system, also causes the breasts to enlarge and feel tender. Most women grow at least one cup size, which is an excellent indication that the breasts are undergoing the changes needed to produce milk. Growth continues through the first month postpartum. There are significant variations, however, among women in how much their breasts enlarge. It helps to know that breasts come in all shapes and sizes and it is rarely an issue that affects the milk supply. Wear a supportive bra to carry the extra weight. Sorry, but it is pregnancy, not lactation, that causes the breasts to sag (Walker, 2014).

The areola, which is the shaded circle around the nipple, enlarges and darkens. Little bumps that look like pimples, known as Montgomery glands, enlarge and secrete an oily substance that will later attract the baby. Nipples that seem flat may become more erect. There is no need to rough up your nipples to prepare for breastfeeding. What you can do, however, is a self-pinch test to check for inverted nipples because this has been known to cause infant-attachment issues. Face a mirror in a manner that allows you to see where the nipple joins the areola. With your thumb above the nipple and index finger below, gently pinch. A truly inverted nipple will then bury itself into the breast tissue. A flat nipple will become more erect. If this self-test leads you to believe your nipples are inverted, consult a lactation consultant or obstetrician about ways to help the nipples protrude.

Observe Your Breasts

Before you learn to watch your baby, take a good look at your body. Your breasts should appear symmetrical, full, and spaced not too far apart. Any variation of this does not mean that they won't make milk but that they should be checked by your doctor or lactation specialist.

With the exception of underdeveloped breasts (see hypoplastic breasts), breast size is not important for making milk, as it is merely related to the amount of fatty tissue contained in the breasts. Research shows there is no correlation between the amount of milk a mother produces and the size of her breasts or the number of milk ducts she has (Ramsay et al., 2005). The most important components for lactation are situated within just a few inches of the nipple. Surgical breast reductions can reduce ducts or sever connections, but some may reconnect over time. It is important to know that it is not unusual to have one breast that is slightly larger than the other, or one that appears different in shape. Ultrasound imaging of lactating breasts has shown that despite differences, there is relative symmetry of the ductal system inside (Ramsay et al., 2005).

Some women may be surprised to discover what they believed to be moles are actually extra nipples or breast tissue that are suddenly growing and swelling from the hormones of pregnancy and lactation. Have your doctor examine these areas. In about 2 to 10% of females, extra nipples and/or breast tissue formed on the milk-line during fetal breast development and did not regress (Walker, 2014). Women also can develop breast tissue in the armpit area. When the milk comes in, these areas swell and may even excrete milk. While concerning, realize that it is completely normal. If you don't stimulate it, the swelling will eventually go away.

Anatomy of the Lactating Breasts

Breasts consist of fat with interwoven glandular tissue that contains the milk-producing cells (Walker, 2014). Breast tissue reaches to the borders of the armpits. There is a blood supply to transport nutrients; lymph-nodes to transport waste; and nerves that send the messages to the brain to release hormones targeted to cells in the breast to produce milk. New research proves ducts and milk cells are intertwined in the breast fat and end at the areola with more than half of the milk-producing cells packed closer towards the lower half of the breast (Ramsay et al., 2005).

The milk-producing cells are called alveoli. Each alveolus is surrounded by muscle cells. The alveoli contain special cells called lactocytes that absorb all the nutrients, protective immunoglobulin, vitamins, and hormones from the mother's blood to make milk. They also have tiny receptor cites that receive prolactin when the baby suckles. Surges of prolactin stimulate the cells to enlarge and multiply until the mother reaches her full milk supply. The alveoli appear in clusters, like grapes with connected branches, known as ductules, which lead to larger ducts that end at the nipple. Genetics determines how many ducts a woman develops. The nipple, made of smooth muscle, easily expands to mold in the baby's mouth. The center of the areola has many sensitive nerve fibers. Each nipple may have as little as four or as many as 18 openings, known as nipple pores (Ramsay et al., 2005). Milk ducts at the tip of the nipple are very superficial and easily compressed. This may be why babies who are not latched on correctly get very little milk.

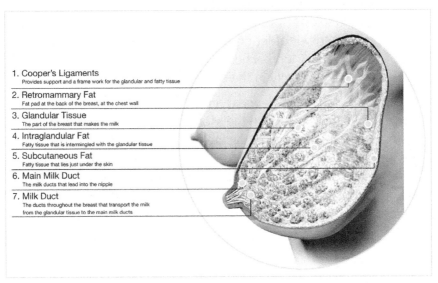

1. Cooper's Ligaments
Provides support and a frame work for the glandular and fatty tissue

2. Retromammary Fat
Fat pad at the back of the breast, at the chest wall

3. Glandular Tissue
The part of the breast that makes the milk

4. Intraglandular Fat
Fatty tissue that is intermingled with the glandular tissue

5. Subcutaneous Fat
Fatty tissue that lies just under the skin

6. Main Milk Duct
The milk ducts that lead into the nipple

7. Milk Duct
The ducts throughout the breast that transport the milk from the glandular tissue to the main milk ducts

ILLUSTRATION 2.1 - Internal Anatomy of Lactating Breasts.
Source: ©Medela 2018. Used with Permission

What Happens During Breastfeeding

Adequate stimulation of the nipple and areola is critical for breast-feeding success because it is responsible for triggering milk ejection (let-down). Without milk ejection, very little milk can be removed from the breast (Geddes, 2007). And if a good amount of milk is not regularly removed, milk production will slow down.

Let-Down

Before nursing or pumping, a small amount of milk flows by gravity to the nipple and areola. When the baby starts nursing, you will notice quick small sucks with intermittent swallows. Suddenly, the baby's eyes open, and the sucks and swallows become slower and longer. This means your milk has let down. Nipple stimulation during breastfeeding tells the posterior pituitary gland in the brain to release oxytocin into the bloodstream (Geddes, 2007). Oxytocin then causes the muscle cells that surround the milk cells (alveoli) to contract, ejecting the milk into little canals that lead to the nipple (Geddes, 2007). When the milk comes down, the ducts expand (dilate). Some mothers release a small amount of milk in pulses, while others have a flood of release. As the baby suckles, pressure increases and so does the flow of milk, triggering multiple let-downs. The average number of let-downs during a feed is 3 to 4, but the range is 1 to 17 (Mohrbacher, 2010). Only the first let-down is typically felt and usually in the opposite breast.

Bubbles of milk may appear on the areola during let-down. It is thought that this, along with the Montgomery glands, are designed to be a scent attraction, enticing the newborn to find the breast with his strong sense of smell (Walker, 2014). These glands also serve to lubricate the areola to withstand the friction from the baby's mouth. Not applying any creams or ointments in the early days of breastfeeding will protect this feature.

BRINGING IN THE MILK

Whether a mother chooses to breastfeed or not, her body is programmed to bring in a milk supply. During the second half of pregnancy, the alveoli become more active and begin to fill with colostrum. After the 16th week of pregnancy, she can produce milk. This is called Lactogenesis I, when milk or colostrum can be produced and released. In the past, when a mother chose not to breastfeed, she was given an injection to help her dry up. It was later discovered that this caused dangerous side-effects, such as strokes and heart attacks (Wambach & Riordan, 2016). What will further influence milk being made is the mother's health, hormones, fluid balance, breast storage capacity, stimulation during breastfeeding, and degree of fullness.

In the beginning, the body drives the milk production. The delivery of the placenta triggers a drop in hormones, stimulating copious milk production, known as Lactogenesis II. While it happens 30 to 40 hours after birth, most mothers don't feel it until their breasts become full 50 to 73 hours postpartum (Walker, 2014). Around 2 to 4 days after birth, you will know that your milk supply is beginning to increase because the breasts will become noticeably firmer, larger, and heavier. If you are lucky, your milk production will kick into high gear while you have an alert baby who is eager to nurse. However, many women awaken to the feeling of tenderness and discomfort, only to discover hot breasts under their hospital gown, and swollen veins, visible through their stretched skin. This is known as engorgement.

Many hormones are involved in milk production. During the milk building phase, there are critical times. In the first 10 days after delivery, the mother's milk-making hormone, prolactin, is at its highest. Breastfeeding frequently in conjunction with a vigorous, awake infant that has a strong suck, stimulates the cells that make and hold milk to multiply in number and grow larger. Surges of prolactin occur with infant sucking or breastmilk expression. Oxytocin, the milk-releasing hormone, is stimulated by physical interaction, such as nursing, cuddling, skin-to-skin contact, and stroking or kissing the infant's soft skin. When he begins to gulp, and his eyes widen, the opposite breast may leak as the milk releases. After Lactogenesis II, the baby becomes the dominating force behind the production of milk, and the breasts enter Lactogenesis III. From here on, the more milk the baby drains from the breasts, the more the body replaces.

Encouraging Your Milk to Arrive

You can ensure a plentiful supply of milk arrives between 48 hours and 4 days after giving birth by bringing your baby to the breast often, at least every 2 to 3 hours or 8 to 12 times in 24 hours. Keep your newborn near you so you can feed him each time he shows a desire to suck. If this is not possible, you'll need to use a hospital-grade pump that is strong enough to mimic newborn suckling (more on this ahead). At each nursing session, offer one side until the baby comes off or falls asleep. Once he wakes up and begins to show feeding cues (see Chapter 6), offer the other breast. If you can only interest your little one in taking one side, switch breasts at the next feeding. Once the milk comes in, it is necessary for the baby to nurse strongly, frequently, and long enough each time in order to soften the breasts for more milk to be produced. Wake the baby and nurse whenever your breasts feel full and uncomfortable. The more milk the baby takes from your breasts, the more milk you will make. This process is called "supply and demand."

Building the Milk Supply

Once the milk arrives, frequent breastfeeding continues to activate milk-producing cells. For most women, the supply will be fully in by 2 weeks (Kent et al., 2016). Other mothers need more time and reach their full volume of milk for that pregnancy by 40 to 60 days after delivery (Allen et al., 1991). Your body's signaling will direct you to build your milk supply. When the breasts feel full, hard, tight, or uncomfortable, your body is communicating that it's time to feed.

There are two factors that control your milk supply: the degree of fullness (the fuller the breast, the slower the milk production), and a whey protein, called feedback inhibitor of lactation. The fuller the breasts, the more of this whey protein is released and the less milk the breasts make. In other words, a fuller breast replaces milk slower. Because of this supply and demand milk-building relationship, when your baby begins to root, fuss, or suck on his hands, offer the breast before the pacifier or any artificial nipple. Be sure that the hunger need is met because, as you can see, this sucking demand is for more than comfort. Its purpose is to develop a sustainable supply of milk for now and the future.

Storage Capacity

Women differ in how much milk their breasts can hold. The range of breastmilk storage for exclusively breastfeeding mothers is 81 to 606 ml (2 2/3 to 20 oz) (Daly et al., 1993). Some women with large breast storage capacity can nurse less often, whereas women with smaller capacity need to nurse more frequently. Storage capacity is not necessarily related to breast size (Ramsay et al., 2005). A mother's capacity may increase when she becomes engorged (Kent, 2007). It decreases with the introduction of solids and weaning (Kent, 2007).

Factors that Affect the Milk Supply

Certain situations can negatively impact the normal development of a mother's milk supply. For example, a long, difficult labor and delivery impacts her ability to handle her newborn and respond. It may also influence the baby's sucking ability, leading to insufficient breast stimulation. This can hinder their start initially. In the absence of a vigorous baby, a hospital-grade pump with a correctly fitted flange (the plastic part you put to your breast) and proper technique is needed to bring in and maintain a milk supply (Meier, 2016). In Part IV of the book, we will discuss how to use a breast pump and what to do when you need to provide additional milk for your baby (supplementation).

There are many other factors, including maternal prenatal conditions, perinatal factors, medical and maternal management, and infant factors that can postpone or prevent the normal development of a milk supply (see Real Causes of Milk Supply Problems on page 351). Seek extra attention from a medical professional skilled in lactation if you find yourself in one or more of these situations. Parents need help and support until everyone recovers. For most healthy women, their bodies will heal, and they will be able to feed their baby. They just need to feed and give it a tincture of time. If you really dedicate yourself during the first couple of weeks to breastfeeding, you can take advantage of the surge of hormones that nature gives you to get the best start for your milk as possible.

PROTECTING YOUR MILK SUPPLY

To guarantee the safety and adequacy of your milk, keep the following in mind, and you will accomplish this very important task: nurse on-cue, avoid scheduling feeds, wait on artificial nipples, check medications, limit caffeine and alcohol, and avoid streets drugs and smoking.

ACTION PLAN

Protect Your Milk Supply
(1) Nurse On-Cue
(2) Avoid Schedules
(3) Wait on Artificial Nipples
(4) Take Care with Medications
(5) Limit Caffeine & Alcohol
(6) Avoid Street Drugs & Smoking

Nurse On-cue and Avoid Scheduling Feeds

One of the most important ways you can build and protect your milk supply is by choosing to feed your baby on-cue (on-demand). On-cue feeding is when you bring your infant to the breast to nurse whenever he shows hunger. The alternative is scheduling feeds every so many hours. Evidence-based studies support on-cue feeding over scheduling. Human newborns are biologically intended to feed frequently and quickly, despite cultural practices that favor scheduling. Putting all those social and primordial arguments aside, let's look at the most crucial point relevant to the modern breastfeeding mother; your milk supply is on the line.

Frequent feeding and emptying are crucial for building the milk supply, which varies with the amount of milk left in the breasts. Not feeding frequently enough will leave milk in the breasts, signaling the body to produce less. Nursing less than your baby demands risks reducing your potential milk supply overall. Consequently, you may wind up needing to supplement with formula or introduce solids sooner than you plan to meet your baby's growth needs. Studies show that if you don't nurse your newborn at least 8 to 10 times every 24 hours, then you will likely wean much earlier than your goal (Walker, 2014). In summary, if it is important to you to breastfeed for a full year, then be careful about limiting breastfeeding in the early months.

Abiding by a strict nursing schedule is also not conducive to the fact that young babies cluster-feed (short, frequent feedings) as many as several times a day. This pattern, common in the evening, is not fully understood. Sometimes it has to do with a baby being tired and overstimulated, furthermore needing more comfort and contact with his mother. Other times, it has to do with calibration. In the evening, the breasts typically have a lower volume of milk than at the start of the day, but a higher fat content because the emptier the breast, the higher the fat. Breastmilk production is designed to be an infant-driven system, and sometimes babies call for higher-fat milk, further demanding short, frequent feedings or cluster feeding. This feeding behavior is common for the first 3 months. Regardless of the reason, a baby's need to cluster-feed would surely sabotage any schedule or cause a power struggle where the baby's needs would be pitted against the mother's—a scenario where someone would be left disappointed.

It's very difficult and probably not a good idea to control a newborn baby's feeding pattern to meet the parents' needs. Infant nutritional needs take precedence. A newborn baby is learning to regulate, learning to feel safe, and adjusting to a very strange world after being inside a protective womb. Parents are tasked with making them feel safe so that they can begin to adjust, interact, and love.

Wait on Pacifiers and Bottles

Pacifiers and bottles can be useful tools in a mother's kit, especially for premature infants who need extra help developing the oral motor skills to breastfeed. For full-term infants, however, early use has been associated with less successful breastfeeding (AAP, 2012).

Pacifiers

The most immediate concern with pacifiers and newborn babies is that artificial nipples displace breastfeeding, which can impact the mother's milk supply and the baby's weight gain, potentially delaying the newborn's return to birthweight. To comprehend this rationale, it helps to understand normal newborn behavior. For the first few months of an infant's life, most babies require 30 to 40 minutes of suckling to be satisfied before going back to sleep. At a typical breastfeed, a newborn will suck for about 20 minutes, then rest for 15 to 20 minutes before wanting to suck for another 20 minutes. If you put a pacifier in his mouth in between breasts during the rest period, it's like ending a two-course meal before all the food has been served. A baby whose needs are met with a pacifier instead of the breast may be too sleepy to nurse or lack the motivation to empty the breast and place the "order" for a full milk supply.

If you want to err on the side of caution, wait until your supply is secure (after the first month). If a pacifier is introduced, try to discontinue it or cut back use once your baby is 6 months old (Sexton & Natale, 2009). Besides challenging breastfeeding, pacifier use has been associated with increased risk of ear infections, fungal infections, latex allergies, and dental problems (Mohrbacher, 2010; Sexton & Natale, 2009).

Bottles and Artificial Nipples

A baby who becomes accustomed to drinking from a bottle may be challenged to breastfeed, and vice versa, because the oral motor skills (mouth, jaw, and tongue movements) required are different. For one, artificial nipples encourage babies to close their mouth and bite down, using their gums instead of the wide-open jaw movements that are needed to milk the breast (Mohrbacher, 2010). The hard, artificial nipple stimulates the baby's tongue to hump back in the mouth rather than cup around the nipple. When a newborn breastfeeds, his tongue stays forward over the lower gum and cups around the mother's nipple, drawing it back deep into his mouth. This forms a teat from the nipple and areola that elongates while it is drawn back (Mohrbacher, 2010). Bottle nipples are firmer and more stimulating. Milk or formula flows immediately from a bottle, whereas, at the breast, a baby must work for it until milk ejection. These factors combined may cause the baby to take preference to the bottle over the breast. Over time, bottle-use weakens a baby's sucking muscles, making it even harder to switch from the bottle to the breast (Mohrbacher, 2010; Walker, 2017).

Considering the supply-and-demand paradigm of breastfeeding, bottle use can lessen your milk supply if protective measures are not taken. You can reduce the negative effects bottle supplementation has on breastfeeding by emptying the breasts using a hospital-grade pump before or after bottle use. A paced-bottle feeding technique can also help mimic the breastfeeding rhythm (see Paced-Bottle Feeding on page 246).

Nourish Your Body

The average breastfeeding mother will produce about 25 ounces of breastmilk per day (Butte & Stuebe, 2015). During the first 6 months postpartum, exclusive breastfeeding will take and burn about 500 nutritional calories (kcal) per day (Butte & Stuebe, 2015). While it sounds like a great weight-loss plan, it's important that you give your body what it needs to make quality milk. Depending on your age, weight, height, and activity level, the body will need about 450 to

500 kcal more per day (AAP, 2012). You'll need even more if you are nursing multiples. A tall, young, and active woman will need more total calories per day than a shorter, older, less active woman who weighs less (Butte & Stuebe, 2015). While the mother's diet does not significantly affect the amount of lactose fat and protein in the baby's milk, it can affect some vitamins and minerals (Smith in Mannel et al., 2012). There is a relationship between the mother's diet and the content of vitamin A, B vitamins, vitamin D, selenium, and iodine found in breastmilk (Smith in Mannel et al., 2012). Taking prenatal vitamins may help you ensure the right amounts, although the body's ability to absorb nonfood sources of vitamins is variable.

To account for the fluid loss, drink when you are thirsty, which will likely be more than normal. Always have a bottle of water within reach when you set out to breastfeed because, often, when the milk begins to flow, it triggers an insatiable thirst. It is not necessary to overdrink. Know that it's not drinking water that causes your body to make milk, but rather, emptying of the breasts. You'll know you are not getting enough to drink if the color of your urine is dark, the urge to go is infrequent, and your mouth is dry.

Consumption of vitamin D and calcium are important while breastfeeding because pregnancy and nursing cause a temporary loss in bone mass (Butte & Stuebe, 2015). A diet that includes 1,000 mg of calcium per day will help (Butte & Stuebe, 2015). Dairy products and green vegetables are excellent sources of calcium. Note: An adequate level of vita-

ACTION PLAN

Enhance your daily diet with:
450-500 kcal of healthy foods
water and milk
1,000 mg calcium
600 iu vitamin D
200 to 300 mg of DHA
Ask your doctor about B12 and iron

min D is needed for your body to absorb calcium. Most women need about 600 international units per day (Butte & Stuebe, 2015). While not the most ideal source of these vitamins and minerals, supplements and fortified foods can offer some benefit to meeting these nutritional requirements.

A maternal diet rich in Omega-3 fatty acids is critical for fetal brain development and continues to be important for your growing baby, who can get it through your breastmilk (Greenberg, 2008). About 200 to 300 mg of the Omega-3 fatty acid DHA daily is recommended (Carlson, 2009). You can meet this need by eating one or two servings per week of small fish, such as canned light tuna, salmon, or herring (AAP, 2012), but there is risk that fish contain contaminants. Avoid large predatory fish (e.g., swordfish, mackerel, tilefish) that can have high levels of mercury (Butte & Stuebe, 2015). Vegetable oil, fish oil, and supplements are also good sources of DHA (Greenberg, 2008). Go to USP.org to search for dietary supplement brands that are verified as contaminant free, such as Nature Made and Kirkland Signature. If you are anemic or have a special diet, such as vegetarian or vegan, talk to your doctor about additional ways you can meet the minimum nutritional needs. For example, a vegan diet may require a B12 supplement, and anemia may call for additional iron (Butte & Stuebe, 2015).

Take Care with Medications

You'll need to protect the safety of your milk supply. First, the greatest concern is preventing contamination of toxins that could get into the milk in concentrations that could harm the baby—think quality. Secondly, you want to avoid drugs that could affect your neurochemical system (secretion of hormones), which largely controls milk let-down. Make sure the medications you are prescribed are safe to take while breastfeeding (go to infantrisk.com). When possible, take pain medication immediately after feeding the baby to reduce the effects of the medicine on your baby (Naumburg & Meny, 1988). In the case of a low-intervention childbirth, ask your doctor about taking ibuprofen for pain relief; several studies have found it to be safe for breastfeeding (LactMed, 2016). Pain should be managed to prevent disrupting milk-producing hormones.

Avoid birth control methods that contain hormones in the early postpartum period, especially if you have risk factors for insufficient milk because these contraceptives have been known to decrease a mother's milk (Berens et al., 2015). (See Starting Birth

Control and Other Medicines on page 354). Cold medicines that contain pseudoephedrine should be avoided. Even a single dose of decongestant can significantly decrease the milk supply, likely due to how it affects the mother's prolactin secretion (Aljazaf et al., 2003). The Infant Risk Center (infantrisk.com) or LactMed can verify whether the medication you need is safe to take while breastfeeding (see Appendix) and may provide therapeutic alternatives. First consult your medical provider.

Limit Caffeine and Alcohol

Nursing mothers should be aware of their caffeine consumption and manage it so that it does not affect their baby or milk supply. There are numerous concerns with high intakes of caffeine, which is found in coffee, cola, energy drinks, yerba mate, and other teas. In studies where mothers consumed 10 or more cups of coffee daily, their babies suffered from jitteriness, poor sleep patterns, and fussiness (LactMed, 2016). Within about an hour of consuming caffeine, it usually appears in breastmilk at its peak (Stavchansky et al., 1988). Caffeine is metabolized slowly in newborns and preterm infants, so it should be avoided for the first month at least (Oo et al., 1995). After that, do not take more than 300 mg of caffeine daily (LactMed, 2016) and try to time it with breastfeeding. Figure a cup of home-brewed coffee has about 95 mg of caffeine. Be careful with energy drinks that do not have the caffeine content labeled. The beverage could contain anywhere from 0 mg of caffeine to well over 475 mg (Caffeine Informer, 2016). Go to www.caffeineinformer. com to check the caffeine content of your beverages.

If you have an occasional glass of wine (4 to 5 oz) or a beer (8 to 12 oz), wait 2.5 hours per drink before nursing. The amount of alcohol that gets into breastmilk closely resembles that of your blood alcohol levels, which peaks about 30 to 60 minutes after drinking or later when consumed with food (LactMed, 2016). Time to metabolize and eliminate alcohol in breastmilk is based on your weight and the number of drinks. Infants exposed to alcohol in breastmilk may take in less milk, have poor sleep, and have agitated behavior (LactMed, 2016). Heavy alcohol use is problematic, especially if the baby was exposed during fetal development (i.e., fetal alcohol syndrome). Alcohol decreases milk production and let-down after five drinks (LactMed, 2016). Babi̇‍   ̇rly exposed to alcohol may develop hȯ   ̇w excessive sedation, and/or fluid retentioṅ   ̇rs who have a family history of alcoholism mȧ   ̇in response with milk production (LactMė   ̇ts have disproven the old wives' tale that bė   ̇k (Wambach & Riordan, 2016).

Avoid Street Drugs and Smoking

A mother who uses illegal drugs, such as coċ   ̇ clidine (PCP), and methamphetamines, sḣ   ̇ breastfeed. Marijuana (cannabis) is also problematic and should not be used while breastfeeding. LactMed's review of available research also shows concerns about smoke inhalation in babies, causing an increased risk of sudden infant death syndrome (SIDS), and retarded motor development. Infants exposed to marijuana tested positive when drug tested. This may have criminal and custodial legal ramifications for parents who expose their baby to marijuana or other illegal drugs.

Women should quit smoking before becoming pregnant or setting out to breastfeed. However, the benefits of breastmilk, even with a mother who is not able to quit, have been found to outweigh the downside of not breastfeeding (Mennella et al., 2007). Never smoke near your baby or allow others to (clothes should be changed after smoking too) because exposure to second-hand smoke increases the risk of SIDS, asthma, pneumonia, ear infections, and bronchitis (Butte & Stuebe, 2015). Nicotine from cigarettes does appear in breastmilk, making it taste like cigarettes. The short-term effects of nicotine exposure include disrupted wake and sleep patterns, where these babies get less sleep overall (Mennella et al., 2007). Research shows tobacco use can also decrease a mother's milk supply (LactMed, 2016).

CHAPTER THREE

. . . .

Understanding Normal Newborn Nursing Patterns

Chapter Goal: Gain an understanding of early breastfeeding dynamics and normal newborn patterns.

NORMAL NEWBORN NURSING PATTERNS

Most healthy babies are awake during the first 2 hours right after birth and have a strong sucking reflex that makes them eager to nurse right away. Take advantage of this first alert time to get comfortable with breastfeeding and give your newborn the colostrum he needs. Let your baby nurse as long and as often as he wants because the more he drinks during the first hour, the more milk you will have later, and the sooner your supply will come in (Parker et al., 2012). Some babies are very fussy and need to nurse frequently to settle down.

After the first 2 hours skin-to-skin with active feeding, the newborn will enter a period of sleepiness for the next 18 hours or more (Wambach & Riordan, 2016). When kept skin-to-skin with his mother, he may arouse drowsily to breastfeed. Around the 20th hour, the baby starts to really wake up (Wambach & Riordan, 2016). He begins a period of cluster feeding, wanting to suckle frequently to keep his blood sugar steady. This can be every 1 to 3 hours until the mother starts to produce copious milk around 2 to 4 days. At times, it may be every 15 minutes during an hour, followed by a good rest. Many parents tell the tale about the long night before the milk came in. This feeding behavior is commonly misinterpreted as an indication that the baby is not getting enough milk at the breast, leading many mothers to feed formula samples they receive. The baby then becomes less interested in the breast, potentially compromising the milk supply.

After the first day, most babies are awake more and nurse often (8 to 12 times in a 24-hour period). The baby fills his tiny stomach, which can only sustain him for short periods, holding less than an ounce at a time. Eventually, babies fall into a pattern of 7 to 9 times daily, depending on the mother's supply and the feeding style of the baby. As your baby grows and your milk supply builds, he will eat less often and seem more content.

A TYPICAL BREASTFEED

A typical pattern at the beginning is 15 to 20 minutes of active feeding, followed by 15 to 20 minutes of active rest before taking the other breast. This routine of both breasts with a little rest in between is normal behavior for a baby feeding on an average milk supply, and is considered one breastfeed total. During a typical breastfeed, the baby latches on and begins suckling intensely. His body is flexed, and his fists are clenched. You would hear rhythmical "suck, swallow, breathe" sounds with little pauses that stabilize the baby's oxygen and coordination. These are known as sucking bursts. Every infant has their own pattern (some have 10 sucks then pause, and for others, 23 then pause).

Once the nursling begins to feel full, he gets a temporary feeling of fullness caused by a surge in the hormone cholecystokinin (Walker, 2017). It has a relaxing effect and slows down his suckling. You will see the baby's hands open and relax. He'll either come off the breast or stay on while his hold of the nipple becomes much lighter. After about 15 to 20 minutes of digestion and dozing, the hormone level decreases, stimulating more hunger. The baby will then seek the breast again (offer the other) and suckle until a second surge of the hormone signals satiation. You may also feel a surge of cholecystokinin and get sleepy (Walker, 2017). What happens next is a matter of the newborn's nursing style. Some eat until they fill their stomach and then sleepily reposition themselves on their mother's chest. Others get their meal and like to hang on. They continue to gently suckle as they drift off to sleep. If you remove the nipple and the baby is not full, he will root again, signaling for more.

During the break, the infant really appears done. Mom, perhaps, will change a soiled diaper and/or burp the baby before offering the other breast. However, many parents commonly misinterpret the break, thinking that the baby is full. They put him down and are surprised when he is ready for more. Some people misinterpret this normal feeding routine as a sign of insufficient milk. Mothers commonly complain that they can't put the baby down. It helps to keep him near the breast for about 20 minutes after nursing. When newborns take their full meal without pause, it can overfill the baby's tiny stomach and result in spit-up.

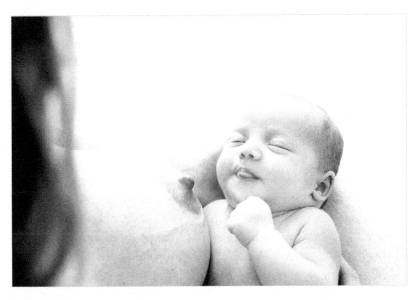

Babies typically rest between feeding on each breast. This baby poked her tongue out sleepily, letting her mother know she was ready for a bit more. The mom fed the second breast, and then the baby took a nice nap.

BREASTFEEDING DURATION

A typical nursing session where the infant takes two breasts lasts 35 to 55 minutes, including a 15-minute break and a happy baby in between. This is not a rule. Focus on watching the baby rather than the clock. Pushing the session to meet a time goal is not necessary. Instead, listen to what the baby's swallows sound like. Some infants eat for 10 minutes, gulp the whole time, and finish happy. Then they go limp and soil their diaper. A timer would tell you that 10 minutes of eating is not enough, but the nursling's cues tell a different story. This is an efficient baby. You can also tell it's enough by feeling your breasts before and after a feed. If the baby relieved the fullness and the breasts feel comfortable, he has probably had enough to eat.

BREASTFEEDING CUES

Following your baby's cues is more important than arbitrary "rules." Understanding cues will empower your parenting intuition and help you develop synchrony with your baby, which will make feedings more predictable.

It's Time to Nurse

Recognizing your baby's signs of hunger is a skill that will help you successfully breastfeed. Newborn babies communicate their hunger or desire to suckle by nuzzling, rooting, and searching. Like the baby, you have your own ways of telling when it's time to nurse by the way your breasts feel. If your baby is very sleepy, due to the effects of labor and delivery or the infant's mere temperament, your breast fullness will signal it is time to feed, driving feedings. Relieve any engorgement (tightness, painful fullness) immediately by breastfeeding or expressing milk because pressure on the milk ducts, caused by engorgement, tells the body to make less milk (see engorged breasts for a treatment plan). After your milk supply is well established (usually around 4 to 6 weeks) and the baby is gaining weight well, you no longer need to wake him up when your breasts tell you it is time to nurse, unless you need to relieve discomfort or protect your milk supply.

Knowing Which Breast to Offer

As the breasts fill with milk, they become firmer, and may leak when too full to relieve pressure. Get to know your "normal" by feeling your breasts before and after nursing. Begin breastfeeding on whichever breast feels fuller, with few exceptions. For one, if the baby has trouble with the flow and is fussy, start on the less full side. If the infant is not gaining weight well, start on the most productive side. Switch breasts when he seems sleepy.

Let-down: Milk Flow

Let-down may cause an uncomfortable tingling sensation for several seconds, often described as "pins and needles." It certainly is a feeling that takes getting used to. It can hurt but several seconds later, it passes, and you feel a sense of relief. Let-down is typically felt in the neighboring breast one is feeding on, leading some women to confuse it with a breastfeeding problem. You can experience the sensation of let-down while nursing, pumping, or even without physical stimulation. Women have long claimed to feel it years after weaning in grocery store settings, set off by a stranger's crying baby. New mothers commonly don't experience the let-down sensation until their baby is 4-to-6-weeks-old, but they often feel it right away when nursing subsequent babies. You can tell your milk is letting down by your baby's cues. You might notice the baby's eyes open wide as you hear loud gulping. The arms and clenched fists relax. You will see suckling slow down to a rhythm of about one suck per second. Newborns choke occasionally or sputter during milk ejection.

Strange Feelings: Effects of Hormones

When you first start breastfeeding, you may feel lightheaded and relaxed. It is nature's way of making breastfeeding pleasurable for you. Responsible for these feelings is the hormone oxytocin, which is the same hormone released during female orgasm. There is no shame in these sensations which are merely a neurochemical reaction.

Oxytocin excretion in the brain is one of the hormones that triggers milk flow in the breasts. It is also common to experience a sudden insatiable thirst during this let-down, so sit down to nurse with a drink in reach. The hormones released by breastfeeding help the uterus return to its normal size and heal faster, hence the cramping you might feel. Prolactin, the hormone that increases your milk supply, also relaxes you.

It's Working

Breastfeed is going well when:

- » About 10 to 30 seconds after the normal intense sensation, you feel a strong pull (not pain).
- » As the baby feeds, he sucks and then swallows without you having to remind him.
- » He stays on the breast long enough to relieve any fullness or engorgement.
- » The baby is content after eating for about 60 to 90 minutes.
- » He is urinating and excreting frequently (during or after every feed in the first 5 to 6 weeks).

Needing to Burp

When the baby abruptly interrupts his meal, pulls off the breast, fusses, and eagerly latches back on, he may need to burp. To help your baby get relief, hold him upright sitting on your lap. To support the weight of his head, hold your hand against his chest and upper stomach, with your fingers spread under his chin in a circle formed by your thumb and four fingers. Gently pat or rub his back in a circular motion, emphasizing the upward stroke. Take care not to bend him forward because this puts pressure on the stomach and may cause him to spit-up. Many babies will burp on their own if they are just held upright for a short time. It's really the upright position, not the pat, that brings up the air. Infants vary in their need to be burped. Some nurse steadily and do not swallow much air. The vigorous baby usually produces a resounding burp in less than 5 minutes. Some need to burp several times during a feed. For these infants, try burping between breasts, or when supplementing, every 2 ounces.

Emptying

While a breast is never empty, it becomes noticeably softer and lighter when a feed is done, or you've expressed substantial milk. You might feel a physical sense of relief or less pressure. The baby will show you cues of satiation, such as a totally relaxed body and open arms.

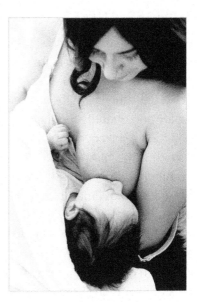

Knowing When to Feed One Breast or Two

Let the baby decide on whether you nurse one or both breasts at each feed. Watch closely for cues. Feed until he relaxes, then wait a bit. If after a short relaxation time, he wakes up and wants more, bring

A new mother cherishes one of the most wonderful breastfeeding moments—when her little one flutter sucks to sleep.

him to the other side, unless the first breast still feels firm. During the early days of milk production, try changing the baby's diaper after the first breast. This usually will wake him up enough to nurse for a while on the second breast. After the milk is in, don't worry if he is satisfied and thriving on just one breast per feed. Later, you may find that the pattern changes and the baby will need to nurse on both breasts to feel satisfied.

Nursing to Sleep

There reaches a point during a feed where an infant is suckling, getting no milk at all, and is perfectly content. This baby is going to sleep. You can tell because he does little flutter-sucks and relaxes his eyes. You no longer hear gulping or notice other signs of let-down. The baby suddenly seems perfectly welded onto your body. Intensity vanishes and the word "angelic" may come to mind. Sit back and relax while you enjoy this beautiful moment in your life.

NUMBER AND FREQUENCY OF FEEDS

As your milk supply builds, your baby will eat less often and seem more content, apart from fussy phases. How often should you nurse? There is no right answer. They say the average baby eats 8 to 10 times a day until they are about 6 weeks old. It's difficult, however, to qualify and quantify feedings. For one, there are multiple definitions for a feed. One such definition is when a baby eats from one breast or both if the baby started feeding from the second breast within 30 minutes of finishing (Kent et al., 2013). In addition, sometimes they eat several times in a single hour, each time seemingly satiated until minutes later, they are rooting for more. Times like this make it unclear as to when one feed starts and the other one ends. Furthermore, when you have a baby who is cluster-feeding all afternoon or waking up several times a night, it is very easy to lose track of how many times you nurse. There is no need to count feeds after your baby has returned to birthweight and is gaining on track. What matters is that you respond to hunger cues.

The main reason the 8 to 10 feeds rule is popularized is for cautionary purposes because studies that show this much stimulation is needed to bring in a milk supply. Once your milk supply is fully developed (around 30 to 40 days postpartum), how often you feed will change. Unfortunately, the widespread "rule" often leaves moms who are nursing more or less than average feeling like they are doing something wrong. Generally, the full-term newborn eats at least 7 to 9 times in a 24-hour period and not on any schedule (figure every 2 to 3 hours during the day and at least twice at night). There are babies that fit the mold, eating on average, but even these infants can have growth challenges. Not every mother-baby couplet has the same physiology. Some babies have a smaller stomach capacity. Also, the mother's milk volume varies, which affects frequency of feedings. Her breastmilk storage capacity may be less and, as a result, her baby may need to eat more often. If your baby is content after one breast and thriving, figure you have a large storage capacity.

If you are breaking the mold, you nurse six times a day, your baby's diaper is getting tighter, he has lots of wet diapers and stools, seems to be growing and gaining weight (you have verified that the baby is past birthweight), and appears content, just realize that your milk supply is getting established early. If you are nursing the average 8 to 10 times a day, and your baby is unhappy and not growing well, then there is something that needs to be checked. A skilled lactation consultant will be able to detect a problem and determine if a change is needed.

Nursing Duration

Eight-week-old Gianmarco took his meals in about 5 minutes, released his hold of the breast, then pushed away. If his mother tried to offer more when he was no longer hungry, he would gag as if utterly repulsed. She was concerned whether her boy was eating enough so she sought lactation help. When the baby tipped the scale with a 5-pound weight gain in only 5 weeks' time, it was clear that quantity was not the issue. Gianmarco's brother Joe had a completely different nursing style. Even after an hour of suckling, he could not bear to let go of the breast.

Nursing sessions with the newborn can easily exceed an hour. If you are worried that a feed is too long, consider his cues and ask yourself if the baby is actively eating the entire time. If you listen closely, you will hear rhythmical swallowing when a baby is getting milk. Once he begins to feel full or the breast softens, the rhythm becomes irregular and the sucks look and feel like little flutters. You can try to take your baby off. If he isn't full, he will protest and cue for more. If the baby is on the breast for one hour and is doing irregular sucks and swallows rather than a consistent pattern, then he may not be nursing correctly. Other possibilities are low-milk supply (see page 347) or sleepy-baby issues (on page 318). If you regularly have one-hour nursing sessions and the baby is still not satisfied, then you should seek lactation help and a medical evaluation.

DEVELOPING A NURSING RHYTHM

After a while of paying attention to your baby's behaviors before and after feedings, you will begin to notice a nursing rhythm that works for the two of you. For example, the baby takes one breast, relaxes for 15 minutes, and has a bowel movement. Then, you change the diaper and he is eager for more. You offer the other side and he nurses until he doses off to sleep. This is a typical pattern. Some mothers have a hard time developing a nursing routine because they are not able to read their baby. If this is the case for you, know that it is not necessarily your fault. Some babies are difficult to read. Developing a nursing routine you can count on will require some experimentation. Before putting the baby down after he has taken the first breast, really wait and see that he is done and is, in fact, sound asleep (see deep sleep on page 93). If you mistakenly put him down to bed when he was intending to take a short rest in between breasts, he could wake up disoriented and upset only minutes later. On the other hand, if he was enjoying a rest in your arms before nestling up to the second breast, he will be very pleased that you are right where he needs you. This response minimizes disruption and builds confidence in your nursing routine.

A diaper change is typically part of the nursing routine because newborn babies often stool each time they nurse, due to the immunoglobulins in the milk and a strong intestinal reflex (gastrocolic) (Lawrence & Lawrence, 2011). If your baby tends to be fussy, a diaper change during the rest period may ruin his whole rhythm. He may prefer to be changed before he goes to sleep or right when he wakes up. Some fussy babies do better if the diaper is changed between breasts. In conclusion, it is very important to look at your own baby and see what makes things go smoothly. Trial and error is how you learn what works for you. In the meantime, you will get to know each other.

COMMON CONCERNS

"Should I wake my sleeping baby for a breastfeed?"

Early on, the baby may be sleepy and difficult to arouse for meals. He may have long stretches during the day where he sleeps 4 to 5 hours. If he is not waking up regularly, then you need to intervene (see sleepy baby). If any of the following are true, wake your baby every 2 to 3 hours:

» The baby has not yet returned to birthweight.

» Your milk has not come in.

» Your breasts are firm and you feel engorged.

» You feel overly anxious and concerned.

» The baby does not regularly wake up on his own to eat.

For the baby not back at birthweight by 8 to 10 days, feed often and see a lactation consultant to evaluate your milk supply.

It is fine to let the baby complete his sleep cycle if the following are true:

» He has surpassed birthweight.

» The baby is at least 1-month-old.

» Your milk supply is well-established.

» Your breasts are comfortable (not engorged).

» Generally, the baby does not sleep through meals; today, he's taking an extra-long snooze.

» Your baby is normally good at showing you when he is hungry.

» When he eats, he is vigorous at the breast.

If you have a normal but sleepy baby, who has frequent wet diapers and stools, does not have jaundice, and is past birthweight, keep a log for a few days to assure seven feeds in 24 hours.

"Is my baby's urine and stool output enough?"

In the hospital, mothers are often told how many dirty diapers their baby should have and are required to log each one, including the type of contents. Then, the nurses meticulously record the baby's output (stools and urine) throughout the day. This tedious tracking is about taking vital care of this precious life to ensure the baby is getting nutrition, passing meconium (first black and tarry stool), thereby reducing the risk of jaundice, among other things, including problem detection. It does not mean that you need to count every diaper thereafter. A simple way to gage the number of diapers is by keeping a garbage pail near your changing area and emptying it once a day. To be sure that the baby is having adequate urine and stool, look at the whole picture—the baby's behavior in conjunction with adequate output (see diaper output on page 269).

Around 6 weeks of age, babies may have a drastic change in their stool pattern, in part because the digestive system becomes more mature and the milk changes. They go from having a bowel movement as much as every time they nurse to once every 1 to 7 days. Stools appear thicker and smell stronger. Less stool output leads some parents to believe that the baby is not getting enough to eat, and perhaps the milk supply is dwindling. It can be alarming and is often responsible for calls to the medical provider. If your baby is receiving breastmilk alone, there is no need to worry about constipation, unless the stool comes out in the shape of hard balls. This is unlikely for a breastfed baby and may be a sign of a different medical problem.

"I'm afraid I don't have enough milk."

Many mothers worry that they don't have enough milk. Unless they do a test weight on an accurate scale after nursing, women are left to follow their intuition and the baby's cues to determine intake. By comparison, the amount a baby drinks in a bottle is easy to visualize. Do have a medical evaluation if your baby appears thin, is not getting heavier, and is regularly discontent after meals. If worried, see a lactation consultant to help you determine whether your baby needs more milk (see perceived insufficient milk supply). At this age, 3/4 ounce to a full ounce is an adequate weight gain per day, or 4 to 7 ounces per week.

NORMAL BEHAVIORS AT THE BREAST

Parents are often blessed with a baby when they have little or no experience. It can be unsettling to take on such a responsibility with a learn-as-you-go approach. Because of a lack of knowledge about newborn behavior, the normal movements, crying, and unsettled behavior during the first few weeks often arouse the parents' anxiety and concern.

Latches On and Off, and Pushes Away

A baby may start to nurse, suddenly let go, fuss, and then latch on again. There are several reasons for this behavior. He could be trying to trigger let-down by working to get a deep enough latch to release milk, he may need to burp, or he may be displeased with the milk flow, which is either too slow or too fast. Babies also appear to be playing with the nipple instead of nursing if the breast is too engorged to grasp (see reverse-pressure softening). Observe what he is trying to tell you. Is he crying because he's getting too much milk? You'll know if, when he lets go of the breast, the milk sprays. Try leaning way back so that he is high above the breast so he'll have more control over the flow of milk. Does he need a burp? Hold him upright. Is he crying because he's not getting enough milk? A lack of gulping at the breast is a sign.

A newborn does not have a lot of control over his limbs and is eager to get a hold of the nipple as he tries to help himself. Hands, meant to help, are in the way. If you find his efforts are frustrating the both of you and preventing latching on, or calming down enough to eat, recline further. If that is unsuccessful or you need to sit upright, assist by wedging his lower arm between your body and his. Place your thumb on his shoulder of the upper arm and apply gentle pressure. This will limit movement of the arm while you help him take the breast.

In general, we don't recommend swaddling for breastfeeding, but there are times when the intense movements of the active baby get in his way. He can't control them and organize himself to feed. If the baby flings his arms and legs when they are free, you may need to swaddle lightly to get breastfeeding going. If a mother is using tools, such as a nipple shield or supplementer, to help with attachment, natural infant movements may become an annoyance.

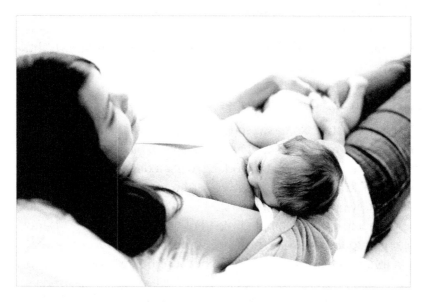

Laid-back breastfeeding helps prevent a number of breastfeeding difficulties.

The Baby's Suction Feels Strong

The baby needs sucking power to maintain a strong hold of the nipple and areola while the tongue and jaw work in tandem to milk the breast. It may seem remarkable how firm of a grasp a day-old baby can have on a nipple. It is very important to check to make sure he is nursing correctly, or the strong suction can cause injury to the nipple within seconds. The nipple and areola should be deep in the baby's mouth. A superficial hold of only the nipple and his gums can cause damage and pain (see nipple pain and soreness on page 271). Not releasing the baby's mouth from the breast properly can also do harm.

Not Feeding on Schedule

Recognize that there is no schedule when it comes to feeding newborns. Some babies barely show interest in nursing on their first day, while others suckle for cumulative hours. Some individual feedings last a few minutes, and others exceed 45 minutes. How a baby behaves in the first 3 days does not determine whether you have an easy or a high-needs baby. Often, the infant is reacting to labor and delivery, and merely adjusting to his new environment.

After the first feed, they want to nurse 2 or 3 more times before taking a good rest. For the next 16 to 20 hours, they may sleep or be sleepy. Breastfeeds are not going to happen on a schedule, such as every 3 hours. Instead, it might be every hour, 2 or 3 times. Then it might be every 4 hours, then a 5-hour period may pass, and the next feed may be just an hour later. If the baby was born in the morning, you may find him wide awake at night, hungry, and seeking the breast. Early on, babies generally do a lot more feeds between 9 pm and 2 am, and fewer feeds between 2 am and 9 am.

Won't Detach from the Breast

Many newborns have such a strong sucking drive that it seems they never want to finish a breastfeed. They are content to be connected to their mother. If the baby is thriving, has lots of wet diapers and stools, and the breasts are softening as you nurse, that baby may just need more suckling. If it's okay with you and your nipples don't hurt, no need to worry. There are normal times when babies are just discontent, needing more holding. If the baby is never happy, however, and does not want to leave the breast, it could be a sign of a milk-supply issue.

Excessive Gas

In breastfeeding support groups, mothers regularly voice excessive gas as a common concern. This normal quirk occurs as the stomach expands and the digestive system develops. Mothers perceive excessive gas as a sign of milk allergy. They eliminate dairy or they stop breastfeeding altogether and switch to formula. If you do limit your diet, see a nutritionist for ways to maintain a balanced diet with the proper amount of calcium.

Excessive gas is likely not a medical problem unless other symptoms are present. Signs of allergy are cradle cap that does not respond to treatment; eczema; clear nasal discharge; vomiting; green, bloody, mucoid stools; and extreme colic that does not respond to holding (see dairy allergy/sensitivity). If your baby has any of these symptoms, consult his medical provider before restricting your diet or using an over-the-counter product. It's best not to medicate "normal." Some anti-gas products contain Belladonna, which has been connected to high blood pressure and stroke (FDA, 2017).

The newborn digestive system is not fully developed and must get used to processing. Meanwhile, the walls of the stomach must stretch and that can lead to discomfort. Babies also take in air while they eat and when they cry. This, combined with regular digestion, creates the natural gas byproduct. If the baby is unfazed, then you can all enjoy a good giggle. If he is experiencing minor discomfort, you can help by holding him on your forearm, so that the side of his face is cupped in your hand, the chest rests on your wrist, the belly lays on your arm just above the inner elbow, and the legs straddle where the elbow bends.

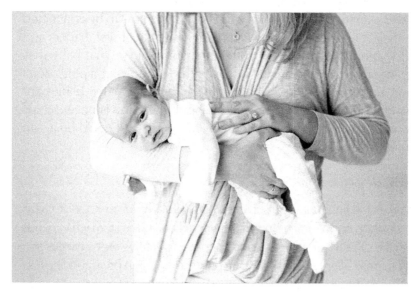

Gassy and colicky babies find comfort in being held tummy down on the forearm.

PART II

Getting Acquainted: A Time for Discovery

. . . .

CHAPTER FOUR

Introduction to Baby Watching—The Intuitive Parenting Approach

***Chapter Goal:** Discover a parenting approach that supports your breastfeeding goals.*

NURTURING OUTSIDE THE BOX

When Casey took her 15-day-old baby to the pediatrician for a check-up, she was surprised to learn that Ella was still 4 ounces below birthweight. The doctor reminded Casey that newborns should be back at birthweight by 7 to 10 days, and should gain about an ounce a day after that for the first 3 months. The new mother thought breastfeeding was going well. Ella cried very little, so Casey relied on a smartphone app to tell her when to breastfeed. Visitors commented, "what a good baby she is." The pediatrician referred them to IBCLC Andrea Herron for insufficient weight gain.

Their lactation consultation included a complete birth and feeding history. Casey had a long and difficult labor, which necessitated many different drugs to help the labor progress and to relieve severe pain. Since she had been home from the hospital, many friends and family were coming over to meet Ella. Casey mentions that Ella sleeps much of the day. "I feed her every 3 hours, like the nurses told me, even if I have to wake her," she said. She seems interested at first, takes the breast, but falls asleep soon after. When Casey lays Ella down, she wakes right up.

It seems that something is preventing Ella from finishing her meals. The next step in the consultation is a physical exam. It reveals that the mother and baby have normal anatomy and the mother's breasts/nipples show no signs of trauma beyond mild irritation. During the feeding observation, Ella eagerly takes the breast with correct attachment, suckles several times, then shuts her eyes and becomes inactive.

Andrea suspects the newborn is shutting-down (habituating). She says, "Let's try reducing the stimulation in Ella's environment to see if she can do better without it." Andrea turns off the lights and encourages Casey to lean way back and bring Ella skin-to-skin. They begin to breastfeed again. Andrea whispers, "Let Ella do her own thing. Try not to stroke her, talk, or move too much. Less is more. Maybe she's not ready to handle a lot of touching while eating." Little Ella begins gulping at the breast and, after a while, finishes her meal before falling asleep. Their test weight shows Ella took in the expected 2 ounces of milk. Casey is pleasantly surprised.

This is a common scenario and solution at the Growing with Baby practice in San Luis Obispo, California, where clinicians are seeing babies who have a hard time getting organized (self-regulating) following long, medicated, difficult childbirths. Breastfeeding literature resonates with these observations (Buckley, 2014). American culture dictates that parents should get their baby used to their home and sleep schedule by keeping the baby awake in the living room. (Most mothers can tell you that they've heard this advice at least once.) But this recommendation fails to consider basic infant development and the neurological capacity of young humans who may not be able to manage eating when all their senses are being stimulated with new experiences. One baby responds to being overwhelmed by shutting down (appearing asleep) while another reacts by crying uncontrollably.

Regardless, the experience after hospital discharge is commonly overwhelming. In some cases, the baby sleeps well in the hospital, leading parents to believe that they have an easy baby, but when they get home, everything seems to fall apart. They either can't wake the baby for feedings, or they can't stop him from crying. Many parents spend their first days home with their newborn, feeling confused by their baby's cues, frustrated by their failed attempts to make the infant happy, and overall, exhausted by the 24-hour care required. They have all their instructions from the hospital, including "feed 8 to 12 times for at least 15 minutes on each breast." In reality, a newborn's feeding patterns don't fit on a rigid schedule. The baby might feed for 5 minutes or an hour. He might seem done, but if the mother does not understand the true signs of satiety, she may put the baby down and lose confidence when he wakes back up, ready to nurse again. Without the clock and smartphones, some parents are hard-pressed to understand when to feed and how to learn what the infant really needs. It can feel like nothing seems to work to keep the newborn calm and satisfied. For the mother, sorting through left brained instructions when coping with her right-brained postpartum emotions puts her clarity of mind at odds.

Meanwhile, pressure coming from well-meaning friends and family members cause further anxiety. For example, they may make comments like, "don't let the baby use you like a pacifier," "Don't give a bottle," "Don't hold the baby too much," and "There should be 'this' number of poops and 'this' many wet diapers." It all means mental distress and conflict for a recovering mother, whose instincts are put on the backburner as she tries to please everyone. Moms coming for lactation help are often confused, frustrated, and hurting. They say, "my nipples are killing me." They ask, "how long should I leave the baby on the breast? I don't know whether to nurse one breast or two at each feeding; They tell me to wait for the hindmilk, but I don't know when the baby gets the hindmilk." Some may begin to blame their body for their baby's fussiness. They say, "I'm sure I don't have enough milk; my baby must be allergic to it. Should I stop dairy?"

Others are clouded with ideas from their 3 am-Dr. Google search, which mistakenly suggested that their baby may be tongue-and-lip-tied or proposed a trial at "block feeding." Without proper diagnosis or professional guidance, some mothers begin to sabotage their own success by making drastic changes to their diet and nursing routine based on this misdirected information and their own desperation for a solution to their baby's fussiness. They have their perfectly recorded logs, detailing the frequency and minutes of their feedings, but all this data has nothing to do with babies being full or feeding the way they are supposed to be feeding.

Rather than following generic instructions and rigid rules of baby care, success comes from watching your baby, listening to what he is saying, reading his unique body language, and responding appropriately. It is pertinent to develop these skills because no two babies are the same. Maybe you have a fussy baby who needs to be held more, or swaddled and laid down in a dark, quiet room. Or, perhaps, the baby is sensitive to stimulation and doing too much results in shut-down instead of sleep, and crying rather than nursing. Then there are infants with subtle cues, like little Ella, who signal (communicate) weakly and shut down easily, causing the parents to miss hunger cues. The result might be insufficient weight gain in the baby.

In Casey's case, she needed skilled lactation assistance to help her understand that the baby's sensitivity to light, sound, and touch was causing a sensory overload that exceeded her threshold. Casey learned how to modify their environment, so the baby could stay awake and finish her meals. The couplet had a rough start, but they got the help that they needed. Casey learned how to read Ella's subtle cues, and she eventually met her breastfeeding goals. If you find yourself relating to Casey and the countless other moms struggling to get settled with their newborn, put the rules and the clock aside. Continue reading, and you will discover a parenting approach that will support your choice to breastfeed and guide you as you nurture your little miracle into a thriving child.

BABY WATCHING

The path to keeping your baby nourished, calm, and happy can come through Baby Watching, a method that helps you quickly learn about your infant and what sort of care he needs. Babies are born with the ability to express themselves to communicate their wants, needs, preferences, character, and basic approach to the world

(Takikawa & Contey, 2010). The parents' job is to decipher theses visible signs and offer a sensitive response—one that promotes healthy growth, development, and self-esteem. Baby Watching will help you identify how your baby communicates each of his needs, preferences, and sensitivities through cues, including sounds, subtle movements, complexion changes, and reflexive actions. By reading these behaviors, whether purposeful or reflexive, you can answer the question, "what does this baby want?" The response will guide you as to how you can tailor your care appropriately for your individual baby, including how to feed and calm him.

How your infant reacts to his environment and each of his activities will give you clues as to his temperament. It will help you see his uniqueness and any strengths, vulnerabilities, or weaknesses that may require extra support. Through this guide, you will begin to unveil his personality and understand the role it plays as you move about your days together. You will discover how you can make each of his activities go smoother, from breastfeeding and diaper changes to play and sleep. The information you gain will reinforce your maternal intuition and help you interpret the ups and downs of your baby's behavior as he passes through normal fussy stages of infant development. With this knowledge, you can make sound parenting choices, despite the inevitable interference bound to come your way. As your observations and responses prove to be correct, your confidence will begin to grow. You'll be able to overcome predictable breastfeeding hurdles, stay on track, and avoid making choices that might otherwise sabotage your success and lead to premature weaning.

The Benefits of Baby Watching

Become a Baby Watcher, and you will become an expert in knowing your newborn. Learning your infant's needs by identifying his initial cues gives you the tools to offer the appropriate response. The right response helps your baby develop good self-esteem and confidence. It shows your newborn love and comfort while building a relationship of trust. By becoming a Baby Watcher, you will be able to prevent a plethora of difficult times, and hopefully, discover a flow that will enable your family to ease into a routine.

There is no recipe for this first task of parenthood. All babies differ in their activity level and the intensity of their reactions to stimuli (input through their senses). They also vary in their ability to adapt to different circumstances. Finally, they are unique in how they regulate themselves to their environment: control sleep, and stay calm and awake long enough to eat, interact, and learn new things. Your infant's personality and temperament are also special, as determined by heredity, maturity at birth, birthweight, and prenatal experience. Baby Watching, although natural, may require a concerted effort to practice. The rewards, however, are worth the effort. Once you become a Baby Watcher, you will be able to anticipate what your infant needs through his facial expressions and behavior alone. You will learn how to tell when your baby is hungry, full, tired, overstimulated, wanting to play, or just needing a break. You will discover the signs of milk flow and identify when he is nursing for nourishment or suckling for security. You will be able to answer, "when am I doing too much? And when do I need to do more?"

The Goals of Baby Watching

There are several main components to putting Baby Watching into practice that the remainder of the book will instruct in detail. Let the following goals be your focus, and you will succeed:

> » **Gain Knowledge**: Understand how healthy breastfed babies behave and develop regarding nursing, sleeping, crying, and attachment.

> » **Have Realistic Expectations**: Based on your infant development knowledge, you learn to adjust your expectations of yourself and your baby during this transition to parenthood and postpartum healing period, so that they are age and phase appropriate, as well as realistic.

> » **Create the Ideal Environment**: Create a physically and emotionally supportive environment that is tranquil and quiet. Keep family

and friend visits short and limited, so you don't miss the chance to observe and respond to your newborn's early-need cues.

» **Identify Your Baby's Cues:** Learn to watch your newborn closely to identify subtle changes in his facial expressions, sounds, skin coloring, gestures, behaviors, reactions to stimuli, and reflexive movements. Recognize that these cues are your baby's "language"—ways of communicating his needs, desires, sensitivities, and preferences.

» **Decipher Cues:** Learn to tell when your baby is hungry, full, tired, overstimulated, uncomfortable, sick, wanting to play, or needing a break. Interpret the cues you've observed and match them with the baby's feelings of hunger, fullness, fatigue, discomfort, overstimulation, ready to interact with you, needing a break, or just wanting to be held.

» **Respond Appropriately:** Try to offer a speedy and correct response to early-need cues before the baby begins to cry. At minimum, a loving response will meet his desire to be touched, acknowledged, and calmed.

» **Unveil Temperament Traits:** To better manage each of his states of awareness and activities, gather clues that will help you discover your baby's individual temperament (personality traits), which explains how he responds to the world.

» **Tailor Your Care:** Learn how you might need to modify your care, your baby's environment, your approach to activities, and the management of visitors to help your baby breastfeed more effectively, learn to interact, and build pathways to healthy sleep habits.

ACTION PLAN

Practice Baby Watching:
(1) Gain Knowledge
(2) Have Realistic Expectations
(3) Create the Ideal Environment
(4) Identify Cues
(5) Decipher Cues
(6) Respond Appropriately
(7) Unveil Temperament Traits
(8) Tailor Your Care

HOW TO BABY WATCH: THE METHODOLOGY

When you observe your infant, you pay less attention to the clock, smartphone apps, and rules, and more attention to how he is communicating with you through cues that signify "I'm hungry," "I'm full," "I'm tired," "I'm wet," "I want to play," or "I need a break." Fortunately, you were born with the tools to practice Baby Watching. The approach uses your main senses and channels your instincts when you stop, look, listen, feel, and evaluate.

THE STEPS

(1) Stop

(2) Look

(3) Listen

(4) Feel

(5) Evaluate

(1) Stop

Slow your pace, cease your tasks, and check-in with your baby often. Breathe deeply—in through your nose and out through your mouth while seeking a state of calm. As you take these moments, completely tune-out distractions and tune-in to your baby. Find your intuitive self.

(2) Look

Watch your newborn closely and observe his level of awareness, whether awake or asleep, and how alert or drowsy he may be. For example, if he appears to be sleeping, consider whether he is, in fact, in a sleep state or shutting down. If he is awake, watch for subtle changes, including how he is moving his body. Is he tense or relaxed, arching away or turning toward you? Look into your baby's eyes. Can you make eye contact, or does he seem unavailable? Is his eye contact intense or superficial? If the eyes are closed, do you see movement behind the eyelids? Watch what he does with his face, such as furrowing the eyebrows or yawning. In general, do you see fatigue, agitation, stress, discomfort, pain, or peace? Observe his skin color above the eyes and on the cheeks. Is there reddening or fairness? Look at the trunk of your baby's body, arms, and legs. Is the skin tone yellow or blotchy? Are the superficial veins prominent? Take a look at how the baby is gesturing. Does he seem to lack control over his movements? Are they jerky or smooth? What sort of behaviors, big or small, is the baby doing? Finally, observe how he reacts to his environment, including sights, sounds, surrounding energy level, and stimulation.

(3) Listen

Since newborns can't use words, we focus on non-verbal communication—early ways babies express their needs. Without close observation and quick responses from their caregivers, they quickly elevate their communication and make noise. Listen for coos, hiccups, spitting-up, whimpering, shrills, fussiness, and crying. Can you hear a certain tone in his cry? Is it high- pitched or moderated, low-energy or high?

(4) Feel

Touch your baby's skin and observe his body temperature. Is the

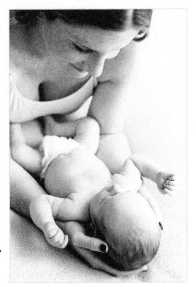

skin warm, cold, or temperate? Does it feel dry, normal, or clammy? Finally, notice how your baby changes when he is brought to your breast. How does he react to your touch and caring response? Does he push away or nuzzle up? Does he feel light, as if molding to your body, or heavy with resistance?

(5) Evaluate

Before you react, look into your baby's eyes again and ask, "what are you trying to tell me, baby?" Since you have informally gone through this process of observing and taking mental notes, your intuition should have gained valuable

Understand your baby better through Baby Watching—stop, look, listen, feel, and evaluate.

feedback. Soon, you'll be able to answer that question with ease. Overall, this is the methodology behind Baby Watching. The next several chapters will give you the knowledge to be able to decipher your observations. They describe the various states of alertness and sleep your baby undergoes, along with each of the behavioral cues that signify that your baby needs you. This information will help you evaluate what sort of response your little one desires.

REACHING DEVELOPMENTAL GOALS

Baby Watching is designed to support babies in reaching four developmental goals of infancy described by late psychiatrist Stanley Greenspan, MD, the world's foremost authority on clinical work with children with developmental and emotional challenges.

ACTION PLAN

Support the Following Developmental
Goals (Greenspan, 1999):
(1) Self-Regulation
(2) Formation of Relationships
(3) Become a Two-Way Communicator
(4) Problem Solve & Develop a Sense of Self

(1) Self-regulation

Greenspan explains: "One of the first goals as humans is that every child is born with a desire to learn 'self-regulation—the ability to feel calm and relaxed (organized), not overwhelmed' by the surrounding environment" (Greenspan, 1985, p. 14). The newborn must gain a sense of control over cycling in and out of sleep and staying alert long enough to eat and interact. The baby must learn to be able to focus on sights and sounds, attending to each one without getting upset or falling asleep, while staying under control.

At the same time, the baby has a codependent desire to become interested in the world through sensory experiences (Greenspan & Greenspan, 1985). Your job is to nurture this desire by responding to your newborn's cues appropriately so that innate curiosity continues to flourish in your baby while you provide him with opportunities to learn. When you respond to the early cues for hunger, satiation, fatigue, discomfort, disengagement, and overstimulation, your baby can more quickly become organized to calmly transfer into his next state of alertness or sleep without getting overly upset. Your sensitive response will help the baby stay awake long enough to eat and interact. Over time, he will learn how to manage his states better and self-regulate. If all goes well, he will enter the first developmentally settled period around 10 weeks, where he will cry noticeably less, stay awake more, smile, and sleep longer stretches at night.

(2) Form Relationships

Greenspan explains the second developmental stage in the human experience as "falling in love." After a baby has learned to self-regulate, he can begin to connect with those around him in a meaningful way. When Dad arrives home and greets his baby with sounds of joy, your little one will start to show his pleasure by looking intently, making sounds, smiling brightly, and waving his arms and legs with energy and delight. This is the beginning formation of a relationship. With support and healthy nurturing, your baby will master this developmental achievement by 5 months (Greenspan, 1999).

(3) Become a Two-way Communicator

The third developmental goal of interacting purposefully and becoming a two-way communicator can only be accomplished after the first two stages have been reached (Greenspan, 1999). This is when your infant's primitive (automatic) reflexes, triggered by feelings, touch, or sounds, will begin to be replaced by purposeful ones—choices and his ability to make movements himself. For example, he might show you that he wants to be carried by reaching out or whimpering. His communication will begin to seem purposeful and clearer. This progress should be apparent by 9 months (Greenspan, 1999).

(4) Problem Solve and Develop a Sense of Self

Once the first three developmental goals have been mastered, your infant will enter a new stage, which will continue past his first birthday, but ideally no later than 18 months. The baby's brain will begin to organize chains of interaction for simple and complex problem-solving (Greenspan, 1999). For example, if he wants a toy out of reach, he will be able to overcome this hurdle by showing you and pointing to indicate that he wants it. He will recognize his sense of self—that he has wants—and will seek to fulfill them.

Baby Watching is the key to success. Soon, you will truly understand your baby's communication and how you can support his goals to develop healthily and normally so that he can suckle, sleep, thrive, and much more.

CHAPTER FIVE

Recognizing Your Baby's States of Awareness and Abilities

Chapter Goal: Unveil your newborn's abilities, strengths, and any vulnerabilities, so you can consider the care he needs to enhance your breastfeeding experience.

FIRST FEELINGS

When Kate looked into her newborn's eyes for the first time, she was surprised by her feelings. She expected intense emotions like sparks—to know him already, but oddly, she felt like she was looking at a stranger. If you feel a lackluster connection of love-at-first sight, it does not mean that you do not love your baby—of course you do, and at this moment, more than anything in the world. Nothing would stop you from protecting your newborn like a tiger with her cub. The actual feelings, however, sometimes seem more like guilt and fear than love. Some mothers find themselves overwhelmed by a sudden sense of burden, a loss of independence, or remorse over no longer being pregnant. If you are shocked or disappointed by your newborn's gender or a physical abnormality, it could make these sentiments even stronger. Some moms feel like they have nothing left to give after laboring for hours and find themselves in a state of total exhaustion and pain. The body just wants equilibrium—for everything to go back into place—for the cervix to close and the wounds to heal. Maybe there are no feelings—just utter numbness.

It is normal not to immediately feel "love" as you know it because you and the baby are new to each other. Those feelings can take time to develop as your infant's personality emerges through your countless interactions with one another. When the emotions of love finally come, they may be so intense that you feel pure joy and a sort of euphoria that makes you instantly crumble to tears. It is all a part of adjusting to parenthood, an expression of your brain changing where cells are forming "motherhood" synapses (connections).

There are sometimes medical reasons for a subdued response. If you had an epidural during labor, you could have suppressed levels of oxytocin, which normally contributes to amorous feelings (Rahm et al., 2002; Stocche et al., 2001). These unexpected emotions could leave you silent with shame, knowing how much you wanted this baby and even more, how long you waited. It's okay. Even among any unexpected emotions, there is no shortage of real love to come. Mothers have described breastfeeding as the most beautiful and fulfilling experience of their life to date—a vehicle for bonding and enduring love. This does not necessarily mean that breastfeeding comes easily, but rather that the joys that accompany it are wonderful.

Your baby's reciprocal love for you may not be apparent until he realizes, around the age of 8 weeks, that he is not literally connected to you and is instead, an individual (van de Rijt & Plooij, 2013). Until he has reached this developmental milestone, he assumes he is a part of what he sees. This realization of individuality and separateness from you will drive an incomprehensible attachment to you. This feeling will grow as he begins to count on your caring response. His sweet smiles on the horizon will be the sparks that ignite this everlasting bond. When his gaze locks with your eyes only, you'll surely feel his reciprocal love.

NEWBORN ABILITIES

Babies are born with certain capabilities that promote the likelihood they will form a responsive attachment to their mother, an innate survival requirement. They have natural social potential and a cuteness that's borderline edible. Research shows that the smell of a new baby sets off reward receptors in the mother's brain in a way similar to how humans respond to the reward of food (Lundström et al., 2013). This may explain the "You're so cute, I want to eat you up" comments people commonly make to babies (cute aggression).

From the beginning, newborns can use all five physical senses. Their senses for hearing, seeing, feeling, smelling, and tasting help them interact and learn about their environment. From the beginning, they have inborn interests like faces, patterns, contrasting colors, and moving objects. They take pleasure in suckling, being held, carried around, rocked, and jiggled. When full and sleepy, they sometimes appear to have a smile. It may take several weeks for the effects of labor and delivery to wear off—even longer for your sleepy baby to "awaken" and his temperament to emerge. In the meantime, you can expect that if he is full-term and developmentally healthy, he will have the abilities of the average newborn baby.

Take the time to bond and get to know your baby. If you watch closely, you can learn a lot about each other early on. You can discover what he is capable of by observing his subtle behaviors and changes. For instance, baby Asher startles and cries when his parents move him too fast. Loud talking shuts many newborns down, which can interfere with being able to finish a meal. Your baby's response to his new world will tell you what sort of care he requires, what he finds stressful, and how he needs you to help him. As you become an expert in understanding your baby, this knowledge will give you a sort of parenting advantage. It will clue you in as to how you can keep your newborn calm so he can eat well and cycle in and out of sleep more smoothly. By having realistic expectations for your baby's natural abilities, you can better meet his needs so that he can develop healthy patterns. In turn, he will learn to feed effectively, gain weight, and succeed in meeting future developmental milestones.

Trained clinicians use an observational method to assess a newborns' capacities, that unveils the baby's particular strengths, temperament style, and needs. It's called the Newborn Behavioral Observation (NBO) system, developed by J. Kevin Nugent, PhD and his colleagues through their work with Harvard Medical School and The Brazelton Institute, which Nugent founded at Children's Hospital Boston. The NBO, derived from the Brazelton Neonatal Behavioral Assessment Scale, includes 18 behavioral observations, where the certified clinician watches the baby in various states of consciousness (awake, sleep, crying), noting how the newborn moves from state to state and reorganizes (calms) himself. The assessment also observes habituation (shutting down) to light and sound, muscle tone, rooting, sucking, hand grasping, crawling response, visual response to face and voice, orientation to sound and voice, visual tracking, crying, soothability, activity level, and response to stress (Nugent et al., 2007). The findings are a window into how the infant's motor and nervous systems work.

Unfortunately, relatively few parents and newborns get the benefits of this assessment because not all doctors are trained to administer the NBO or have the time in a normal office setting. Using what we know about the NBO's goals, strategy, and intent, this chapter will help you do little informal assessments in the form of Baby Watching to help you discover your newborn's capacities in all five senses and more, including self-protection skills. (To see the NBO in action, go to YouTube and search NBO assessment or Brazelton.)

INFANT STATES OF AWARENESS

Before getting into the heart of Baby Watching, uncovering specific infant cues and the helpful maternal responses needed, it is important to have a solid understanding of the six different infant states. In other words, whether a baby is asleep or awake, and how awake or asleep he is. Half of the states are of wakefulness, and the other three are periods of sleep. There is also a wild card, not included in the count, known as habituation, which is often confused with a state of sleep but is certainly no substitute, as you will soon discover. The goal is to understand how your infant's states of awareness affect each of your caregiving activities, especially calming.

State Regulation

The way babies experience the world depends upon how sleepy, alert, or irritable they are. The work of Dr. T. Berry Brazelton tells us that a baby's response to sights, sounds, and touch are influenced by his state at the time, or level of awareness. Brazelton development the Neonatal Behavioral Assessment Scale, which is used internationally to evaluate the physical and neurological responses of newborns, their emotional well-being, and individual differences. He taught us to understand babies by watching how they react to their surroundings. Your baby's responses, in the form of behaviors and cues, will tell you when he is ready for touching and hearing your voice, or when it is time for a break. Your newborn will also show you how he protects himself when he has had too much excitement or input through what's called habituation. Newborns have little control over their state. In other words, they often cannot keep themselves awake or stop themselves from crying. Until they learn to manage their states and reflexes (become organized), they are captive in the state of the moment.

The first goal of the neonatal period is state regulation: the ability to control bodily functions, manage emotions, and maintain focus and attention (Brazelton & Cramer, 1990). Babies learn this control through maturity, the caregiving they receive, and general interactions with their environment. You play a meaningful role in your baby's ability to become alert and interactive. Research has shown that newborns whose mothers were alert, attentive, and provided appropriate physical stimulation were better able to maintain their wakefulness, spent more time gazing at their mother, and showed positive interactions (Gable & Isabella, 1992). Regulation and rhythm are also closely connected. For example, we learn to adapt to the rhythm of the environment, such as waking with the rising of the sun, having dinner at sundown, and then going to bed when it's dark outside (circadian rhythm).

Regulation involves controlling physical, cognitive, emotional, and behavioral responses (Brazelton & Cramer, 1990). Looking away is believed to be one of the first intrinsic behaviors newborns do to regulate their state. The gaze aversion lowers their heart rate and reduces stress, so it's important that parents wait for the baby to pace the interaction (Field, 1981). Recognizing your baby's level of awareness will help you know the best time and appropriate way to respond. Since each state comes with a set of predictable behaviors, you might be able to tell how he will react to your care and for how long. You'll notice when your baby is transitioning to a different state, which alludes to what he might do or need next. The sooner you become an expert in his language, the easier it will be to help your baby stay calm, feed better, become more alert during the day, and sleep well at night, thus reaching the first goal of regulation.

How Personality Affects State

Your infant's innate temperament (personality) influences how smoothly or roughly he handles transitions between states. Some babies rapidly change state without warning. They go abruptly from asleep to alert to full-blown crying. These babies are often labeled "difficult." Other infants have slow state changes and make it easy for parents to intervene quickly before crying begins. People tend to call them "easy." Discovering your baby's unique temperament is covered in Chapter 10, along with how you can tailor your caregiving. By providing your baby with a sort of predictability and rhythm to your tender-loving care, you can help him learn to gain control. By learning the states of awareness, infant cues, and your baby's style of communication, whether subtle or obvious (potent), you will begin to nurture a healthy relationship.

States of Awareness

The following section will describe each of your baby's states of awareness to help you identify them easily. The three awake states are known as quiet alert, active awake, and crying. The sleep states are called deep sleep, light sleep, and drowsiness. The tricky one is habituation.

Quiet Alert

Newborns spend most of their day drowsy or asleep. Other portions of their time are spent eating or fussing. This leaves only a short period of time for being calm while awake and alert. This stage is known as "quiet alert" and usually happens 15 minutes before and after meals. When a baby is in a quiet alert state, his eyes are bright and wide open. He can make eye contact with others. His facial movements are extensive, and he may reach his tongue toward you if you are interacting with him. His body is flexed and alert. He can focus his attention on objects, such as moving fingers, faces, and voices. When in a quiet alert state, babies appear well organized with their arms and legs still. This is the best state and time for teaching, playing, and feeding. By providing your infant with sights, sounds, and food, you can help maintain this state. Taking the time to watch and respond to your baby's "timeout" and "I want to play" cues (described in the next chapter) will help your infant become more able to stay awake to interact with others. Maturity and your help will make these alert periods longer and more frequent. The quiet alert periods are important because, during this window of time, infants have an opportunity to learn and parents fall in love.

ACTION PLAN

Learn States of Awareness:

AWAKE STATES
(1) Quiet Alert
(2) Active Awake
(3) Crying

SLEEP STATES
(1) Deep Sleep
(2) Light Sleep
(3) Drowsiness
*Habituation

Active Awake

You will notice your baby's state shift from quiet alert to active awake when he begins to look away during play, appears distracted, and ceases to make happy sounds or facial expressions. Then the infant might arch his body, increase movements of the arms, behave a little fussy, and perhaps even release gas. The skin may become flushed or blotchy.

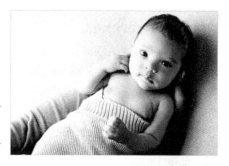

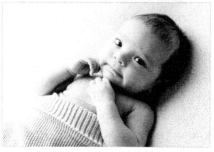

Active awake is a pre-crying state. During this period, babies communicate that they have had enough of the present activity and feel overwhelmed by their surroundings. They become more sensitive to noise, handling, and their hunger. When you notice your baby's fussiness, reach out and intervene before he enters a state of active crying because in active awake, soothing is easier. First, try calming the baby with the least stimulating interven-

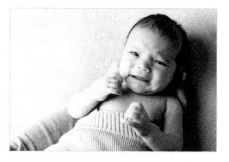

In this photo series you can see the transition from quiet alert to active awake. Notice how the infant's movements become disorganized.

tion. For example, talk to your newborn with a relaxed tone of voice and say, "Mommy's here. How can I help you, my love?" Next, help him hold his arms against his chest. If the fussiness persists, gently pick him up and bring him close to your body. The most effective soothing techniques during active awake include swaddling, holding, cuddling, shushing, and rocking.

Crying

The crying state is characterized by loud screams, shrills, facial grimaces, and increased body activities. The baby's arms flail. He may arch his back or kick. Crying is the final signal that your baby has reached his limit and needs you. A newborn's cries are a reflex—an automatic reaction to any feeling of discomfort or stress. This is a good time for rocking and cuddling. This is not a good time for playing, teaching/ learning, and feeding. For the "easy" baby, the minute you pick him up, he might stop crying. But for the more sensitive or "difficult" baby, once he reaches the crying state, he is stuck there and then the parents are stuck too, regarding solutions. This is where the Baby Watching really comes in handy. It helps to prevent this challenging state as much as possible. Crying will be covered in-depth in Chapter 7, including what's normal, ways to calm the baby, and how to manage it better overall.

Deep Sleep

While in a deep sleep, the baby's arms and legs are still and relaxed. He has occasional startles or twitches about every 5 minutes (Nugent et al., 2007). The eyes are closed, and you don't see rapid eye movements (REM) behind the lids. Breathing is steady and shallow. Any facial expressions cease except for the mouth, where the baby may make suckling movements.

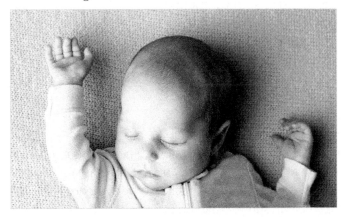

In deep sleep, you can see this baby's relaxed forehead and cheeks which appear to be sinking into her chin. Rapid eye movements are not observed in deep sleep. The hands are open, and the body is still.

If the baby falls asleep in your arms or an undesirable place, you may want to wait for the signs of deep sleep before laying him down in bed to avoid waking him up. While deep sleep is a good time to make the transfer, this is not a good time to try to wake up your baby for any sort of interaction, like feeding, for several reasons. For one, babies in a deep sleep do not wake up easily so you may get a rude awakening, pun intended. And secondly, infants need deep sleep to allow the brain to rest. If you watch closely, you may see your baby cycle into light sleep within a matter of minutes. Sleep will be covered in Chapter 8 and 9, including normal patterns, ways to promote longer stretches, co-sleeping, and sleep safety.

Light Sleep

Like adults, babies cycle in and out of deep sleep and light sleep, and not necessarily in any order. Light sleep is needed for the brain to organize new information, grow, and develop. In this state, infants make some body movements and noises. Even with the eyelids closed, you can see that the eyes are moving or twitching, known as rapid eye movements, or REM. Facial expressions in light sleep include quirky smiles and even sucking. Your baby may make brief fussing or crying sounds as well. The breathing is noticeably slow or fast but overall irregular. Light sleep is also the dream state. The noises your

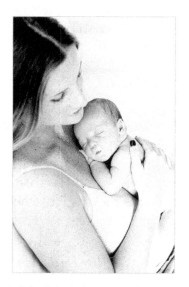

In light sleep, babies can make facial expressions and sucking movements, showing they might be dreaming about breastfeeding.

baby may make during light sleep do not mean he is ready to eat. If you want him to continue sleeping, do not pick him up. If left alone, babies in light sleep can cycle back into deep sleep. If the baby is stimulated, he will surely wake up from light sleep since this is the state that usually comes before waking.

Drowsiness

While drowsy, the body movements are variable, including mild startles from time to time. The eyes are heavy-lidded and open with a dull glazed look, then close. The baby may have some facial movements, like a crooked smile but often, none. Drowsiness is a state between asleep and awake. If you need to wake your baby to get a required feed in or face one of life's other realities, this is the best sleep state to do it. You can comfortably awaken your drowsy baby with gentle strokes to the face and upper body. Placing the baby on your bare chest will arouse him to feed, as his little nose detects the scent of your milk. Undressing, diaper changing, and talking are also effective tactics. If you have trouble waking your drowsy baby, try switching it up. For example, use your voice one time, touching the next, then skin-to-skin time. As you vary these tactics, watch for signs of arousal. If the baby gets sleepier, you may be shifting too fast. Variety awakens (Barnard & Thomas, 2014).

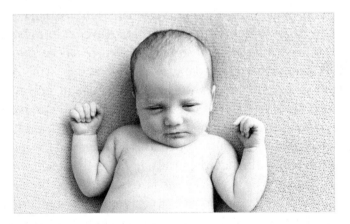

A drowsy baby is not quite awake or asleep. This is an excellent time to help transition the infant to sleep.

The Wild Card: Habituation

In their first 4 weeks, babies have a heightened protective mechanism called habituation, which they use to shut out bothersome stimuli, according to the research of Dr. Brazelton. The habituation behavior allows infants to reduce their reaction to repeated stimuli and essentially, learn to adapt (March of Dimes, 2003). Without this skill, they would react to everything in sight or earshot, leaving very little time and energy for vital tasks, i.e., eating and sleeping. When habituating, the baby appears to be sleeping. However, he is neither asleep nor awake—rather, he's shutting down. When a baby is feeling disturbed by too much noise,

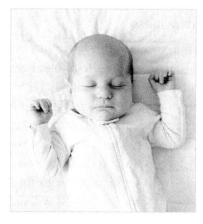

A habituating baby is entering a "sleep protection" mode that looks like sleep. Notice the presence of muscle tone.

motion, light, or other environmental factors that overwhelm his nervous system, it may cause him to habituate.

Just as all babies vary in their sensitivity, they also differ in their capacity to habituate. It is often the easy babies that habituate well, whereas overstimulation causes difficult babies to cry a lot or behave colicky. People typically confuse habituation for sleep. They say things like, "wow, what a great baby. He sleeps through all this noise," or "as long as we're in the car, he sleeps." Habituation, however, is no substitute for sleep, although it sure comes in handy for parents needing a dinner with their infant in tow. Habituating too often is not healthy for babies because it decreases time needed for sleeping and eating. A baby who shuts down all day, rather than taking proper naps, may not sleep well at night because he is too overtired to get good rest. To put it in perspective, try to remember the last time you stayed out far past your bedtime in a very stimulating place like Las Vegas. One could assume that after staying up all night, you would surely hit the sack and rest deeply. But it was probably not a good night's sleep.

The other trouble with habituation is that newborns only have the ability to shut out unpleasant stimuli in this way for several hours a day. By the evening, they lose control and spend much of dinnertime responding by crying or fussing. After the day spent habituating, they are quite simply overtired and fed up. This can be a very stressful time for families, making parents emotional and unnerved. It might seem like Mom keeps the baby calm all day, but when Dad returns home and she needs a break, all he gets are tears from his baby, crippling his confidence and motivation. Throughout the day, ask yourself, "is this baby sleeping or habituating? Is he shutting down in reaction to activities?" In the case of excessive evening fussiness, reflect on the hours prior and try making changes tomorrow.

ACTION PLAN

Limit Habituation. Habituation often happens:
In the car
On long stroller rides
In a noisy room
In a chaotic environment
When there is too much stimulation
When the baby is being passed around to visitors

Balancing State Control

The first day or two in the hospital, some babies shut down in response to noise and activity. They appear to be sleeping but could be habituating. Then they get home to a quiet environment, and they start crying because they are overtired from being overstimulated in the hospital. Also, infants have lost any excess fluids, which then drives their desire to eat more. However, if the delivery was highly medicated, the baby may take up to a month to recover to normal alertness. For example, a baby's state control may be affected by a long epidural with pain medication or a cesarean surgery, where the mother was on a lot of drugs and post-surgery pain medication (Klaus & Klaus, 2010).

State control essentially is the ability to sleep a long time and stay awake long enough to eat, bond, and learn something new. It is so important for parents to know. The goal of the first 2 months is to identify what gets this baby to sleep too much and what makes him cry too often. Usually, the answers have something to do with the baby's environment and our responses to them. Keep in mind what the baby underwent prior to the present place and time. Neither crying too often nor sleeping too long is good at this age. If they sleep too much, they do not gain enough weight. When they cry too much, they burn a lot of calories too, and they wear out their parents. It certainly makes life very stressful for families.

In general, you can help your baby learn regulation by spontaneously spending time face to face during quiet alert states. Take care that this early social interaction is a sensitive exchange. For example, avoid soliciting and forcing your baby to engage when he's not in the right mood or state. Overly enthusiastic visitors tend to make this mistake. When the baby looks away, do not bring your face to his gaze. Rather, wait until he turns back and shows readiness to interact again. Imitating your infant's behavior will also bring favorable results.

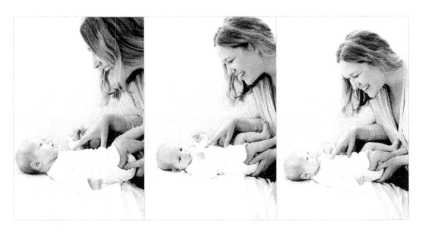

(1) The mother engages her baby to play. (2) When the baby feels overwhelmed, she looks away, giving herself a timeout. Meanwhile, the mother waits patiently. (3) After a short break, she returns her gaze to her mother.

GETTING TO KNOW YOUR BABY

Touch

A sensitivity to touch is a valuable tool in the newborn's sensory repertoire. Touch triggers various involuntary reactions that draw the baby closer to having his needs met at the breast and in his mother's arms. For example, certain ways you touch your newborn will trigger predictable responses. If his cheek is stroked or rubs against something, he will turn toward the stimulus with his mouth open wide. This is a reflex that gives him a readiness to suckle and a way to find the breast, known as rooting, which is most intense when the baby is hungry. Some babies easily root while others need more to respond. Observe the sensitivity of your baby's rooting reflex by touching the skin near the corners of the mouth and seeing whether it causes his mouth and/or head to turn. Is it triggered easily or not? If your baby has a weak rooting reflex, this can challenge your baby's hunger communication. He may have to let you know he's hungry by crying instead of a subtler cue, like rooting.

You can also use touch to help settle your baby. Numerous studies show that gently and moderately stroking the baby's skin has positive effects on his behavior and development. For one, it can reduce heart rate and promote calming in preterm infants (Field et al., 2006). When a newborn's feet are touched from heel to toe, the toes spread out rather than curl in, as they do with a 6-month-old. This is called the Babinski reflex. It stimulates a sucking desire. When a new baby is alert, placing your finger in the palm of his hand will cause the Palmar reflex, where he will close his hand around your finger and hold it tightly. This grasping reflex lasts up to 4 months. In an NBO assessment, the clinician observes the strength and sensitivity of the baby's hand grasp during a quiet alert state. You can try it too.

Reflexive movements are not purposeful. If you see your baby crawl or push his feet on your lap to stand up, it does not mean that he is trying to walk or crawl. Rather, the movements are inborn survival reflexes to help the baby get to the breast on his own. It is the loss of these innate responses that prove your baby's physical development is progressing. Once the reflexes are gone, voluntary movements are possible. In general, a new baby does not know that their little hand that comes out of nowhere and scratches them belongs to their body. Since newborns are not developmentally ready to understand their body is separate from their mother's, they feel the most secure when they are skin-to-skin on her chest (van de Rijt & Plooij, 2013). Skin-to-skin contact with the mother also has been shown to improve the baby's overall weight gain (Ohgi et al., 2002).

Handling Your Newborn

Newborn babies are small relative to those handling them. They can be picked up with a scoop of a single hand. Resist the urge to handle your baby with such ease and advise others to take extra care. Newborns, especially the sensitive ones, need to be picked up with their whole body comfortably held and feeling like it is supported. Bring the baby as close to your body as you can when lifting and be sure the arms and legs are not loosely dangling in the air mid-transfer. Failure to do so could set off a fussy baby very easily.

Newborns are also very sensitive to cold, hence why diaper changes can be traumatic. Rather than removing all the baby's clothes and diaper, exposing the body to cold, be sure to keep at least the belly covered with a blanket or leave an article of clothing on as you deal with cleaning the bottom. Gowns with an opening for the feet are helpful for early diaper changes because they keep the upper body covered. Wipe warmers and white noise machines can also make diaper changes go smoother for new or sensitive babies.

Strength and Movement

From the beginning, was your newborn able to lift his head and peak at the world, or does his proportionally large head seem too heavy to lift? With little strength and coordination, a day-old baby can move his head, arms, legs, and hands. Every day, he will gain more and more control over the position of his head. Observing your baby's neck strength will guide you as to how much support you'll need to provide. Breastfeeding and time skin-to-skin with your newborn, belly down on your body, will help him build muscle strength in his neck. As the first month goes on, his body will uncurl, and movements will slowly appear to be more purposeful. A sudden, startling movement may cause him to quickly extend all four limbs and fingers, then bring them back to his core clenched. This is called the Moro reflex. It lasts for up to 6 months (Gerber et al., 2010). Try to avoid things that trigger the Moro response in your baby.

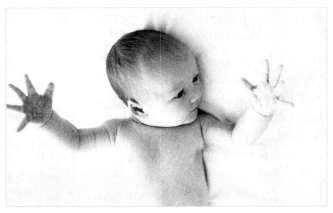

A startling noise or sudden movement can trigger a response in the baby known as the Moro reflex.

In an NBO assessment, the clinician helps parents observe their newborn's muscle elasticity in the arms and legs, first resting the baby on his back in a relaxed and alert state (Nugent el al., 2007). Then, they stretch the baby's coiled legs out as far as they go and release, watching how the legs retract. The same test is done with the arms. A tense and jittery infant may show strong resistance, while a baby with floppy arms and legs shows very little (Nugent el al., 2007). Parents can help their baby build strength by providing tactile stimulation during quiet alert routine play (Nugent el al., 2007). For example, have the baby push his little feet against your hand and offer small rings to tug on.

Vision

From day 1 through 2 months, newborns can see well 8 to 14 inches away from their eyes. They can focus, but everything beyond that is blurry. While a good seeing adult has about 20/20 vision, the newborn has about 20/200 vision (Nugent et al., 2007). While the essential anatomical parts of the eyes are completely constructed, visual acuity is dependent upon further development of the nervous system. The connections and interpretations by the brain are not developed until about 3 months after birth (Nugent et al., 2007). Through experiences guided by you during quiet alert periods, your newborn can continue to develop his visual acuity.

New babies have a preference for patterns that are black and white because their color vision isn't fully developed. They are also enticed by curved objects. Hence, they are innately interested in looking at people's faces and are particularly drawn to look and stare at eyes (Dupierrix et al., 2014). Studies demonstrate the newborn's preference for the mother's face. Researchers found that babies seem to know the difference between their mother and a stranger (Pascalis et al., 1995). Researchers also believe that newborns can differentiate emotions based on facial expressions and find mutual gaze calming (Blass & Camp, 2003). Smile for your baby and make eye contact often to nurture your bond. Breastfeeding will provide wonderful opportunities to gaze into each other's eyes and develop rapport (Klaus & Klaus, 2000).

One way you can learn about your baby's vision capacity is by making different facial expressions and seeing how he responds. For example, stick out your tongue. Your little one may be able to imitate you by pushing out his tongue through his lips. A day-old baby can follow an object, but it takes several weeks for the eyes to be able to make smooth tracking movements. In an NBO assessment, the clinician observes the infant's ability to track by holding a small red ball (ping pong sized) 10 to 12 inches from his face (Nugent et al., 2007). Once the baby focuses on it, the ball is slowly moved within vision range to see how well he follows.

Throughout the first 2 months, mimic this test with a small high contrast object to watch how your infant's tracking ability develops. Note that these assessments should be conducted when the baby is calm and alert. Too much all at once can overwhelm a young infant. When your baby averts his gaze, know it is time to cease. Refrain from offering toys to a baby in a crying, agitated, or drowsy state. The more you feed the baby's curiosity during quiet alert states, the more he learns to interact and grow intellectually. Through these positive experiences, you can reinforce your baby's desire and motivate learning.

Hearing

In the womb, babies begin to hear. By the end of the third trimester, the fetus can hear evidence of a vibrant and noisy world outside the uterus. They distinguish the sounds of their mother's voice and seem to recognize her when they finally meet (DeCasper & Fifer, 1980). While the anatomical parts for hearing are there at birth, development is not complete. The hearing center of the brain has further connections and refinements to make during the first 6 months of age to improve hearing function and the beginnings of language understanding (Nugent et al., 2007). Until then, a new infant cannot hear or localize all sounds and frequencies. At first, they hear sounds and speech with a sort of echo. Their hearing is sensitive, so noise may seem louder and more stimulating than it is for the rest of us.

Babies have different responses for various sounds. They might freeze and cease their own behavior in responses to a sound or look around to see which direction it came from. A loud sound might trigger the baby's Moro reflex, causing the arms and legs to shoot out. A disturbing sound might make him turn away or even shut down (habituate). For a baby who is held upright in a quiet alert state, a pleasing sound would be that of his mother's voice, talking in a soft, slow, repetitive, and high tone. For example, "I love you. Yes, I do. I love you. Yes, I do." We call that "Baby Talk." Numerous studies show newborns prefer the sound of their mother's voice. In one such study, mothers of preterm newborns were able to calm their baby and reduce the infant's heart rate with their voice alone (Rand & Lahav, 2014). Newborns are more responsive to higher tones when awake and lower tones when drowsy (Nugent et al., 2007).

In an NBO assessment, the clinician observes some of the newborn's hearing responses by holding the baby upright in a quiet alert state in a way that allows the infant to turn his head (Nugent et al., 2007). Then, the specialist gently shakes a rattle about 10 inches away from the baby's ear. If the newborn is responsive, he may quiet his body, turn to find the sound, and/or brighten his face with interest, apparent by wide open eyes. Note: A baby with a limited auditory response may not react to the sound, or even try to locate it. This assessment is repeated with the other ear. A baby may not react if he does not like the sound.

Taste and Smell

Newborn babies already have their senses of taste and smell intact. In fact, these senses are even more sensitive than an adult's. Most babies can positively identify their mother's milk and smell from any other person (Cernoch & Porter, 1985). Research also shows a preference to sweetness; infants suck harder and longer as they differentiate between plain, lightly sweetened, and very sweet tastes. They can show you disgust by foul smells and even respond to sour and bitter tastes by turning away, crying, or making awkward facial expressions.

Oral Expression

During the first few days of life, the newborn can make reactionary sounds, but the noises are more reflexive than purposeful. Needs prompt these sounds but soon, people's faces and voices will also trigger oral communication in the form of coos and gurgles. The baby has a readiness to control his cries so that they sound different, say for hunger over pain, but it will take several weeks for most parents to be able to distinguish between the two. Research shows a correlation between sucking behavior and sound where the rate of sucking increases in response to pleasing sounds (DeCasper et al., 1980). Over time listening, you'll notice his unique sucking pattern.

Stress Response

Mother Nature gives newborns a way to alarm their parents, arming them with the ability to produce sounds and signals with nonverbal behaviors. Crying is the most obvious stress response babies have but there are many other lesser-known cues. Subtle signs of stress include grimaces, mouthing movements, changes in breathing, and slight color changes. More obvious stress cues include crying, startles, tremors, rapid skin-color changes, spitting up, and interruption in breathing (Nugent et al., 2007). Begin to catalog what makes your baby feel stressed so you can start to understand what his threshold is for stimulation.

Self-Consoling Skills

A new baby who feels overwhelmed and sets out to cry may search for ways to self-console. A baby with such skills may bring his hand to his mouth and suck to try to calm down. An infant with self-consoling skills may settle down from the overstimulation when put down in his bassinet and left alone for a break. While you may notice some subtle early self-soothing, know that most new babies usually require their caregiver's help to stop crying.

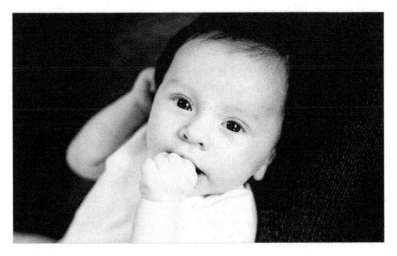

During interaction, this newborn uses his self-consoling skills to help himself stay calm and alert.

You can observe your baby's self-consoling skills when he starts to cry by slowly introducing one tactic at a time, beginning with the least stimulating. Gently set him down to give him a moment, knowing that he may set out to an all-out-cry. In an NBO assessment, the clinician begins by looking and talking to the baby, seeing whether he can use the professional's voice and face to quiet himself (Nugent et al., 2007). If after 10 seconds, the crying continues, the clinician places his hand on the infant's belly while continuing to offer soothing words. Then, he offers the baby more support by holding the arms and legs. Picking up the infant, then rocking, then a pacifier is tried, each one at a time with about 10 seconds before the next. The clinician observes how quickly the baby soothed, if at all, and how much support it required. Some babies calm by staring at something or using their hands to settle. You can conduct a similar test to see whether your baby needs more or less help to maintain organization. If a calm state is not reached, you'll want to identify stress triggers and focus on caregiving that prevents crying.

Sleep Protection

Babies can protect their sleep from noises, light, and other stimulation in their environment, but the extent to which your baby can shut out sleep disturbing stimuli depends on his unique capacity for self-regulation and sleep protection. His level of reaction to sleep intrusion can tell you a lot about how he responds to stress. For example, a trained clinician conducting the NBO shines a flashlight for a brief second or two on the eyelids of a sleeping newborn. The parents and clinician observe any reaction the baby makes, such as a startle or any other sign of stress (see stress response). After 5 seconds, the clinician shines the light again, looking for the baby's reaction and whether it has increased in intensity, like crying or decreased, like a facial grimace. This test gets repeated every 5 seconds, up to 10 times.

Some babies can protect their sleep better than others and may simply turn away and stop responding, reducing their response (habituating) within the first five shines of light. A baby who adapts, but with difficulty, may finally be able to overcome the challenge after six exposures to the flashlight. Other infants display great sensitivity to the light and rather than protect their sleep by habituating, they awake and cry.

This simple test has great implications for caregiving. If you have the baby that does not habituate well, you'll need to help him protect his sleep until he develops the skills to do it on his own. You can support this special need by putting your baby to sleep in a dark and quiet place in your home, where his sleep will be less likely disrupted. If you have a baby who has a wonderful sleep-protection capacity, you'll need to watch closely to make sure he doesn't spend too much time shutting down. Because habituation burns more calories than sleep, limit stimulation (lights, noise, guests handling the baby) in the home.

Interaction During the Early Days

Newborn babies are, in many ways, captive to their state of the moment, whether asleep or awake. Too much stimulation will turn them down. If you are hoping to get their attention, you may need to darken the room, get down by their face, and talk quietly for a response. During the first few days, babies have short windows of alertness before they get drowsy again and need you to stop the stimulation so that they can drift off to sleep. In the coming chapters, we will discuss the environment for success and how you can further tailor your care based on your baby's individual sensitivities and temperament. Like a sweet Maui onion that can draw tears in an instant, you are beginning to peel away the layers on this intimate journey of discovery. The sooner you understand this new member of your family, the fewer tears will be shed. The next step is identifying your baby's early cues, designed to alert you to a pressing need. Soon, you will have passed the first hurdle of parenthood. Your baby will be alert and interactive: someone you are beginning to understand.

. . . .

CHAPTER SIX

Knowing Your Newborn:
How Your Baby is "Talking" to You

Chapter Goal: Learn to identify each of your baby's cues that signal his needs. Understand what your baby is trying to tell you so that you can offer responses that help him breastfeed effectively, stay calm, and sleep soundly.

BABY TALK

Babies communicate using special body language, known as cues, long before they can speak. In the womb, the fetus develops the ability to enact physical behaviors that after birth attract reactions from the caring adults they rely on to meet their needs for growth, development, safety, food, and comfort. Most importantly, babies can tell their parents exactly what they need by using these special motor behaviors. There is meaning behind their subtle behaviors and facial expressions, like when they purse their lips and turn their head, open or close their hands, and/or arch their spine, among many other movements often triggered by inborn reflexes or feelings of discomfort.

Ultimately, these reflexes help them interact and bond with their caregivers in the hope of having their needs met. For example, even the slightest brush of the mother's skin against her newborn's cheek can trigger an insatiable drive in the baby to search for the breast and respond with behaviors that show hunger. If the mother is paying attention and is responsive to her baby's needs, she will bring him to the breast for nourishment and comfort. This interaction is designed by nature to build her milk supply and meet her baby's biological needs.

Babies differ in how they signal. Some are more transparent, predictable, and regular than others (March of Dimes, 2003). They vary in how clear their communication is. In other words, whether their cues are often subtle (mild signals) or obvious (potent signals), this readability will either challenge or help you understand your baby. For example, the communication of a placid or easy-going infant will likely be unclear, whereas a baby with frequent potent cues will be more obvious and may give parents a sense of urgency with each cue, making them feel rushed. Luke quickly goes into a loud cry the minute he wakes up. Addison wakes up, sucks her hand, and if the mother doesn't notice, she misses a meal. Addison isn't gaining weight while Luke is very chubby.

Just as readability varies, so does predictability. Some infants quickly develop a sort of regularity regarding sleeping, waking, and eating cycles (March of Dimes, 2003). They are often labeled *easy* babies. If you have a predictable baby, you will be able to learn how to anticipate what your baby is going to do next based on the prior behavior (Stratton, 1982). A predictable baby might eat every 3 hours before dozing off to sleep each time. Still, a predictable baby may not respond consistently in all activities. Hence, learning your baby's cues is a suitable strategy to understand and care for the need of the moment. The parents of an unpredictable infant, with little regularity and unclear cues, will likely be the most challenged to figure out and anticipate what their baby needs. In Chapter 10, you'll be able to learn how to unveil the unique characteristics that define your baby's personality.

How your baby moves his hands or tongue, and how relaxed or tense his little body looks, will tell you something about what he needs. For example, before a breastfeed, the baby might flex his arms, bob his head, open his mouth wide, fuss, or suck on his hands to show a desire to eat. Recognize that crying is a late, more desperate (potent) way of communicating, and typically follows one or more earlier subtle cues.

THE IMPORTANCE OF A MATERNAL RESPONSE

Newborns are innately programmed to brighten their face when you look at them. That's how they get your attention. It's from years and years of evolution. When you look into your baby's eyes, you also brighten your face, and perhaps comment. If a parent is in touch with her child, when the baby looks away, the mother will give him a timeout as not to overwhelm him. If the baby keeps looking, the mother stays engaged. The more you respond in this way and build the bond, the more you enforce interaction (parent-infant communication) and the sooner the baby will get organized. Again, being organized means not being stuck in a state of sleeping or crying, but rather, being able to stay awake and alert so longer periods of interaction can take place.

Unfortunately, nature gives us consequences when we don't pay attention. If you misread your newborn's early "I need something cues," i.e., "I'm hungry," or ignore them all together, the infant will likely go from rooting to crying in a desperate attempt to get someone's attention. His state of calm becomes disrupted. The next time he needs something, he may become anxious, sensitive, and consequently more apt to cry (Greenspan & Greenspan, 1985). This miscommunication delays the newborn's ability to self-regulate and may interfere with his sense of trust when needs are not being met (Greenspan & Greenspan, 1985; Leach, 2010).

Babies must feel recognized to have trust. They generally start off equally in their potential to grow, learn, and be accomplished. But, if the environment does not nurture that and find a way to say, "Yes, you are worthwhile. Yes, I want to listen to you. When you look at me, I want to look at you," then they turn off. If this continues, then the shutting-down reaction is reinforced (Vorster, 1980). Without trust, young infants find their job of learning to self-regulate more difficult.

In extreme cases, babies whose needs are regularly unrecognized may begin to lose interest in the world around them, which can hinder the child's normal, healthy development, according to a body of research produced by Greenspan and Leach.

There are differences, however, in how well babies adapt. Greenspan explains, in *First Feelings*, "When feeling internal disharmony, some people can easily return to a state of focused attention and deal with the challenge at hand. Others, when faced with anxiety or internal conflict, immediately panic and their fragile sense of 'organization' is upset" (Greenspan & Greenspan, 1985, p. 15). This disharmony challenges bonding between the mother and child. Not understanding the baby's cues, nor providing the right response can delay the baby's ability to reach the first settled state at 10 weeks (Nugent et al., 2007). When babies are not recognized, they feel stressed, and this disorganization interferes with the beginning parent/child relationships and attachment.

A baby who fails to develop a secure attachment, and repeatedly reaches a state of crying or withdrawal when his needs are not met, may develop emotional characteristics that carry on into adulthood, including how the person deals with stress (Vorster, 1980). He may become overly anxious and insecure (Leach, 2010). But when you go to your baby and react to early need cues before crying begins, your infant will gain more confidence and advance in his development. It will help make your baby more secure and capable, while giving him a feeling of self-worth.

DECIPHERING YOUR BABY'S CUES

Your baby is *talking*. While you are still discovering what he is trying to tell you, what you've probably discovered by now is that the baby's needs are many and confusing. One thing is certain; you undoubtedly want to fulfill these needs, and anything that conflicts with that will likely make you feel very uncomfortable. That's your instinct *talking*. However, interpreting your baby's non-verbal communication might sometimes feel like a frustrating game of charades. Be a good detective. When your baby cries, look at his body and listen to the rhythm and tone. At first, your newborn's cries will all seem to sound the same. However, with time (about 4 to 6 weeks), many parents say they can tell what their baby needs by the specific sound or tone of the cry. Before then, body language cues are keys to unlocking doors of misunderstanding.

Using the Baby Watching method (stop, look, listen, feel, and evaluate) will help you start to meet and overcome this common challenge. Take the time to identify what your baby does when he feels hungry or full (satiated), wants to be social (interact) or be alone (disengage), is ready for sleep, and needs comfort or calming to manage discomfort or overstimulation. Most likely, several cues or behaviors will happen at the same time, showing you what your baby is trying to tell you, just as we use many words or phrases to communicate. Furthermore, it is important that you combine observations of clusters of cues to get an overall picture of what your baby needs (NCAST, 2003). This chapter describes potential groups of cues (clusters), beginning with the most subtle and initial ones before progressing to potent and later cues. It will also show you how your baby might respond when his cues have been missed. Ways to quickly rebound will be provided, so you can calm your baby and fulfill the needs you've identified.

ACTION PLAN

Recognize My Baby's Cues for:

Hunger

Satiation

Time-out

Overstimulated

Fatigue

Discomfort

Engagement

Hunger Cues

Newborn babies have a distinct sucking drive, triggered by a decrease in blood sugar levels (Mohrbacher, 2010), which makes them seek their mother's breast. This is interpreted as hunger or thirst—a need for nourishment, essentially telling them that it's time to eat. The sucking drive makes them wake up and fuss to attract their mother's attention. Newborns give clear signs of hunger. By learning what those signs are and watching your baby, you can initiate feeding before crying begins. It is especially important to respond to your baby before he cries because trying to nurse a crying infant is frustrating. Crying babies need to be calmed so that they can coordinate breathing and breastfeeding mechanics (correct tongue movements). Remember that your body also gives off cues when it is time to feed. Your breasts may feel uncomfortable or a tingle. If your baby's communication is unclear, you will need to listen to your body and respond to its signals.

Early Signs of Hunger

When newborns are hungry, they give off initial engagement cues that show an interest and readiness to eat, like cooing or sucking sounds. Most early signs are subtle—mild messages, like looking at Mommy with wide-open eyes. They wake up, stick their tongue out, look around, then they bring their hands up to their mouth and perhaps suck or gum their fingers. You will notice rooting, which is when a baby opens his mouth wide, purses his lips, and moves his head from side-to-side. Some babies make

HUNGER CUES

Mouthing Movements
Tongue-Smacking Sounds
Rooting
Reaching Out
Hand to Mouth
Hands Held Together Under Chin
Hands Grasped Over Belly
Arms Tightly Flexed
Turning Toward Breast
Fussing
Crying
Back Arching
(Adapted from NCAST 2003)

smacking noises. When cues go unnoticed, the baby may become restless. An infant several weeks old may begin panting with excitement when picked up, as if anticipating what's to come. If in the lying position, a hungry baby will turn his head toward the body of his caregiver, as if looking for the breast. If he makes contact with the warmth of a neck or arm, he may even attempt to suckle. If close to the breast, he might try to help himself, bobbing up and down until he hits the bullseye.

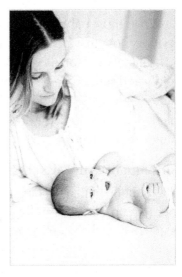

You can confirm this hunger hunch by bringing the baby to the breast when he shows you readiness cues. If he latches on eagerly and begins sucking vigorously, you can be sure of his thirst. If he gave you the cues, then keeps letting go of the breast, burp baby. Once the baby starts nursing, he will attend to business and reward you with focus and attention. Infants

A mother conducting Baby Watching observes one of the earliest hunger cues: the baby's arms come up and she roots from side-to-side.

are sometimes relaxed at the beginning of a feed and show engagement cues while suckling gently in the hunger posture (NCAST, 2003). For example, the baby will bring his hands together underneath his chin with open or closed fists and look at his mother's face with wide, bright eyes.

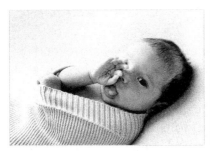
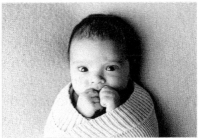

This baby is showing her mother several hunger cues before she sets out to cry, including holding her hands under her chin, tightly flexed arms, hands to mouth, tongue smacking, and mouthing movements.

While most babies' "I want to eat" cues are easily interpreted, there are those that are more difficult to understand. It really depends on the infant's personality. Coming from a sleep state, some wake up rapidly and scream desperately to be fed. They give the impression that they are not getting enough to eat. Others awaken slowly and quietly, casually looking around and waiting for their mother to recognize that they need to be fed.

Consequences of Missed Cues

When subtle initial feeding cues go unnoticed, babies naturally increase the intensity of their communication by crying, arching, or even pushing away. These are considered late feeding cues. The fussy or more difficult baby will start screaming, with no intention of giving up. Once this persistent infant reaches a crying state, it is very difficult to settle him down, especially to eat. Crying babies have a hard time breastfeeding. When crying, the tongue goes toward the roof of the mouth. With the tongue up, the baby cannot take the breast.

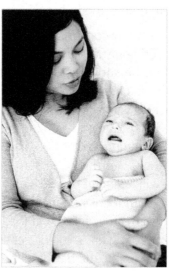

When crying, the tongue goes toward the roof of the mouth. With the tongue up, the baby cannot take the breast.

Easy newborns sometimes fuss quietly until they are tended to, or they shut down and go to sleep, consequently skipping a much-needed meal. Infants that make a habit of habituating at meal times may not gain enough weight. In summary, you may have waited too long to breastfeed if the baby is crying loudly, arching his back, and having trouble latching on. Or, you may be missing your newborn's hunger signals often if he is breastfeeding less than 7 to 9 times a day, waking up and going back to sleep before he eats, or sleeping a lot (more than one 5-hour sleep period in 24 hours).

How Breastfed Babies Signal

Humans are mammals with mammary glands that can produce milk with the birth of a child. Some mammals are spaced feeders, meaning that they feed infrequently (Dewar, 2008-2014). Their milk is high in protein and fat, designed to sustain their offspring for long periods (3 to 4 hours) while the mother forages (Jenness, 1974). Space feeders leave their babies behind in the nest and when they return, the animals feed vigorously and quickly (Dewar, 2008-2014).

We are continual feeders (Tilden & Oftedal, 1997). Our milk is low in fat and protein, and changes throughout a feed and during a 24-hour period (Jenness, 1974). Newborn babies count on their mother for frequent feeds that not only nourish but help them reduce stress and maintain their body temperature. Without proximity and frequent skin-to-skin contact with the mother, early humans risked death. Babies are required to signal frequently to develop normally, form attachment with their mother, and build the milk supply.

Bottle-feeding practices have human infants imitating spaced feeders (Dewar, 2008-2014). Formula takes longer to digest. They commonly overeat, leading to increased risk of obesity. Scientists are just beginning to understand the implications of changing the feeding paradigm, not to mention the food contents. For one, this model may be affecting human cognitive and psychological health beyond infancy, as attachment issues and lower IQs are being observed in bottle-feeding populations. In a UK study of over 10,400 children, babies who were schedule-fed at 4-weeks-old had poorer cognitive and academic outcomes between age 5 and 14 compared to those fed on-demand (Iacovou & Sevilla, 2013).

How to Rebound: Help your Baby Get Organized

If you think you often miss hunger cues, and your newborn is not gaining enough weight, breastfeed every 2 to 3 hours or sooner, even if you must wake him from sleep. If you missed the early hunger cues and your baby is now crying, you can help by gently and slowly picking him up. Hold him upright and close to your body. Talk softly, then make shushing sounds. You may need to swaddle him. Some babies will calm down quicker if the room is dark and quiet. You can try offering a clean finger or pacifier to suck on just long enough to calm him before bringing him to the breast. When he calms down, express some milk to the nipple tip to arouse his sense of smell, then try to breastfeed.

Satiation Cues

Watch your baby's body. It will tell you when his hunger is satisfied. When he first starts to eat and is famished, his fists will be tightly clenched and held close to his face. His body will be tense. He will suck hard and gulp. He may sometimes gasp and choke. As he fills up, you will see his body begin to relax. He will continuously swallow with a little rest every 10 to 20 sucks. As his hunger is satisfied, his entire outer arm may relax and drop down to his waist while his hands open. When completely full, some babies gently release the nipple and let go of the breast, or push away. Others like to hold on, lightly sucking (doing flutter sucks) until they drift off to sleep. From his fingers to his toes, his little muscles will become so relaxed that it's as if he is molding into the contours of your body (your baby's nest). You may notice very little, if any, facial expression. Be aware that babies who are sensitive to the environment, or perhaps

SATIATION CUES

Arms Extended
Arms Limp Alongside the Body
Relaxed Fingers
Decreased Muscle Tone
From Vigorous Eating to Flutter Sucks
Gently Releasing the Nipple
Pushing Away

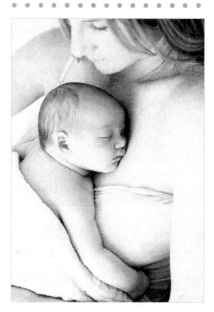

After taking the second breast, this baby showed she was content and full by gently releasing the nipple and resting herself on her mother's chest where she fell asleep. Her arms fell limp alongside her body, showing she had a good and satisfying feed.

are not having a deep enough hold of the nipple, may appear this way very quickly into the feed. It might make you think the baby is done, but the minute you put him down, he will wake up and cry. For hard-to-tell infants, listen for sucks and swallows.

Consequences of Missed Cues

If you misunderstand your infant's satiation cues, you may wind up ending a feeding session too soon. If this becomes routine, it is like offering snacks rather than full meals. If your baby is not filling up his stomach during feeds, he could be hungry sooner than if he had completed a meal. This may also lead to insufficient weight gain and for you, confusion regarding your milk supply. Feeding more often than what you expect to be normal may lead you to believe that you don't have enough milk, when in fact, it may be as simple as misunderstanding satiation cues. Many new babies eat for 10 to 20 minutes, rest for 10 to 15 minutes, then want more. This pattern should be expected and does not signify a problem.

Just as you can shorten a meal, you can miss the "I'm full" cues. Babies that are forced to eat when they've had enough may push away from the breast or arch their back. For an eager baby that takes in too much milk too fast, it may cause him to spit up the extra milk that does not fit into his stomach. If the spit-up resembles breastmilk just as it went down rather than partially coagulated or digested milk, this may be the case. Eight-week-old Gianmarco, who suffered with silent acid reflux, known as GERD, gagged if he was brought to the breast when he wasn't hungry or was pushed to nurse to a time goal. Mom was confused because the baby took his meals in less than 10 minutes, far shorter than her expectation and the instructions she received. In this case, the baby's cues communicated several things: the mother had an abundant, established milk supply; Gianmarco was an efficient nurser, getting enough to eat despite the short feeds; and he had a medical condition, GERD, that required extra care.

Some babies will continue to suckle softly, long after their meal is complete in a light sleep state. Gianmarco's brother Joe needed to suckle for about an hour at each feeding, preferring to sleep attached. His patient mother, who enjoyed breastfeeding and watching her nursing bundle, behaved liberally and enjoyed this peaceful time.

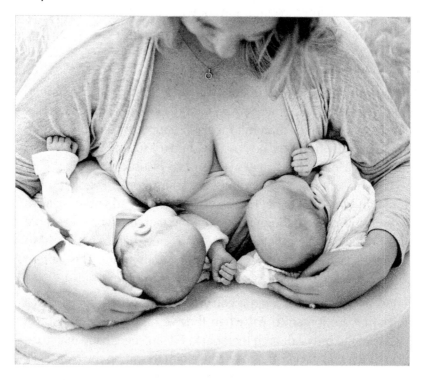

These twins show how different the cues are for a baby who is full and content (left). Notice the infant's relaxed arms compared to the sibling (right) who is hungry. Her body is tense as she actively feeds.

How to Rebound

Rather than watching the clock to determine when to end a breastfeed, allow your baby to tell you when to stop. If he is relaxed, appears satiated, and you no longer hear milk-flow, you can choose to release him from the breast by breaking the suction. After a few seconds, if you see that your baby is eager to feed again or cries, continue nursing. If not and he is content, try laying him down to sleep. Try not to force a feeding session to reach an arbitrary time goal or you may find yourself wiping up spit-up from overfeeding. Breastfed babies are auto-regulators. They ask to eat when hungry and settle when full.

Engagement Cues

Babies naturally want to interact with their caregivers and learn about their surroundings. If you pay close attention, your infant will tell you when he is ready to socialize or play by showing you engagement cues. For him, "ready to play" also means able to look, listen, and learn. It's your opportunity to talk and teach.

Early Subtle Cues

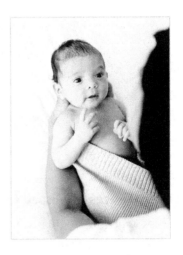

A nursing baby wanting to interact in a focused and purposeful way shows engagement cues. During breastfeeding, these signals happen when the baby stops sucking and makes eye contact. When a newborn wants to interact, he shows his mother by being calm and alert. When he moves, his muscles are relaxed, not tense. When your baby wants to interact with you, he might lift his head, direct his eyes at you, and follow your voice or face. His eyes open wide as he gazes intently at you or a toy brought in sight. Other mild cues may be as simple as raising

This baby is in a quiet alert state, showing a readiness to interact, play, and learn. Her bright eyes and gaze are strong engagement cues.

the eyebrows and crinkling the forehead. These early engagement cues are subtle, making Baby Watching essential.

Later Potent Cues

Other engagement cues are more obvious. He might stretch his fingers and toes toward you or a toy. You may even hear the sounds of cooing and squeals of delight. An infant ready to engage will brighten up his facial expressions by smiling and looking into his caretakers' face. If you reciprocate and match your baby's intensity, you two will be able to share a long mutual gaze and may even get *lost* in each other's eyes. Enjoy this moment to bond and experience a sense of timelessness.

ENGAGEMENT CUES

Mutual Gaze
Eyes Wide Open & Bright
Quiet Alert State
Raises Eyebrows
Slows Sucking to Make Eye Contact
Lifts Head & Searches for Your Face
Reaches Toward You or an Object
Smiles and/or Coos

Consequences of Missed Cues

Babies who are regularly ignored when they signal their desire to interact may shut down, lose interest in others, and become increasingly withdrawn or antisocial. Parents lose opportunities to appreciate their baby and bond while the infant is in a calm and alert state. Newborns lose opportunities to learn.

How to Rebound

Try to talk and play with your baby during these alert periods. Walk around the house and show him new things, faces, and pictures. Go outside and give him the words for the sounds he hears and objects he sees. This is a wonderful time to fall in love with each other because a baby who is ready to engage is also tranquil. It means his needs have been met and you can expect a period of calm before he transfers into his next state. If you miss an opportunity to interact, dedicate yourself to play the next time your baby shows you he is ready to engage. Mutual gaze and response are one of the simplest and earliest forms of play. Just look into each other's eyes and smile.

Timeout Cues

Just as infants have cycles for paying attention, they have windows for needing a break. It is of tremendous value to the baby when his parents are responsive and sensitive to the communication cues that signal the need to stop stimulation (disengage). New babies are sensitive to what they hear and see, and can be easily overwhelmed. The hyper-sensitive ones may respond by doing too much sleeping or fussing. Others have an innate capability to calm themselves by sucking on their tongue, listening to voices, or finding a light to focus upon.

Early Subtle Cues

So, how do you tell when your baby needs a break? Initial timeout signals may include burping or passing gas, hiccupping, drooping eyelids, drowsy or glazed eyes, and yawning. He will begin to look away from you (gaze aversion) and appear disinterested in the rattle or distractions you offer. His face will have little expression—a closed mouth, lowered eyebrows, or a wrinkled forehead. He will generally appear sober or unfocused, and may even pout his lips. Pay attention to what your baby does with his hands. He will begin to do all sorts of inconsistent behaviors when he's signaling a timeout, such as grab an ear, pull on his clothes, bring a hand to his mouth, clasp his hands together and intertwine the fingers, and rest them on his belly (NCAST, 2003).

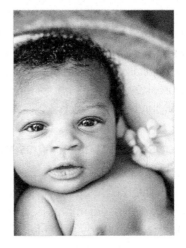

If a baby is breastfeeding and needing a break because he feels full or has to burp, he may extend one or more fingers outward, away from his body, or splay his hands (NCAST, 2003). He may also become very restless and latch on and off the

This baby is showing by her hand movements and glazed eyes that overstimulation is setting in. She went from quiet alert to active awake and is ready for a timeout.

breast repeatedly. During socialization or activity, a baby wanting to disengage might put his hands behind his head or do what's called a cling posture, which is when the baby pulls his arms to the side of his body and bends at the elbows (NCAST, 2003). An older baby might grimace at his caregiver or curl his lips inward as he holds his mouth shut. He can lower his eyes and head in avoidance. When he's tired and needs to disengage, he may even rub his eyes.

Later Potent Cues

If these cues are missed, the infant will increase his communication to more potent signals. He will cease to make eye contact and turn his head away. He may attempt to withdraw. An older baby will be able to push away or increase the distance between himself and his caregiver or an object, or signal "stop" with a raised open hand (NCAST, 2003). You will notice the arms and legs become restless. Squirming or extreme arching of the back will be a telltale sign that this baby needs a break. And if that's not enough, he will surely begin to cry.

TIMEOUT CUES

Burping, Hiccuping, Passing Gas
Heavy-Lidded, Drowsy, Glazed Eyes
Looking Away (Gaze Aversion)
Wrinkled Forehead
Little Expression, Sober Look
Closed Mouth, Pouting
Yawning
Pulling on Body Parts or Clothes
Brings Hand to Mouth
Clasps Hands
Extends Fingers
Cling Posture (NCAST 2003)
Fussing or Crying

Consequences of Missed Cues: Overstimulation

Babies needing a timeout may become irritated, upset, and overstimulated if their early cues are ignored repeatedly. When timeout cues are missed, infants become agitated, and their discomfort leads them to cry. They may clench their hands into fists, become red in the face, and tighten into a rigid or arched body. Overstimulated babies look stressed and may even have a frown in between their eyebrows. Agitation causes increased heart and breathing rates, which accelerate with further interaction. During agitated crying, infants prolong their breathing, which may cause them to choke.

An overstimulated baby can mimic colic behavior in the sense that the crying can be difficult to stop once the baby works himself up into a frenzy. It can go on for hours.

OVERSTIMULATION CUES

Disorganized Body Movements
Wide Eyes that Look Scared
Not able to Fall Asleep or Alert Calmly
Fussing
Crying
Body Arching
Passing Gas
Calming Techniques are Not Working
Excessive Crying/Colic-Like Behavior
Seems Spell-Bound
Cluster Feeding

How to Rebound

By learning your newborn's timeout cues, you can avoid these problems. The best-case scenario is to respond to the early timeout cues before he gets fussy by reducing stimulation, then limiting it altogether. If you missed this window of opportunity during the early cues, you have your work cut out for you. Dr. Harvey Karp, author of *The Happiest Baby on the Block*, recommends a technique to trigger the baby's calming reflex. Try swaddling your infant, arms down. Lay the baby on his side on your forearm, tucked close to your body, then gently move, causing the head to slightly wobble, while making shushing sound (Karp, 2002). A white noise machine that makes the sound of rain, water flowing, or crashing waves can substitute shushing.

For the very sensitive, difficult baby stuck in a wailing state, despite your every effort, you may have to let him cry for short periods and alternate with holding. First, swaddle the baby in a dark, quiet room to reduce stimulation. Then, as Dr. Brazelton's literature recommends, hold the infant for 5 minutes, put him down for 5 minutes, and continue this cycle. This is not considered "crying it out," but rather, decreasing and eliminating stimulation. Some parents find success by laying the crying baby on their chest while reclining. Don't move or pat. Understand that even calming tactics can overstimulate the baby, so the infant and parents are merely getting a break. During the periods of holding, try not to bounce, but instead, visualize yourself floating, and rock once per second while holding the baby's whole body against yours in a tight and secure fashion. The goal is to imitate the feeling and movement your baby had in utero.

"The Witching Hours"

Be aware that zero to 2-month-old babies develop tense feelings (stress) as we do. Until they are about 10 weeks old, many babies are unsettled. A baby who is overstimulated by the experience of the day will cluster-feed during the evenings, wanting to nurse several times an hour. This time, typical for babies 3-to-10-weeks-old, is commonly referred to as "The Witching Hours." It is a frustrating and challenging time for parents and infants alike.

Understand that crying and suckling are ways the baby feels more relaxed and works off the stress of the day. Know that fussing in your arms is one of the most caring ways you can help calm your baby. If feeding and holding are not enough, try swaddling arms down. Then bring your baby to your chest and relax into a rocking chair. Rock back and forth while shushing loudly and holding him tightly. His tense little body should begin to relax into yours. Fussy times like this also call for baby wearing. Walk around the house and yard together. Give each attempt 5 minutes before changing your calming method. You may be able to trigger the baby's calming reflex (Karp, 2002).

If these evenings become the norm, try something different the next day. For example, rather than putting the baby down for naps in the living room, seek out a crib or bassinet in a dark, quiet bedroom. Also, try eliminating all stimulation (light, sound, movement) once your infant is asleep, even at nap times. Remember, babies who rest well during the day, rest better at night.

Fatigue Cues

It's important to watch your baby and determine his fatigue window—how long he can stay awake and alert without getting overstimulated and going into a crying state. During the first 10 weeks, it is typically 60 to 75 minutes. Catching the early signs of fatigue are the trick. A glance at the clock should confirm what you already know—it's time for bed. Fatigue cues and timeout cues are sometimes one in the same. However, with timeout cues, sometimes the baby just needs a moment to look away, whereas with fatigue, the baby needs to be soothed to sleep. A baby that is getting tired goes from looking around happily to, maybe, hiccupping. His sounds go from joyful to fussy. His movements go from smooth to jerky. The skin looks blotchy and lacy, resembling the impression of a web where the superficial veins are prominent. One of the most obvious cues of sleepiness is the redness in the eyebrow area. Older babies rub their eyes.

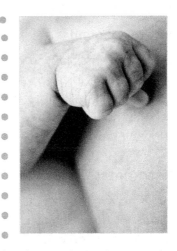

FATIGUE CUES

Hiccuping
Heavy Lidded & Drowsy Eyes
Redness Around the Eyebrows
Lacey Skin Complexion
Jerky Movements
Fussing or Crying
Yawning

Skin complexion changes, such as a marbled appearance, is one of the earliest and most subtle cues for fatigue, allowing astute parents to intervene and easily transition their baby to sleep long before crying begins.

Consequences of Missed Cues

Stimulating a baby who is ready for sleep may cause agitation, over-stimulation, and crying. (See the Consequences of Missed Cues: Overstimulation above in the Timeout section.) A flustered baby is very difficult to reorganize and settle to sleep.

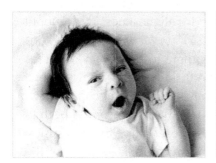 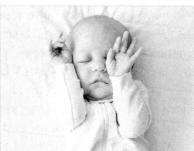

A cluster of later cues before crying beings undoubtably shows fatigue, such as yawning and rubbing eyes. Redness in the eyebrow region is another sign.

How to Rebound

As much as possible, you want to catch a sleepy baby and respond before he starts to cry. Swaddle the baby in a darkened, quiet place. Follow the suggestions for responding to an overstimulated baby if this does not immediately help him fall asleep. The more you can help your baby stay calm, the more he will learn not to cry.

Discomfort Cues

Babies may wake up or become quickly agitated for several reasons that do not include hunger but shear discomfort. Such needs include being too hot, too cold, sick, or soiled. Your baby may be uncomfortable if his body is cold to the touch or if you notice perspiration. Wiggling, groaning, and crinkling of the face may also signify discomfort. Fussiness or crying are more obvious cues that may accompany one or more of the others.

DISCOMFORT CUES

Core too Cold or Hot to the Touch

Perspiration

Wiggling

Groaning

Crinkling of the Face

Fussing or Crying

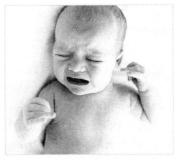

A newborn crinkles her face to show her parents that something does not feel right. She is in an active alert state.

How to Rebound

If you suspect your baby is not tired or hungry but simply uncomfortable, check to see if he is sweating or if the body is cold. If your infant is moist, remove one layer of clothing at a time to see how he responds. If there is more reason to be concerned, take his temperature to make sure he is not ill. If the core of the body is cold, add a layer of clothing and a hat. A lot of heat is lost through the head, since it accounts for a proportionally large surface of the baby's body.

Your baby may seem uncomfortable when needing a diaper change. Some infants are sensitive to the sensation of being soiled. Typically, these babies are also sensitive to light, sound, touch, and temperature. The good news is, they are usually the ones that are easy to potty train as toddlers. It all depends on the nine temperament traits, which will be discussed in Chapter 10. Other children do not seem to be bothered by a dirty diaper. The solution is to check the diaper to eliminate this factor and keep the baby dry.

Unidentified Cues

If you are still learning the meanings behind your baby's cries, experiment by bringing him to the breast each time he wails. His response will teach you what he needs and help you identify the cries. For example, when you try to feed a tired baby, he will nurse for a short time and quickly fall asleep. A hungry baby will nurse strongly and for longer. Match the response with the behavior and take note of the tone of his cry. The more you watch your baby, the easier he will be to read and the more confidence you will have in your ability to meet his needs. After a while of making this conscious effort to identify your baby's cues and assess his behavior, you will gain the experience to make this an automatic way of interacting. As you work through this learning curve, your tool kit will continue to fill, and you will be amazed by how quickly you can calm your baby.

There will be those times, however, where you will face confusion as the baby cries. Nothing you do seems to be working. If you feel overwhelmed, put the baby in a safe place and take a break for a few minutes. Breathe it out as you try to calm yourself. Then, take your baby into your arms, look into his face, and try to read his emotions. Say, for example, "Mommy is here. How can I help you?" Your baby can tell that, even when you don't solve his problem, you care. This response alone will bring him comfort and a love that is far-reaching. World-renowned child development psychologist Penelope Leach emphasizes that it isn't crying itself that's damaging but crying that gets no response (Leach, 2010). If nothing you do is helping your baby calm down, realize that your attempt and closeness is still attachment and support.

Getting Organized

Responding to your baby's early need cues and offering the appropriate response supports his potential to reach the first wonderful settled period around 10 weeks of infancy, where a baby can begin to organize himself and self-regulate his states. The writings of the late Dr. Stanley Greenspan, MD, the world's foremost authority on clinical work with infants and young children with developmental and emotional problems, tell us that at the very foundation of the human emotional experience is the security we feel when we are recognized, organized, and regulated (Greenspan & Greenspan, 1985). When things fall apart, we feel anxious and out-of-sorts. But as soon as we develop a new harmony by using our adaptation skills to deal with it, we feel regulated again, and our life is back in order. A great example is the disharmony we feel in the home after the birth of a new baby. Hopefully, over time, using adaptation skills and support, we can adjust and reach a new level of organization. Once we are successful, we are rewarded with a new sense of confidence and trust in our marriage and family.

It is essential that parents learn their infant's cues so they can monitor things that might bother the baby and affect his ability to calm and interact. Not doing so could deter his speed of development, ability to learn, and desire to breastfeed. Let this be your main goal for the first 10 weeks of your baby's life. Discover "what is this baby trying to tell me?" and answer "what does my baby need?" As you succeed at understanding his cues and responding to his communication, a rhythmic interaction begins like a waltz that lets him know he is important and loved.

PART III

Parenting with Appropriate Expectations for YOUR Breastfed Baby

CHAPTER SEVEN

Crying Defined:
A Time for the Baby to Talk

Chapter Goal: Understand crying and discover techniques for coping, calming, and managing these difficult times.

WHY BABIES CRY

The very first time your baby cries, sighs of relief are heard throughout the room. Later, the same sound brings quite different feelings—perhaps anxiety or at least a sense of urgency as the cries unearth your most primordial instincts—the call of motherhood. To the pediatric nurse, who examines your nude baby, the lusty newborn cry tells her that all is well. When a newborn baby doesn't react to this handling, the nurse is alerted to look for illness.

Pediatric Nurse Andrea Herron describes what young baby cries meant to her when she worked as a triage nurse in the busy UCLA Pediatric Emergency Room. There, parents arrived at the height of concern with their fragile infant in hand.

"I knew the crying baby was vigorous and less ill," Andrea says. "The lethargic, quiet baby got my attention. These babies were prioritized to be evaluated by the doctor. Of course, if what I heard was a spasmodic type cry and I saw the baby holding his breath in between screams, I knew that baby was in pain and needed immediate attention."

Babies cry at birth and during the early months in reaction to both feelings inside their body and sensations they experience. This is the young infant's main way of communicating and is one of the six states of awareness. Newborns have little control when they reach a crying state and often need help to calm. Until they develop the ability to self-regulate, they can rarely do it on their own. At first, the sound of the baby's cries are nonspecific, except for the pain cry, which sounds alarming, is high-pitched, and comes in waves.

Any change in the infant's surrounding or sensations he feels in his body can result in a cry. A gas bubble or change of temperature can set off the baby because he cannot process or understand these new experiences. Over time, babies learn to change their tones, creating different sounding cries that express their various needs. Around 6 weeks of age, the hunger cry becomes more distinguishable. It's desperate and continuous. Babies also cry when lonely because they are not used to being isolated and separate. Regardless of the type of cry, we are tasked with trying to figure out how to calm them as quickly as possible.

How We Respond: Instincts vs. Interference

A baby's cry raises our heart rate and blood pressure. In response, the body releases stress hormones. It's nature's attempt to spark a reaction. But sometimes, our brain makes us feel conflicted about whether we should respond to crying. This is caused by our life experiences, cultural norms, and social teachings we receive through the advice of peers, elders, and media. This bombardment of conflicting information spurs ideas expressed through our inner voice, causing us to ask, "is my baby trying to manipulate me? Am I going to spoil him by holding him too much?" It may make us worry before we act, potentially interfering with our innate response.

The parents' own childhood experiences can affect how they respond to their crying baby. For example, if you were often left to cry as an infant, you might respond to your baby in one of two ways: it could cause you to be oversensitive to the crying, and in response, you react to even subtle whimpers. Or, it could result in the opposite, causing you to be distant and less responsive. It is important to develop awareness of this influence because it may impact your baby's future emotional health and development. If it's something you cannot overcome on your own, consider talking to your medical providers for a referral to a psychotherapist.

Parental response to crying is also culturally programmed. For example, in some indigenous tribes, the babies are put to the breast upwards of 50 times or more a day for nourishment and comfort (Barr et al., 1991). This is a norm—a socially acceptable response to the baby's cues. This parenting style results in little crying outside of normal developmental crying (Barr et al., 1991). In comparison, Western mothers are advised to breastfeed 8 to 12 times a day, or even fewer, because they value less-demanding feeding routines. Unfortunately, scheduling and delaying responses results in more crying overall (Barr et al., 1991).

When the infant cries at night and can't fall back asleep, we worry that we will be holding this baby, forever. Day breaks, and we can count on relatives to confirm this belief when they observe and comment on the following scenario; your newborn cries. In response, you groan, look pained, then rush to your baby. The relative will either state, or imply by their behavior, that you are going to spoil the baby if you always pick him up when he cries. In an attempt at being gentle, they might say, "are you sure he's hungry again? Didn't you just feed him?" It may cause you to worry, "am I spoiling my baby or am I meeting his needs?"

Since you've made it this far into the book, your instincts are likely telling you that regularly comforting your crying newborn with whatever means possible is meeting needs and building trust, and not spoiling. You would be right. You can never spoil a baby by responding and helping him calm down. These cultural and personal expectations have long-term developmental and psychological effects on our children. A parent's habitual way of responding to their baby's cries can affect bonding. The infant's cry and early reflective smiles begin the interaction. The adults' engaging and excited response encourages the baby to attach.

Sandy Jones, the author of *Crying Baby, Sleepless Nights*, writes, "Research has shown that parents who are the most afraid of spoiling their babies are the most likely to produce children who act spoiled." Rather than responding promptly to their baby's early need cues, they tend to wait until the crying escalates, sounding louder and more urgent. This may create distance in the relationship. "The baby's trust in her caregivers begins to erode, which makes her quicker to cry and harder to soothe," Jones says. "Eventually, she grows into a clingy, overly demanding, and insecure toddler" (Jones, 1992, p. 15).

During the early months of your infant's life, it is essential to respond to your baby's call, crying, rooting, etc. This developmental phase is not a time to be concerned about boundaries. When you respond to your baby's early-need cues without fears of spoiling, you are teaching him, through positive reinforcement, to regulate into a quiet alert state or restorative sleep. Once your baby has developed a secure attachment, helping your child grow patience can be your next goal. An older baby that has had his needs met will believe you when you say, "I'm coming; just let me finish." These next chapters will guide you through the moments of desperation when your baby is crying instead of sleeping. You will learn how to tame those tears and feel more confident in handling your baby's crying and sleeping issues by adding this understanding of normal infant patterns and sleep development to the wonderful instincts you already have. Remember that there is no perfect way to parent. The best way is the one that feels right for you.

MISPERCEPTIONS ON CRYING AND CALMING

There are widespread ideas that have been around for decades, busily pitting breastfeeding mothers against their instincts. Although science has disproven many of them, culturally based beliefs that undermine breastfeeding are alive and well. Remember that just because the advice comes from well-meaning people in your life, it does not mean you need to follow it. Besides spoiling claims, the following are some of the most common misperceptions about crying and calming, which we will refute to help you distinguish between facts and fiction.

"Your baby is crying to manipulate you," said Fiction.

Despite what you hear, child development research psychologist Penelope Leach explains in *The Essential First Year* that "being manipulative requires sophisticated thinking that depends on a brain chemical called 'glutamate' working in the brain's frontal lobes (or neo-cortex). That glutamate system is not established in a new baby's brain, so she isn't capable of thinking much about anything—let alone how to control you" (Leach, 2010, p. 78).

"Babies cry to exercise their lungs," said Fiction.

Crying interrupts breathing, reduces the amount of oxygen that gets into the blood, causes raised blood pressure and dilated pupils (Jones, 1992). Babies cry to communicate a need that has not been met. If left to cry, they may lose control and get stuck in a crying state. When this happens, it makes calming and settling much more difficult.

"Holding the baby too much is bad for the spine," said Fiction.

Nature meant for newborns to be carried by their mother most of the time. We know this because of the positive effects mother/child skin-to-skin contact has on the newborn, such as temperature regulation, reduction of startles, and slowed heart rate (Moore et al., 2007). Unlike other mammals that can walk hours or days after birth, human infants take upwards of 9 months to a year or more to walk. This immaturity leaves them dependent upon nurturing adults and/or older siblings to carry them and keep them safe.

"The baby needs to know that you are the boss," said Fiction.

A baby does not cry to control you. Rather, it is his only verbal way of signaling a need. They can't say, "I'm scared, I don't know where I'm at. I'm so tired, but I can't fall asleep. I'm hungry, where are you?" When the mother says, "Oh, you are hungry," she is teaching the baby the language that later replaces the cry. Attending to your baby leads to the schedule and predictability you want because it helps you learn his cues and communication. For example, when you pick up your crying baby and try to breastfeed, but at times, find he quickly falls asleep, you start to learn that this type of cry is a tired cry. Soon, you will memorize this sound and recognize fatigue, so instead, you will know to put the baby down for his nap.

ON "CRYING IT OUT": STRESS ON THE BRAIN

It is a common Western practice to make a baby "cry it out," with the goal of teaching the infant to fall asleep, independent of his caregivers. Babies, however, are too young to be left to cry themselves to sleep. Considering the latest brain and psychological research, we advise against "crying it out" sleep-training methods. Purposeful crying is not healthy for young infants and, in fact, many experts argue it can still be damaging for babies up to 1-year-old (Leach, 2010).

Child development research psychologist Penelope Leach, the author of *The Essential First Year,* says, "Too much crying is too much stress, and stress is never good for babies." She explains that acute and continued stress stimulates the baby's adrenal glands to release the stress hormone, cortisol. "High levels of cortisol that build up over time can be literally toxic to a young baby's rapidly developing brain. Repeated episodes can permanently affect his response system so that it becomes hypersensitive and he overreacts to minor stress with major fear and anxiety, not only as a baby but as a child and an adult too," Leach writes (Leach, 2010, p. 112). Her startling summary is worthy of further explanation.

Current radiology techniques and PET scans have unveiled dynamic growth and development of the brain during infancy and early childhood. This technology has allowed neuroscientists to study how early experiences influence brain development. What they discovered is how incredibly vulnerable the newborn brain is and how important maternal bonding, touch, and responsiveness are for healthy psychological development. At birth, a newborn's brain is only one third the size of an adult brain. By age three, the brain is 90% an adult size (Jackson, 2002). This growth is critical for emotional and intellectual development.

The newborn brain is made up of billions of neurons. Neurons are programmed to make circuits by joining with other neurons through synapses. One neuron can eventually develop thousands of these connections (Jackson, 2002). The potential for synapses (connections) by age 3 when it peaks is incredible (in the trillions), but it is dependent upon both positive and negative experiences. Scans of a 12-year-old brain show remarkably fewer synapses than that of a 3-year-old. This is because the brain essentially prunes away synapses that don't connect to neurons while other areas expand. At birth, many cognitive neurons are not yet in their final place in the brain and must migrate like inchworms to the frontal lobe during the first 3 months of life (Paredes et al., 2016). If this migration is disrupted, it can lead to defects.

Each part of the brain is responsible for various functions. Maternal responsiveness to crying may affect the limbic system and the prefrontal lobes, the areas of the brain that control emotions. These parts develop and connect by the first 18 months (Jackson, 2002), with further maturation needed. During intense crying, the brainstem can be damaged and affect the person later in life (Perry, 1997).

Another scientist, Dr. Allen Schore, from the UCLA School of Medicine, studied the effects of prolonged crying and found it causes trauma on the development of the right side of the brain (responsible for emotions and attachment), further affecting the infant's mental health and ability to regulate (Schore, 2001). Dr. Schore discovered that during periods of intense crying, the brain of the infant is flooded with so much cortisol (stress hormone) that it can shut off, stunt, or destroy brain connections in this area. When this happens chronically, stress hormones reduce the number of synapses in the brain. Damage to this region of the brain can lead to depression later in life (Schore, 2001). It is thought that a baby left to cry will eventually stop calling for his parent but will continue to have high levels of stress hormones (Middlemiss et al., 2011). Later, it may make the toddler clingier and more irritable. The more resilient child may be less affected. A reminder; we are talking about purposeful crying that gets no response, not normal, developmental crying.

The Development of Trust

The good news is neuroscience has found that a nurturing environment actually increases brain connections and can be protective against many emotional problems later in life. Through breastfeeding, Baby Watching, and responsive caregiving, a baby can form a healthy emotional attachment with his mother by building a foundation of trust.

In the 1950s, psychologist Erik Erikson discovered that the development of trust or mistrust is the first of eight important psychological milestones babies achieve, influencing their interactions for the rest of their lives (Erikson, 1950). Positive, nurturing experiences develop the baby's sense of trust in his mother and his environment. When a baby emits a hunger cry, the prompt transfer to his mother's warm breast, where he soon begins to satisfy his hunger, tells the infant that when he feels hungry, nourishment will be provided. When she watches her baby and acknowledges subtle cues, the baby learns that his needs will be met. This interaction cements the bond, creating an attachment that is an essential component of normal psychological development (Bowlby, 1970).

Many mothers are pressured by family, friends, peers, and even media to let their baby "cry it out" to make the baby fall asleep independently. Leaving a baby to cry until he exhausts himself so much that he goes to sleep robs the infant of hope and replaces it with a sense of mistrust in people, his self, and the world. People fail to understand that sleep is a learned behavior (see Chapter 8). Strengthen your own family values and present a united front to relatives so that you can better deal with the people that object to your parenting methods or those that make you question your choices. Have a discussion with your partner. Use the questions in the box as prompts. Realize that your responses during pregnancy could differ greatly when you answer the same questions after your baby is born.

Strengthen Your Value System

Ask the baby's father or your partner ...

(1) Is scheduling our baby's care important to you?

(2) How do you feel about letting our baby's cues show how to meet his needs?

(3) Are you worried that comforting our baby when he cries or feeding him on-cue could spoil him?

(4) How do you feel about co-sleeping (bedsharing) with our baby?

(5) Where do you stand on letting the baby cry to sleep?

(6) Has anyone made you feel uncomfortable about our choice to breastfeed?

(7) How can we support each other and make sure we are on the same team?

(8) Add your own:

_____

NORMAL CRYING: FAIR EXPECTATIONS

In response to unexpected crying, many mothers wean and begin bottle-feeding formula because it is often interpreted as hunger. Excessive fussiness often leads the mother to believe that her milk supply is insufficient. Other factors, however, may exacerbate a baby's normal crying patterns, such as temperament and/or the infant's environment. It is important that you understand normal crying patterns so you can have appropriate expectations for your baby. Armed with this knowledge, you hopefully won't find yourself questioning your body's milk supply or your parenting when hearing covert remarks from well-meaning relatives.

The Development of Crying

Most newborns start out relatively quiet during the early postpartum hours and days in the hospital. During the next few weeks, they begin to *awaken* and make themselves heard. Research shows that the amount of time babies spend crying tends to increase from birth until 6 weeks, when it peaks and then begins to decrease

(St. James-Roberts, 2001). What follows is a decline progressively after that (Brazelton, 1962). In general, a normal 6-week-old infant cries for about 2.4 hours a day (Brazelton, 1962). By 3 months of age, crying is significantly less—half of what it was at its peak (Wells, 2003).

During the first 3 months of life, about 40% of the crying clusters in the evening. After that, it is more evenly distributed throughout the morning, afternoon, and evening until the baby hits 9-months-old, when nighttime crying becomes common (St. James-Roberts, 1993). This evening crying has to do with the baby's developing nervous system (Brazelton & Sparrow, 2003). With the parent's comfort and attention, crying often reduces itself to fussiness that goes back to crying when the parent ceases calming efforts. Dr. Brazelton studied this crying behavior. One study involved surveying 80 mothers. He found that there was a predictable fussy period at the end of each day. It involved a cyclical crying that stopped with holding but the babies were more jittery and easily went back to crying with any change in stimuli (light, sound, etc.). The babies ate and slept more soundly after this 3-to-4-hour crying episode.

Understanding this predictable fussy period helped the parents to accept and take the behavior less personally. Dr. Brazelton concluded that this fussy period is an organizing process. The baby is letting off steam from an overloaded nervous system. The baby takes in stimulation all day long, and it's too much. He then fusses, purging the stress and reorganizing to get ready for the next day. Brazelton further explained that through his parents' responses, the baby attaches better and knows who his mom and dad are after this phase (Brazelton & Sparrow, 2003).

CAUSES FOR NORMAL CRYING

For most infants, crying and irritability has no underlying medical cause (Hiscock & Jordan, 2004). But it's not meaningless. Babies cry because they have a need and, biologically, it is their tool to get their parent's attention for care, nourishment, bonding, and above all, to ensure their survival. Using Baby Watching techniques, learn to stop, look, listen, feel, and evaluate to gather clues and decipher the meaning of the cries so you know how best to respond.

Hunger

When a baby first begins to cry, parents shift through their jumbled brain for their handy checklist, where at the top, it says *hungry*. If you bring your baby to your breast and what follows is a long, satisfying feed with lots of gulping, *BLING, BLING*, you were right. If the baby latches on and begins suckling only momentarily, then either lets go and burps, or falls asleep, chances are that there is a different, possibly benign, reason for the crying. Watch your baby. Does he have his hands up near his mouth with his arms tucked close to his face? Meanwhile, is his little face twisting with his mouth open wide, eagerly trying to find the teat in the sky? Does his cry sound desperate? You will hear panting: "Aha, aha, aha." If this sounds like your baby, feeding is likely to be the best response to this cry.

If excessive crying is on your list of top complaints, suspect your baby is not getting enough to eat as a cause if he regularly breastfeeds several times an hour and the minute you put him down, he cries and roots again for the breast. Also, he has poor weight gain, and you have reason to believe your milk supply may be low (see Risk Factors for Insufficient Milk Supply on page 352). Note: A baby whose feeds are scheduled will likely have frequent bouts of hunger crying.

You might sometimes feel like your baby needs more than you can give. This is normal. Biologists have a theory that human offspring are designed to demand more resources than the mother can necessarily provide and signal, not only for nourishment, but to prove their worth (Wells, 2003). Through crying, the infant tells his mother, "pick me. I am worthy. I need you." Through natural selection, demanding offspring have an increased chance of survival, which advances this behavior to future generations (Wells, 2003). During this period, frequent suckling increases milk production. The establishment of the milk supply coincides with a decrease in crying. Hopefully, it helps to understand that a certain amount of crying and fussing is a normal part of infant development—one that supports bringing in an ample milk supply.

Changes and Transitions

Newborn babies often cry during transitions, everything from sensation changes to activities. For example, from being warmly clothed to undressed, held to put down, or asleep to awake. Many cry when they go from their mother's soft and pliable chest to a firm or crinkly changing table. They cry when they go from the feeling of security, tightly held in a swaddle, to the unfamiliar freedom of having their limbs out in the wide-open air. One baby might enjoy sheer nudity while the newborn with a low sensory threshold screams when submerged in a bath. A baby who startles easily is more likely to cry during these transitions.

Take care in handling your baby. Move slowly and keep him close to your body. When you undress him, he may start to scream if he feels too cold. Keep in mind that young babies don't regulate their temperature well on their own and need to be protected, especially if they are born early. If your baby often cries during transitions, keep him covered during changes, removing one article of clothing at a time while not exposing the whole body to nudity, even when bathing. Make sure your baby is close enough to see your eyes and use your voice to explain what you are about to do together. For example, "Mommy is going to change your diaper now. Let's go clean you up."

Fatigue

Babies exhibit many behaviors to show you that they are tired. For example, the skin becomes blotchy, and a halo of redness appears around the eyebrows. Crying begins when those cues go unnoticed and un-responded to. While this is normal crying, avoid making a habit of waiting until your infant is upset because it becomes increasingly difficult to resettle the tired baby the longer you wait. When crying presents itself to be a problem as you go about your days together, suspect that you are missing your baby's sleep cues if your baby's total sleep duration falls more than an hour short of the average (Hiscock & Jordan, 2004). For a baby less than 8-weeks-old, that would mean anything less than 15 hours of sleep. However, if your baby only sleeps 10 to 12 hours a day and is happy, that may be all the sleep that he needs. A 2-to-3-month-old should be getting a cumulative of 14 hours every 24 hours. If you are struggling with reading your baby's cues, see chapters 6 and 8 for techniques.

Overstimulation

Most newborns are only able to be awake for about 75 to 90 minutes. Infants who stay awake longer than their body can tolerate become overstimulated. They become increasingly disorganized by the minute until they "lose it." Newborns count on their parents to help them relax into sleep before they become overstimulated. If instead, they are passed around, played with, changed, etc., they will surely begin to fuss to express their unease.

Once the baby is overstimulated, it can seem impossible to put him to sleep. Overstimulation can trigger a crying spell, which can take upwards of an hour to stop. A baby who is frequently overstimulated may mimic colic behavior. Anthropologists have yet to find a world culture that escapes peak crying phases that occur in early infancy. It seems to be worse in the evening after the baby has been stimulated all day. Needing to release stress, many new infants fuss and cry for hours. Unable to be totally soothed, they seem spellbound, hence the coining of "The Witching Hour."

Overstimulation can also occur independently of fatigue. For example, many parents find that their well-behaved baby who "slept" through a noisy event later cries for hours. Mothers often suspect that the baby is reacting to that food she ate. In reality, the baby habituated to shut out the disturbing stimuli. He cried later because his brain was overwhelmed by too many experiences to process. While you can't always isolate your baby from stimulating events, just realize that when you play, you pay.

Pain, Discomfort, and Illness

Listen closely to the tune of your baby's cry. A high-pitch cry is a way to express pain or severe discomfort. The pain cry will alert you to respond quickly. Does the baby's face appear pale? If he is also arching with a shrill cry followed by intermittent breath holding, undress him, and check from head to toe for any areas that may be swollen. Blanket sleepers or footie pajamas sometimes have excess string from the seam that can wrap around a toe and cut off circulation.

There are times when the baby cries simply because he is sick or doesn't feel right. Signs of sickness include fever, low body temperature, rash, stuffy or runny nose, cough, and clammy skin (see When to Seek Professional Help on page 154). If your baby has blood and mucus in his stools, is lethargic, and you notice that the soft-spot on the top of his head appears puffy and pulsing or sunken, call your healthcare provider and take your baby to the emergency room immediately.

Sickness, especially a stuffy nose, can challenge breastfeeding since coordination of breathing is essential during a feed. Babies are nose breathers, so if the nasal air passage is blocked or congested, they are forced to interrupt suckling and let go to mouth breathe. Ask your health practitioner about using saline solution in conjunction with a bulb syringe. It will loosen the mucus, making it easier for him to nurse. Also, try breastfeeding in a room with a cool mist humidifier. A word of caution; mothers commonly develop plugged ducts when their baby is sick. Pay attention to your breast fullness, and hand express or use your pump whenever you feel uncomfortable or notice firm areas that do not soften by the end of the feed.

Separation: Needing to be Close

Babies often cry just because they need to be attached to their mother so that they can be fed. While it may not fit into the Western culture, it is biologically imperative. Humans are one of 4,000 species of mammals. Mammals are divided into various categories, depending upon the maturity of the baby at birth, the amount of contact they need with their mother, and the amount of fat and protein in the maternal milk. The categories in descending order of those demands are cache, follow, nest, and carry. The more mature the type of mammal is at birth, the more protein and fat there is in the mother's milk, so they require less contact and frequency of feeding (Gert et al., 2001). The less mature baby needs continuous contact with the mother and nourishment. Humans are carry mammals. They are among the least mature at birth, helpless with underdeveloped brains. Our biology dictates that our newborns need constant contact with the mother and skin-to-skin touch to maintain their body temperature. Human milk is the lowest in fat and protein of all mammalian milks, necessitating frequent feeds for our babies to grow, develop their brain, and be content.

Because of the human biological dependence on closeness and nurturance, nature programmed a distress cry, triggered by separation, likely to promote infant survival. Research shows that even newborns less than 2-hours-old recognize physical separation from their mother (Michelsson et al., 1996). In one study, babies who were separated from their mother 90 minutes after birth and placed in a cot cried nearly 10 times more than the ones who were not separated (Michelsson et al., 1996).

Developmental Crying

Throughout your baby's first year and beyond, you will notice crying with no apparent cause. But not all signals of distress mean that there is something truly wrong. When the cause of your newborn's crying seems to be a mystery, the reason may be developmental (Leach, 2010). Parents are most concerned with their baby's crying within the first 3 to 4 months of infancy, particularly notable peaks of crying at 3 and 5 to 6 weeks of age (St. James-Roberts, 2001). The experts agree that the most intense part of the day when much of the fussing and crying behavior occurs is the late afternoon and evening hours (St. James-Roberts, 2001). Unfortunately, it's also the hardest to deal with because parents are tired. Research finds that much of these crying spells that cause parents to worry are due to normal "developmental processes that occur in babies" (St. James-Roberts, 2001). Changes happening in the brain are sometimes difficult for your baby to manage. He has feelings and experiences new sensations that he doesn't yet understand (more in Chapter 17). It is all a part of adjusting to the world outside the womb. Bringing him to your body or your breast will offer him comfort, love, and security.

Crying Related to Temperament

Some babies cry and fuss more than others with longer bouts and have a harder time stopping once they've begun. If that's your baby, try not to be discouraged by your friend's child, who you've never heard make a peep. It's easy to assume that you either have the best baby in the world or the hardest. Some babies are quite frankly more challenging than others, and it could be a matter of temperament. Research shows infants with "difficult" temperament cry more often and longer than those with an "easy" temperament (Barr et al., 1989). (More on this in Chapter 10.)

The sensitive child is easily bothered. The infant with a high intensity of reaction cries instead of whimpers. The baby with low adaptability shrills when faced with a new experience rather than widen his eyes with curiosity. The baby that cries and fusses a lot will likely continue to be demanding past the first 3-month peak of crying. Babies also cry when they are bored. Repetitive, rhythmic motion, or white noise can help (see Calming Techniques ahead). Parents with intense and difficult-to-soothe babies may be deterred from group play or social gatherings with other families due to fear of judgment and embarrassment. Public humiliation is the part of parenting many people are not warned about. It's a humbling experience for sure. One mother described being asked to leave an infant-support group because her baby was irritable. If you find yourself in a similar situation, seek other groups that are more supportive and understanding.

Crying Associated with Breastfeeding

If your baby begins to nurse, then starts to cry, it's time to use your Baby Watching eye again. The tears may be due to frustration as he impatiently struggles to trigger milk flow. Listen closely. If there is an absence of swallows and gulps, this is likely a cause. If your baby goes from vigorous gulping to coming off the breast abruptly and screaming, you can suspect that he needs a burp. Hold him upright and give him a few pats to help expel the air in his belly that's causing him to be so upset. When the milk lets down, the flow can be quite fast. If this seems to be bothering your baby, he will appear stressed and gulp loudly. Elevate the baby above your breast so gravity can give him more control over the flow.

A baby that cries after being brought to the breast may also be trying to tell you that he's not hungry after all. It will be apparent by his disinterest. He may even push you away. You've got your work cut out for you. It's time to investigate what has him so unsettled. The infant will also push away if his latch is not deep enough to start a good sucking and swallowing rhythm (see breast attachment). If this happens often and you feel nipple pain, seek skilled lactation help.

Crying After Nursing

If your baby regularly cries after breastfeeding and arrival of the spell is as punctual as a Swiss train, there may be an underlying cause. Once digestion is well underway, 10 to 15 minutes after the meal, babies having an uncomfortable reaction to the food may start a high-pitch cry. If this behavior continues for more than a week, get an assessment from a medical and lactation professional. In a minority of infants who suffer from frequent irritability and excessive crying, a reaction to cow's milk or other food allergens may be the cause (Hiscock & Jordan, 2004) (see dairy allergy/sensitivity on page 332). If the baby also vomits frequently, about five times a day, gastroesophageal reflux may be to blame (see GERD on page 333). Rarely, a fussy baby who vomits forcefully has a condition called pyloric stenosis (see pyloric stenosis on page 335).

EXCESSIVE CRYING: COULD IT BE COLIC?

For countless mothers, just after they establish breastfeeding and begin to feel confident about parenting, colic takes them by storm. In order not to be confused with other potential clinical conditions or normal fussy developmental periods, Wessel's Colic is defined as periods of crying that last for 3 hours or more a day, 3 days a week, for at least 3 weeks (Savino, 2007). Remember the "rule of three." It helps to keep a diary of the crying spells, if you suspect colic.

Since there is an absence of disease associated with most infants who go through colic, colic is not so much a condition. Rather, it's something young infants do (Barr, 2001). Typically, sudden and inconsolable crying begins in the late afternoon and evening hours. It is fair to call them episodes because there is a clear beginning and an end. The crying is characterized by a high pitch, redness in the face (flushing), the release of intestinal gas, and curling of the arms and legs into the fetal position (Savino et al., 2014). Babies going through a colicky spell appear to be having difficulty passing stool or gas. They may even hiccup and burp. They clench their fists and sometimes arch their back, seemingly in total despair, but researchers are not certain these babies are in pain. Regardless, in search of comfort, they demand to eat frequently, barely giving the mother a rest between feeds, often leading to nipple soreness.

Colic is widespread among infants, being observed in approximately 10 to 30% of babies (Lucassen et al., 2001). It initiates around 2-to-3-weeks of age and suddenly diminishes in 12-week-olds (Asnes & Mones, 1982). It has been known to cause anxiety and pit one spouse against the other as they both face a sense of helplessness. It can chip away at your confidence, and certainly, the harmony in your home. Despite the major disturbance of a household held hostage to colic, researchers consistently believe the behavior is benign because babies who go through colic are otherwise healthy.

While parents find themselves bewildered by what suddenly has overtaken their sweet baby, so has the medical field because even though colic is easy to determine, the jury is still out on the actual cause, and the sure solution continues to elude researchers, even after decades of studies (Savino, 2007). The latest theories and available evidence to this disturbing behavior shows colic may be manifested by food hypersensitivity or allergy, immaturity of gut function and muscle movement, or behavioral causes, such as inadequate maternal-infant interaction, anxiety in the mother, and difficult infant temperament (Savino, 2007).

So, what can you do if your baby has colic? First, stay calm. Rest assured that the colic is likely not due to a disease nor anything that you have or have not done as a parent (Savino, 2007). One important scientific finding is that parental inexperience does not seem to be a cause of excessive crying (St. James-Roberts, 2001). (It doesn't just happen to firstborn babies.) Secondly, try to break the *spell* by deploying historically effective baby calming techniques. Popular methods are described ahead. Special care should be given to assure that your efforts to calm your baby do not further stimulate him (less is usually more), so it's okay to take timeouts. Thirdly, try not to be too discouraged when your efforts fail. Research found that 1-to-3-month-old "high criers" may be difficult or impossible to soothe (St. James-Roberts et al., 1995). It helps to take turns with the other parent or helper as you try calming techniques. Finally, be patient because there is hope. Just as suddenly as colic

ACTION PLAN

Managing Colic
(1) Stay Calm
(2) Deploy Baby Calming Tactics
(3) Reduce Stimulation
(4) Take Turns
(5) Be Patient
(6) Ask for Help
(7) Inform the baby's physician to rule out an underlying cause.

comes on, so does it spontaneously disappear. Parents typically see an end to these crying episodes by 3 months of age (Savino, 2007), when the baby naturally reaches a developmentally settled period.

WHEN TO SEEK PROFESSIONAL HELP

If your baby's crying concerns you, or you are reaching the end of your coping strategies, pay attention to your mommy-warning light. It certainly warrants further consideration in case there is an underlying medical condition or reason. Your medical professional can examine your baby and identify whether more can be done, whether it be further reassurance that everything is normal and on track or, potentially, intervention to treat any medical condition. Your practitioner may also suggest ways to survive the colic period. If you notice any of the following red flags, take your baby immediately for emergency care (Karp, 2002):

» A lethargic baby that does not wake up regularly to nurse over an 8-to-12-hour period

» Unusual body temperature, such as a thermometer reading over 101 degrees F. or lower than 97.0 degrees F.

» A high-pitch shrill cry, unlike his normal crying

» Green, yellow, or bloody vomit, or vomiting more than 5 times a day

» A bulging or sunken soft spot on the head

The following symptoms indicate that a medical office visit is necessary (Karp, 2002):

» Extreme fussiness while breastfeeding that regularly starts soon after nursing begins

» Constant irritability with hardly any calm periods throughout the day

» Poor weight gain (growth of less than half an ounce a day) averaged after about 5 days

» Fever or any signs of illness

» Excessive crying that continues to get worse

» Changes in stool, such as diarrhea, stool that resembles pebbles, or contains blood

» A rash on the baby's body or inside the mouth

Call your obstetrician or midwife if you:

> » Cannot tolerate advice from others,
> » Regularly feel angry, anxious, and/or depressed, even after the crying has stopped, or
> » Have thoughts of hurting your baby.

If your baby cries excessively and no medical issues are identified, try to gather a team for support and assistance. All parents need help with this issue. Breaks are essential. Know that there are resources and skilled professionals trained to help you overcome these common newborn issues, including your local health department and department of social services. Excessive crying and irritability that does not improve over time may be a sign of a sensory-processing issue (how we organize and understand information we receive from our senses). Other signs include breastfeeding issues, long feedings, excessive gagging when taking objects deep in the mouth, and intense frustration at the breast when feedings don't go well (Mohrbacher, 2010). Early intervention can help lessen these challenges and give you tools to manage different cognitive styles of thinking and learning. Never be afraid to ask for help. It is your job to be concerned and to give your baby a voice.

CALMING TECHNIQUES

During the first 10 weeks of their baby's life, all parents are busily working to find out exactly what calms their little one. From singing to rocking, often, it requires many efforts. Sometimes, it only takes bringing the baby to your chest and holding him close. The usefulness of each calming technique will depend upon your baby's sensitivity to light, sound, and motion, and whether he finds those stimuli pleasing (Jones, 1992). For example, one baby drifts off to sleep with the pleasure of a swing while another finds the movement traumatizing. Discontinue any efforts that your baby finds disturbing. As you use trial and error, start with the least stimulating intervention, such as picking him up and bringing him to the breast. If he has already completed his meal, try swaddling. Give each tactic a few minutes before moving on to the next while taking care not to further excite or stimulate the baby.

Limit Separation

We know from research that newborns find separation from their mother biologically disturbing. Research shows that spending 3 to 4 hours a day carrying your young infant can reduce the overall time he spends crying and fussing by as much as 43% at 6 weeks of age (Hunziker & Barr, 1986). Calming begins with your presence. Being "there" for your baby when he awakes and cries during the night can help him return to sleep faster (Mao et al., 2004). Room-sharing at night will help you achieve this goal. Breastfeeding often and babywearing will help you maintain this attachment.

There are many wonderful products available for moms to literally wear their baby, including soft fabric slings that are made to carry the newborn horizontally while enabling ample air flow. Using a baby sling in the home may free up your arms and get you used to using one for future outings while giving your newborn the comfort he needs. Follow manufacturer instructions for safe babywearing, such as making sure the infant's head is out of the cloth, and the neck is straight. Your baby's face should be visible (close enough to kiss) so that you can protect his breathing by keeping the nose and mouth airways clear of any fabrics. The chin should be up and not flexed into the baby's chest. There should be support for his head and neck to prevent the whiplash a sudden movement could cause. Also, check to make sure the way the baby is positioned in the carrier against your body is correct for safe hip development. His weight should be supported by the buttocks and thighs in a frog-like posture, rather than straight-legged.

Swaddle Securely

Newborn babies, for the most part, lack control over their large muscle movements, which are often triggered by automatic reflexes and sensations that come within their body. In response, their arms and legs flail about, and as they become tired, their movements become increasingly disorganized. This can make a nap-ready baby feel uneasy—a sure trigger for a crying spell. Without feeling "under control," the baby is distracted by his lack of coordination and is hardpressed to focus on calming down. You can calm him by recreating a womb-like sensation of being tightly contained in a warm environment. With a Velcro or zipper swaddle, wrap the crying baby from the shoulders down. Then, bring your little bundle into your arms. Lay your baby onto his side over your forearm, facing outward so he can look around while you walk around. Swaddling is most effective when combined with rhythmic motions and/or sounds described next.

Repeat Rhythmical Sounds

Newborns are also used to a loud womb. As a fetus, he heard the muffled noises of the outside world, and the percussion of the mother's beating heart, whooshing of blood flowing through her arteries, and gurgling of her active digestion. This is why, after birth, they often find droning, monotonous (white noise) sounds that are repetitive and rhythmical soothing. With white noise, you can distract your baby from minor discomforts that are causing him to cry. By tuning into the repetitive sound, he may be able to "tune out" what's bothering him and relax into a lower state. Before environmentally friendly white noise machines, parents reported creating repetitive sounds to stop crying by running water, finding static on the radio, running a hair dryer or vacuum, or putting the baby near an operating dishwasher or dryer. Avoid placing your cellphone white noise app close to the baby's head. The jury is still out on the harm of this practice.

Some babies instantly calm or soothe to sleep when they hear humming or lullabies sung from their mother's endearing voice. It is important to talk to your baby for language development and soothing. Research shows that newborns prefer sounds from a human voice over a rattle or toy, and that of their mother's over any other voice (Goodman, 1992).

Make Rhythmical Motion

During 9 months of gestation, the baby became accustomed to few hours of stillness nestled in their active mother's womb: those she reserved for sleep, which even then, was disrupted by frequent bathroom trips and tossing and turning throughout the night. Science shows that when the baby's head moves due to motion, it stimulates the vestibular system located deep within the ear, telling the brain the body's relation to gravity (Jones, 1992). These signals to the brain develop the baby's nerve pathways. Note: If your infant was born premature or finds motion uncomfortable, it may take months to enjoy.

Many babies are calmed by rhythmic walking, slight jiggling, gentle swinging, and rocking. If you are having a hard time settling your baby to sleep, hold him upright against your body so that his head can peak over your shoulder and walk around the house or yard. As his head gently wobbles from the movement while still supported, he may begin to relax. Consider a walk in the stroller. Many parents tell of the times they went for a drive or circled the block continuously until their baby finally fell asleep. Whatever type of motion you choose, try to keep it smooth and one movement per second. Stick with the same movement for at least 3 to 5 minutes before changing. Of course, there are many contraptions on the market designed to create motion for the baby while keeping him secure in a 5-point harness—some reportedly "move like Mom." If you need to take care of your personal hygiene, prepare a meal, or are desperate for a break, reserve your device for this time. Realize though that, overall, no technology can replace the benefits of human touch.

Offer Fresh Sights

When you step outside, you may notice your baby at least momentarily respond to the atmospheric change with silence. Young infants enjoy looking at faces, and high contrast shapes and patterns. Hold your baby upright over your shoulder, and move around the house and yard. Often, fresh sights are just what it takes to settle his crying. Just a simple change will help the infant's brain shift from crying to a quiet alert state.

Induce Sucking

Once your baby ceases to wail, thanks to your many efforts, he may still be fussy. Fussiness is essentially reduced crying behavior that escalates again when the caregiver stops trying and puts the baby down. While the infant is still upset, he may be settled enough to breastfeed. Suckling without hunger can still help. Show him that he can comfort himself by bringing his hand to his mouth. Avoid using newborn gloves or sleeves. He needs his hands to self-soothe and experience the world. Touch develops nerve connections in the brain. If you are concerned about sharp nails causing scratches, use a fine file to gently remove any edges. Once your baby is gaining weight on target and breastfeeding is going well, you can introduce a pacifier after a meal. Do try to limit pacifier use to the most demanding time, such as the evening. Early pacifier use can reduce the milk supply because it replaces suckling at the breast, decreasing demand (ABM, 2010).

Reducing Crying Overall

You can frequently help prevent crying by practicing a baby-led philosophical approach to your parenting. Dr. William Sear's Attachment Parenting (breastfeeding, cue-reading, baby wearing, co-sleeping), Baby Watching, and Biologic Breastfeeding are all methods that can help reduce crying overall. When a mother adopts this responsive style of parenting, it will help her to be more sensitive to her baby's needs and often curb crying spells before they even begin. Research finds that feeding on demand and picking up babies before they cry in the first few weeks of life reduces the amount of time the baby spends crying by as much as 50%, compared with babies whose parents schedule their routine and delay their response to crying (Barr et al., 1991).

The optimal response time to a baby in need is 60 to 90 seconds (Jones, 1992). After that, the amount of time needed to calm the baby increases three, four, and in some cases, 50 times (Jones, 1992; Thoman, 1975). Learn to anticipate when the baby is ready to eat through Baby Watching. Anticipate infant needs by identifying the early cues for hunger or needing comfort and bring him to the breast. If you have a predictable baby, this will be easier. If you have an unpredictable baby, creating a routine can help you establish a rhythm.

COPING WITH CRYING

Coping with crying is difficult for parents (and anyone in earshot). We are programmed to be disturbed by it, so we respond to our young. Crying averages 84 decibels at close range (10 inches from the infant's mouth), which is 20 decibels louder than ordinary speech (Jones, 1992). If the baby is inconsolable and does not quiet, this continuous noise can be quite disturbing. If we are not able to soothe our baby, we can become anxious and depressed (Murray et al., 1996). Over time, we may lose confidence and develop feelings of inadequacy. This natural reaction was coined by social psychologist Martin E. P. Seligman as "learned helplessness" (St. James-Roberts, 2001). Once we reach helplessness, we respond less to the crying, often resulting in internal feelings of guilt. Yes, parenthood is an emotional rollercoaster.

Since much of crying is normal and often inconsolable in the early weeks, researchers recommend parents form realistic expectations for their baby's crying and sleep patterns, and find ways to cope by simplifying household tasks and accepting help from family and friends (Hiscock & Jordan, 2004). (See coping with the adjustment to parenthood for more tips on page 377.) When you reach your wit's end, put the the baby down in his safe place for a few minutes at a time (Brazelton & Sparrow, 2003). When you pick him up, you can try helping him burp. It's not "crying it out," but rather, reducing stimulation and giving you a critical break to maintain sanity. Accept that this is a difficult time of your life and know that it will soon pass. While it seems like time is moving at a snail's pace, in retrospect, it will be remembered as happening fast. During the childrearing, they say the days are long, but the years are short.

CHAPTER EIGHT

How Breastfed Babies Sleep: All Things Considered

Chapter Goal: Gain realistic expectations for your baby's sleep, how it develops, and what you can do to support it.

ALL THROUGH THE NIGHT

For the first time in your memory, you might experience the dark of night at every hour as you startle into consciousness to tend to your little one. As you bring your newborn into your embrace, hopefully, you will cherish this peace and quiet—not a single text distracting you from enjoying these precious moments alone with your sweet baby. Or, maybe you feel lonely waking up to breastfeed when the only sounds in earshot are the hum of the refrigerator and the suckling of your baby satisfying his hunger. Realize, though, that you are not alone. Mothers everywhere are drowsy-eyed—awake, feeding their babies, and hoping for some Zs.

After you adjust to the surges of oxytocin breastfeeding triggers and the feeling of euphoria subsides, sleep deprivation will surely set in. For many parents, their own well-being becomes a state of chronic neglect as newborn care takes precedence. After a while of sleepless nights, the yearning for a block of uninterrupted sleep becomes desperation, which leads many parents to wonder whether they are doing something wrong or should be parenting their breastfed baby differently to promote longer sleep. Family members, or the mother herself, may even start to speculate or fear that she doesn't have rich or sufficient breastmilk. Fears are compounded by unsolicited outside criticism and casual advice (social interference). It seems that everybody is asking, "how is your baby sleeping?" While it might be meant as small talk, this casual prompt plants a seed of doubt, leaving parents to believe that there is something wrong if their baby is not sleeping through the night. In response, parents commonly supplement the baby's diet or wean from the breast (Ball, 2003).

This chapter will help you understand normal sleep development and answer how you can encourage sound sleep for your baby with his uniqueness in mind. Hopefully, by learning about your baby's biological rhythm and capabilities, you will set up an environment conducive to building good sleep habits. We all want our babies to sleep but we must start with realistic expectations to reach that goal.

COMMON SLEEP MISPERCEPTIONS

Most of the unrealistic expectations parents create for their babies stem from cultural norms and Western trends for infant care (Ball, 2014). They hear an earful of common misperceptions disguised as good advice. When parents hear from their peers who claim that their baby is already "sleeping through the night" (even if it was one time, parents still brag), it makes them think everyone else's baby sleeps more than theirs. "Maybe you should try letting him cry it out," they advise. This barrage of pressure can influence parents who are desperate for sleep and willing to try anything to get it, despite their better instincts. Let's address some of the most common misperceptions about sleep before they seep into your consciousness and cause you to create unrealistic expectations for your baby.

Fact or Fiction?

"Your baby should be sleeping through the night by now," said Fiction.

Note that this phrase is often disguised as a passive-aggressive question, such as "Is your baby sleeping through the night?" The answer should be, "Of course not." First, do you envision a baby that goes down at 9 pm and wakes up at around 6 am? In reality, this does not typically happen until after the first birthday. For an infant, "sleeping through the night" has been defined as a 5-hour stretch from midnight to 5 am (Moore & Ucko, 1957). In reality, only about half of babies sleep this well but not until 5-months-old, and the others just don't (Henderson et al., 2010). The study that defined our modern idea of "sleeping through the night" was done in 1957, based upon the results of 160 parent surveys. Parents reported that 70% of the babies slept 5 hours at 3 months. Things were different in the U.S. during the 1950s. Fewer than 9% of mothers breastfed because parents were told formula was superior to human milk (McKenna & McDade, 2005). Also, babies slept apart from their parents in separate rooms. They likely stirred and fussed without waking their parents. Parents ignored their infant's cries at times because, back then, they were warned that there would be psychological consequences for co-sleeping and frequent nighttime feedings (McKenna & McDade, 2005). This "normal" for sleeping through the night is out-of-date and arbitrary.

The fact that so many people comment on newborn sleep is a symptom of the Western value that babies should sleep for long stretches and be able to achieve this pattern early in infancy (Ball, 2014). In other societies, such ideas are unusual (Ball, 2014). The Euro-American expectation that a "good baby" sleeps through the night is not realistic when you know how normal human sleep develops. And when expectations are too high, we, as parents, are sure to face disappointment and uncertainty that causes us to question our competency. The fact is, the circadian rhythm, which regulates a person's ability to distinguish night and day, doesn't begin to develop until about the third month, along with the ability to sleep longer stretches (consolidation), which occurs between 6 to 12 months (Meltzer & Montgomery-Downs, 2011).

Additionally, for the first few months, babies need to nurse every few hours to optimize growth. Their stomach empties within 2 hours, digesting breastmilk in about 90 minutes (Lawrence & Lawrence, 2011), so breastfed babies feel hungry every 2 to 3 hours. A mother who boasts to the pediatrician that her baby is sleeping through the night will likely draw more concern than praise if her infant is not gaining weight as expected. If she is not waking herself to express milk or nurse and she becomes engorged, she could potentially decrease her milk supply or develop complications, such as plugged ducts, and/or mastitis.

If the baby is sleeping through the night by 3 months and is reporting good growth, he is likely a more mature baby who can take big volumes of food, combined with a mother who has an abundant breastmilk supply. Remember, it is essential for your little one's health and that of your milk supply to have a baby that wakes throughout the night to breastfeed.

"The baby has his nights and days mixed up. If you keep him awake during the day, he will sleep better at night," said Fiction.

Many new babies seem to sleep much of the day, then wake for feeds all night. Remember that newborn babies are not yet capable of distinguishing night from day because their circadian rhythm is undeveloped (Ball, 2014). Be leery of those who advise you to keep your baby awake all day so he learns to sleep through the night. The contrary is true; sleeping better during the day improves night sleep. The better rested your baby is by the evening (not overstimulated, took his naps), when normal fatigue starts to set in, the easier it will be for him to fall and stay asleep. Keeping a tired baby awake is bad for the developing brain. For one, it can negatively impact learning. Infants rely on frequent naps for the formation of long-term memories, such as new behaviors (Seehagen et al., 2014). When overtired from nap deprivation or general fatigue, the body releases stimulating stress hormones that interfere with night sleep and subsequent naps.

"You need to let the baby cry it out so he learns to go to sleep on his own," said Fiction.

Young infants wake because they have needs that must be met, whether it be hunger, thirst, a want for comfort, a soiled diaper—the list goes on. Behavioral sleep interventions should not be applied before the baby is 6-months-old, if at all. After, instead of forcing the baby to "cry it out," try techniques described ahead. A systematic review of "cry it out" methods found a risk of unintended outcomes, such as premature cessation of breastfeeding, increased maternal anxiety, and increased risk of SIDS (Douglas & Hill, 2013). We patiently wait for our babies to crawl, walk, and talk. We would never let our baby who can't walk yet sit there and cry until he stands and puts one foot in front of the other. Yet, we are encouraged to let our little ones who can't self-soothe, cry until they wear themselves out and give up. (For more, see "crying it out".)

"Giving your baby a bottle of formula or rice cereal before bed will make him sleep longer," said Fiction.

Your grandparents might swear that giving your baby a bottle of formula mixed with rice cereal before bed will surely make your little one sleep better. This advice was dogma in the early 1960s but has since been proven to be harmful. Researchers studied the effect of cereal on sleep and found that adding it to a bottle did nothing at all to speed up the age of sleeping through the night. That first uninterrupted 6-hour stretch of sleep came no earlier in those who received cereal in their bottle (Macknin & Medendorp, 1989). There are other reasons not to give cereal in a bottle. The baby may choke because he is not ready for solids. It can also lead to obesity because it increases caloric intake.

Despite popular belief, supplementing with even a bottle of formula before bed will not improve your night's sleep either. Advice that hails the bottle as a quick fix to get the young infant to sleep through the night should be recognized as breastfeeding sabotage for the vulnerable mother who is trying to cope with sleep deprivation (Doan et al., 2007). One study showed that not only did giving a bottle of formula not improve parent sleep, but it resulted in sleep loss of more than 30 minutes per night (Doan et al., 2007). It further found that while exclusively breastfed babies woke up more frequently, they slept more overall per night, returning to sleep faster after waking to breastfeed.

REALISTIC EXPECTATIONS: LOOKING FORWARD

When you are asked if your newborn is a good sleeper, don't allow this inquisition to lead you to question how you are doing as a parent or whether there is something wrong with your baby or your breastmilk. Rather, to prevent unnecessary grief, it is important to modify your expectations to match normal infant sleep patterns.

Nearly a third of parents have a significant problem with their child's sleep behavior (Armstrong et al., 1994). When parents don't understand what's normal, it can lead to perceived insufficient milk supply, supplementation that does, in fact, reduce the maternal milk capacity, and other breastfeeding interference. In a study of over 3,200 parents, researchers also found that not understanding "normal" sleep patterns leads to misdiagnosis of gastroesophageal reflux (GER) and overuse of sedative medication (Armstrong et al., 1994). A whopping 31% of 25-to-38-month-old children were disciplined, including spanking, to get them to settle to sleep. About 27% of parents reported that they let their child cry, 11% at less than 1-month-old. Many concerns can be resolved with a better understanding of how the breastfed baby normally behaves through-out the night—what his patterns are like for sleeping, waking, and feeding as he grows. Focus your efforts on coping strategies rather than supernatural sleep goals.

Sleep Defined

Our common knowledge and expectations about sleep are based on adult patterns but it takes time before infant sleep resembles adult sleep. There are two major categories of adult sleep: rapid-eye movement sleep (REM) and non-rapid-eye movement sleep

(NREM). REM is also referred to as active sleep or light sleep. During this sleep stage, the brain is very busy, organizing memories and consolidating the experiences of the day. If you observe someone in light sleep, you might see the face twitch, smile, or frown. During REM, people make noises: talk, cry, or whimper. While the eyelids are closed, underneath, there is movement back and forth, showing that the active brain may be in a dream state. To protect you from physically acting out your dreams and harming yourself, the body is temporarily immobilized.

The other main category of sleep is NREM, also known as deep sleep. During NREM, your blood pressure decreases, heart rate and breathing slow, and body temperature drops. The body is in a restorative state, working to repair muscles, boost immunity, and reenergize for the next day. In NREM, the brain is resting in a deep slumber that progresses through various stages, with each stage getting deeper.

Adult Sleep vs. Infant Sleep

When first falling asleep, adults go into deep sleep (NREM). Adult sleep changes from deep sleep to light sleep in 4 to 6 cycles throughout the night with increasingly more light sleep as we get closer to the latter half of the morning hours. During light sleep, the body can shift positions and resettle back to sleep. Ambient noise and activity can easily arouse a person. You have probably experienced being awoken in the middle of a dream. Furthermore, we do not sleep through the night, but rather, we wake often. It is when we are awake for about 3 to 5 minutes or more that we register this awareness. Overall, 20 to 25% of adult sleep is spent in REM, and 75 to 80% is spent in NREM deep sleep (Carskadon & Dement, 2011).

During lactation, the normal distribution of light sleep, deep sleep, and REM sleep changes in women. In one study, mothers who were exclusively breastfeeding spent significantly more time in slow-wave (deep) sleep than bottle-feeding mothers (Blyton et al., 2002). Researchers believe the altered sleep is attributed to an increase in the relaxing prolactin hormone that circulates the body during lactation.

Infant sleep is different from adults (see Sleep Comparison Chart). There are three types of sleep referred to as quiet sleep (similar to NREM), active sleep (similar to REM), and indeterminate sleep (Davis et al., 2004). While the adult cycle is about 90 minutes, the infant's is 50 to 60 minutes. The length of the sleep cycle stays relatively stable during the first 5 years of a child's life until it reaches the mature level of 90 minutes at about 8 years of age (Barnard & Thomas, 2014).

In quiet sleep, there is little movement, and the baby cannot easily be aroused, even for breastfeeding. Deep sleep develops as the baby's brain matures. At first, the newborn spends about half his total sleep time in active sleep (Barnard & Thomas, 2014). This is known to be protective against SIDS. By about 3 months of age, the proportion is more quiet sleep than active sleep. For the fetus and young baby, rapid-eye movement sleep is the period of maximum brain activity that makes it critical for the rapid brain development that is occurring, including the sensory systems (Graven & Browne, 2008). Over the first few months of life, periods of deep sleep become longer, and the cycles of active sleep become shorter. In the beginning, young infants are not capable of sleeping more than 2 to 3 hours at a time. As the brain further develops over the first 3 months, changes enable babies to be more organized about their sleep.

Early in life, while the brain is rapidly developing, it's very important for the brain to regularly start and complete the sleep cycle in the natural pattern. Research shows that deprivation of REM sleep can result in behavioral problems, permanent sleep disruption, decreased brain mass, and more than normal nerve loss (Bergman, 2007). During a sleep cycle, brain wiring occurs, which is essential for the formation of long-term memories and cognitive development. REM is characterized by fast brain waves. As the brain enters deep sleep, short-term memories, sensory inputs, and new knowledge retained during the baby's experiences awake are gathered and transferred to another part of the brain where consolidation of memories occurs (Graven, 2006). During consolidation many irrelevant short-term memories, like details of the day, are discarded, while more important memories are retained. Brain scans show that in the final stage of REM sleep, the knowledge the brain retains is returned using brain waves, organized in the form of long-term memories (Graven, 2006).

TABLE 8.1 - Sleep Comparison

SLEEP CYCLE	BEGINNING	MIDDLE	END
ADULTS **90 minutes**	Non-REM (Quiet/Deep Sleep)	Non-REM (Quiet/Deep Sleep)	Non-REM Then REM Light Sleep
NEWBORNS **50-60 minutes**	Active Sleep (REM)	Quiet Sleep 20 minutes	REM

Circadian Rhythm: The 24-Hour Sleep/Wake Pattern

In mature adults, there is a center in the brain that controls the release of hormones that wake us up and let us sleep. This center keeps us in tune with the 24-hour cycle. When the sun rises, daylight detected through the retina of the eyes activates this internal "clock." The brain center makes the body temperature rise and then releases cortisol to energize the body for wakening. When darkness falls, the brain center tells the body it's time to wind down and go to sleep by lowering the body temperature and releasing the melatonin hormone, which makes us feel sleepy. You might notice that exposure to bright lights and screens elicited by smartphones and digital devices at bedtime interferes with falling asleep. Overall, this brain center gets us in rhythm with the 24-hour light cycle, known as circadian rhythm.

In utero, the fetus largely follows the mother's circadian pattern. Her hormones, temperature, and movement influence activity in the womb. Once born, he begins the development of his own circadian rhythm. Circadian rhythm develops throughout childhood with variations during growth spurts. Sleep architecture changes throughout one's life (Institute of Medicine, 2006). An inconsistent lifestyle and lack of wake/sleep routine can delay normalization and create problems.

Researchers discovered a biological sequence of events in the infant's development of circadian rhythm that goes as follows: The first biological rhythm emerges between 6 and 18 weeks of infancy, led by the secretion of cortisol and initiation of nighttime sleep consolidation (Joseph et al., 2015). The scientists suspect that this maturation represents the infant adapting to his external environment and gaining a sort of balance. A week after cortisol appears in the body, the sleep hormone (sulfatoxy melatonin) is produced. Then at 10 weeks, there is a maximum decrease in deep body temperature associated with darkness. Finally, at 11 weeks, they noticed the expression of a clock-controlled circadian histone gene (H3f3b) in the saliva of infants.

So, as much as you want to control how well your new baby sleeps at night, much of it is out of your hands. You can help him adapt and not do things that interfere with this unique development, but sleep consolidation is predetermined through genetics, biological development, and temperament.

Although there are statistical times a baby's own day/night rhythm develops, it will differ depending upon the infant's neurological maturity. For example, premature infants take longer to obtain circadian rhythm. Some babies' temperaments are influential as well. For example, a sensitive baby who reacts more to light and sound may have a harder time developing a predictable circadian rhythm if that environment is not modified for the baby's sensitivities (i.e., darkening the room). The caregiver's routine also affects how the baby's rhythm forms.

During this time, families will need to reestablish a new routine, which will also help the baby get a rhythm. Turning down the lights and winding down activity in the home after dinner is one way you can create environmental prompts that will help your baby learn to quiet and regulate into a lower state for sleep. It is also important to note that your breastmilk has the hormones that cue the baby. Morning milk has stimulating hormones. The peak amount of sleep-promoting hormones contained in breastmilk occurs around 3 am (Cubero et al., 2005).

Research shows that these middle-of-the-night feeds are important for the development of good nocturnal sleep rhythm (Cubero et al., 2005).

Normal Patterns as Sleep Organization Develops

Newborn

After birth, patterns of awakening and feeding are usually dependent upon hunger relief, the infant's blood sugar levels, the baby's feeding skills, and the mother's milk supply. The typical newborn baby sleeps an average of 16 hours per day, with a range of 10.5 to 18 hours (Barnard & Thomas, 2014). There are numerous sleep periods with an erratic pattern, ranging from 1 to 4 hours each, but as little as 30 minutes. If your baby has a 5-hour stretch of sleep, he may demand a cluster of several hourly breastfeeds afterwards to make up for missed meals. Do not allow more than one 5-hour sleep period in 24 hours because it can decrease your milk during this critical time and impact the baby's weight gain.

For newborns, the longest stretch of sleep usually occurs during the first part of the day while the nighttime is characterized by frequent waking. Rarely are newborns on their parent's schedule, being more awake during the day than at night. Parental expectations reinforced by babycare books often say that babies "sleep from feeding to feeding" (about every 2 to 4 hours), but this discounts all the crying, burping, changing, and bathing that goes on. You can count on the fact that most newborns get the amount of sleep that they need, which varies widely from baby to baby.

One to Three Months

Between 6 weeks and 3 months old, the baby is more awake during the day and beginning to sleep longer at night. He begins to develop circadian rhythm and self-regulation. This trend continues until it stabilizes at about 6 months. You will notice that there are episodes of fussiness, crying, or agitated wakefulness in the evening hours during the second month of life. This fussy period peaks at about 6 weeks of age, or 6 weeks after your baby's due date, if he was born early. Babies begin to make social smiles at about this time, and afterward, the fussiness begins to decrease. The onset of social smiles followed by a decrease in fussiness reflects maturational changes within the baby's brain. The brain can tolerate more noise and environmental events. The baby is more able to console himself, which permits him to fuss less and calm down, especially at night. Because of these biological changes, a full-term 6-week-old infant may be able to develop night sleep organization. This means that the longest sleep period (4 to 6 hours long) regularly occurs at night.

If you are co-sleeping but don't plan to bedshare much longer, about 3 months is the age to move your baby out of your bed because sleep associations are forming. Once the baby develops attachment and memory of his sleep environment and routine, it will become more difficult to transition him after this period. You can tell memory is forming when your baby, who used to sleep anywhere, suddenly resists change or refuses the occasional bottle.

Three to Five Months

Between 12 and 24 weeks of age, day sleep organization develops. Most babies still take about three naps per day. Some infants take long naps while others are very short. Daytime sleeping can be unachievable if there is too much stimulation (light, noise, or motion). Babies begin to sleep about 8 to 10 cumulative hours at night (Barnard & Thomas, 2014). Improved motor skills enable the baby to thumb-suck and self-soothe. The startle reflex that disrupted sleep is gone. Some infants calm themselves by wrapping their arms around their body in a self-embrace. Sleep patterns become much more predictable, and the baby is becoming more capable of going to sleep on his own without a lot of support. However, since memory has formed, whether your baby can go to sleep without being rocked or breastfed will depend on whether there has been variety to get there, regularly. For example, a parent who always uses motion to put her baby to sleep may have a baby who depends on motion to go to sleep. Countless mothers easily and comfortably put their baby to sleep at the breast. If this is the case for you, understand that he may require sucking to fall back asleep at night when he cycles into light sleep.

For many parents, just when they think their baby has mastered sleep, there is a rude surprise in the form of a new behavior. That sweet baby that you easily nursed and rocked to sleep is suddenly waking often and calling for you throughout the night, more than the usual number of feeds you adapted to. It's so common, that if you Google it, you will find pages of articles titled the 4-month-sleep regression. If you co-sleep, expect to nurse more at night than peers who are not bedsharing or breastfeeding.

The goal, by 18 weeks, is to develop a routine and understand your baby's uniqueness (i.e., what does he need to have a more peaceful sleep at night?). Understand that by this point in time, your baby has enough maturity to start developing habits. Note that it is important to create habits that you can live with. Even more, make sure your expectations of your baby are appropriate for those lifestyle choices. For example, do you want to sleep next to your baby? A normal pattern and realistic expectation for the co-sleeping 3-month-old is that after a 3-hour sleep, the baby will potentially wake every 60 to 90 minutes and probably need to nurse a little bit before going back to sleep. If you don't mind and it works for your family, then don't worry about it. However, if your goal is for your baby to be an independent sleeper and in his own bed by the time he's 6 months old, then at about 18 weeks is the time to try to put the baby down when he is drowsy without nursing, rocking, or holding. Keep in mind that your baby might not adapt well to this because of his individual sensitivities. Some babies fall easily into that routine, and you can gently nudge them in the direction you want, while others may have a stressful response to this change. So, you need to adapt your goals and family boundaries to your baby's temperament (explained ahead).

Five to Nine Months

Between 5 and 9 months, the baby's daytime sleep decreases to two naps per day. Usually, one nap lasts around 1 hour, and the other is about 2 hours long. The range for uninterrupted night sleep is

1 to 12 hours per night. In one study of 640 babies, where parents were surveyed, only 16% of babies were sleeping through the night at 6 months old and had no regular sleeping pattern, meaning 84% were not sleeping through the night (Sadler, 1994). Parents reported that their baby's number of night waking ranged from 2 to 8 times a night (Sadler, 1994).

The 5-to-9-month-old is undergoing remarkable advances in motor development. Babies practice their skills all through the night while asleep. If you bedshare, this can be a very challenging time (see Sleep Safety). Needing comfort due to teething pain or separation anxiety and hunger are also a few of the many reasons babies stir awake. A little time nursing makes the baby feel better, helping him relax and drift back to sleep. This is a quick fix and works well for many parents without problems. Be aware that if done every time the infant awakes at night, it can result in a habit that leads to excessive night waking until the baby is weaned (more than 5 times a night). To prevent this, make sure your little one is truly awake and not merely making noises and movement in light sleep before you pick him up. If not co-sleeping, when he wakes up all the way, go to him but try not to take him out of bed. Offer comfort, like rubbing his back or singing a lullaby. Breastfeed if you think your baby is hungry or thirsty, or if your breasts feel full. Rotate soothing methods so that you are not breastfeeding every time the baby wakes up, or he will learn no other way to get back to sleep. Many mothers tell the tale of having to get up every 60 to 90 minutes to either breastfeed or rock their baby back to sleep. By this age, the goal for the family that wants an independent sleeper is to help him learn ways to return to sleep (sleep associations) without becoming overly reliant on parent intervention.

About One Year

A one-year-old will likely be sleeping about 13.5 hours in a 24-hour cycle, but the range is 9 to 18 hours. If your baby has developed good sleep organization, the bulk of those hours will be nighttime sleep. Many 1-year-olds start transitioning from two naps per day to one. When the baby's naptime is changing, and the family is trying to identify when to find the right times for the nap and lunch, the whole sleeping schedule may become erratic. In the nearby chart, you'll find sleep parameters from the National Sleep Association. Note: These are recommendations. If your baby's sleep falls out of the range of normal, but overall, he is happy, growing, and thriving, then most likely, your infant is meeting his own sleep needs.

TABLE 8.2 - Sleep Recommendations from the National Sleep Association

AGE	HOURS RECOMMENDED	APPROPRIATE RANGE OF HOURS	HOURS NOT RECOMMENDED
NEWBORNS 0 - 3 MONTHS	14 to 17	11 to 13 or 18 to 19	Less than 11 or more than 19
4 - 11 MONTHS	12 to 15	10 to 11 or 16 to 18	Less than 10 or more than 18

DEVELOPING HEALTHY SLEEP HABITS

As you can see by the typical sleep patterns at each age, the amount of sleep babies and parents get is a huge range. Research shows that the total amount infants sleep can vary widely from day-to-day with a difference as great as 12 hours (Wooding et al., 1990). The type of sleep associations a baby develops has an important role in the infant gaining the ability to cycle in and out of sleep independently without needing your help.

There are many different books and techniques, some research-based, and others built upon personal experience, that preach dogma about quick fixes to get the baby to sleep through the night. Of course, we all want the magic bullet, but ask most experienced parents, and they will tell you that learning to sleep through the night takes time. Understanding normal sleep patterns and following research-based techniques will help you handle your baby's sleep development with more skill.

Help Your Baby Develop Focus and Control

Most young babies are not capable of falling asleep on their own, nor can they control their emotions and bodily functions, or pay attention for very long. Over time, they gain control over these behaviors with the help of their caregivers and make great strides in accomplishing their first developmental goal of state regulation (i.e., staying awake longer, and lengthening independent sleep). You can support your baby in this task and further promote the formation of healthy sleep habits by having predictable routines. Babies must have a present mother who is attentively providing sensitive responses to what the baby needs at the moment. This is called synchrony. For example, when your baby gazes at your face, a synchronized response is to look into his eyes. When the baby looks away, a sensitive response is to not seek his gaze by following his head but to give him a break. Learning the baby's signals for sleep is a part of this. By being present and watching your baby, you recognize his fatigue signs, and you give it a name. For example, you might say, "Sleepy eyes. Let's go nighty night." And then you gently put your baby to sleep. So rather than following your agenda, you synchronize with your baby's rhythm, which helps him develop a more predictable and regular schedule. Over time, by paying attention to the baby's cues and responding, he will become more regular and regulated.

> **ACTION PLAN**
>
> Pathways to Healthy Sleep Habits:
> (1) Develop Focus and Control
> (2) Identify Early Sleep Cues
> (3) Capture Windows of Opportunity

The parent's routine can help the baby transition smoothly through his six states of awareness (modulate his states), so he can get better sleep. Know that light influences the development of the circadian rhythm (Harrison, 2004). Research found that exposing 6-week-olds to light in the home during the early afternoon correlated to better sleep at night (Harrison, 2004). The household rhythm can also affect the baby's ability to regulate his states. For example, too much activity can make it difficult for him to manage to stay awake because it causes habituation, resulting in evening crankiness and crying fits. If you can, it helps to plan your week so that activities happen at the same time each day. Keep stimulating visits brief for your newborn, so it does not disrupt the natural cycle. Too much activity can cause parents to miss their baby's early sleep cues, causing agitation and crying spells.

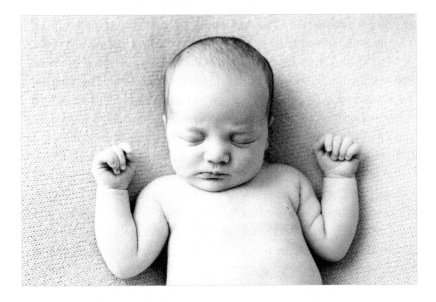

While habituation looks like sleep, it does not replace it. Too much habituation can lead to excessive fussiness and crying spells in the early evening hours. New babies often habituate in a loud room and on a long car ride.

A patient was referred to Andrea Herron for a feeding assessment due to extreme, "colic-like behavior." The mother was desperate and exhausted. She felt like she could never put her baby down without him screaming. Because of the symptoms and extreme irritability, the doctor prescribed medication for reflux. The breastfeeding evaluation revealed that the mother was missing the baby's timeout and sleep cues. Andrea taught her Baby Watching techniques so the mother could understand how to anticipate naptimes. Within 24 hours, their struggle and weeks of irritability were resolved.

Learn to feed your baby with the arrival of early hunger cues, and the same goes for sleep. Creating healthy sleep associations will help your baby be better organized about sleep. Sleep associations are habits we form that help our body calm so that we can transition to sleep (Sadeh et al., 2010), such as reading before bed, or snuggling with a pillow or blanket.

Babies frequently arouse during the night. If the parents spent a long time to get the baby asleep initially, then the baby may require the same intense effort to go back to sleep throughout the night. Infants who find their own way of relaxing into sleep may be able to self-soothe back to sleep following each sleep cycle. Their higher arousal state may require little parental intervention. Others might make you doubt your parenting response to your baby's nighttime behaviors but know that it is not your fault. These habits all begin with the infant—their intensity, maturity, and innate reactions to the world. The way the baby acts will cause parents to be more involved. For example, Daniel showed clear fatigue cues and could easily be laid down to sleep. His cousin Paul couldn't sleep unless he was nursed, rocked, and held until he was in deep sleep. In general, trying to help the baby develop self-soothing skills will lead to less calling to parents during the night. Try the following techniques:

» Occasionally lay your baby down to sleep while drowsy.

» Babies often drift off to sleep with the pleasure of nursing, but many become reliant on breastfeeding to fall asleep. If your family choice is to co-sleep and you easily drift back to sleep, enjoy yourself, and benefit from this easy technique. Many working mothers who chose not to co-sleep change their mind when they realize it is the only way they get sleep while making up for time apart.

» If your baby often nurses to sleep but you don't want this to be a part of your routine, alternate the ways you put him to sleep. For example, rotate between cuddling, rocking, singing, massage, taking a walk, white noise, etc.

» Wait until the baby is really awake and showing feeding cues before picking him up during the night to breastfeed. Recognize that the movements your baby does during light sleep do not always lead to waking and needing to nurse. You can allow your infant to finish his sleep cycle. Otherwise, you may have more night wakings and nursings than necessary.

» Practice Baby Watching. During the day, soothe your baby back to sleep as soon as you notice fatigue cues, or after he has been awake for no more than 60 to 90 minutes.

Capture Windows of Opportunity

There are times during the day and night when your baby's brain will become drowsy and less alert. This is called "sleep pressure." We all experience this throughout the day. For us, we may stay awake by standing up, walking around, having a snack, or drinking a caffeinated beverage. For infants, signs of sleep pressure are the best and easiest time to promote sleep. Seeing signs of drowsiness is a window of opportunity for you to easily soothe your baby because the sleep process begins to overcome him, naturally facilitating this transition. Once again, Baby Watching will help you identify the signs of drowsiness. Typically, a young baby will become drowsy again after completing his feeding, changing, and quiet alert routine every hour and a half or so. Once he starts crying excessively, stress hormones rise and further stimulate the brain and body, preventing sleep. If you reach this point, you may want to stop sleep efforts and wait until your baby is drowsy again. Mothers have complained of episodes where it has taken upwards of 2 hours to soothe their baby to sleep once stress kicks in.

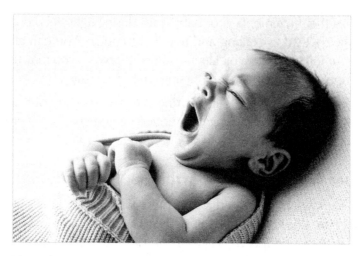

It's much easier to settle a baby to sleep with the onset of early fatigue cues that are windows of opportunity before crying begins.

Identify Early Sleep Cues

Babies are not automatic sleepers. They are too busy learning and processing everything that is new. We can usually identify new sounds and ignore them, but babies cannot. If they hear it, they must process it. It can take up to 30 minutes to get some infants to sleep. If you can begin to identify your child's signs of fatigue, you will start to learn how to help him transition to sleep more smoothly. When tired, your baby may exhibit one or more of the following behaviors:

» Decreases movements or quiets down

» Stops looking at you or his toys, or begins yelling at the toys

» Eyes become glazed

» Starting at 3 months, the baby will begin to rub his eyes

» Yawns (early sign), then fusses

» Skin becomes mottled (a marbled appearance)

» Redness appears around the eyebrows.

If you miss the signals of fatigue, your baby becomes stressed, and his body releases cortisol. This makes him irritable and hyper, thus, unable to sleep. It is also more difficult for infants to fall asleep or stay asleep when the brain is not in a drowsy state. As the brain matures, these biologically determined periods of drowsiness will become more predictable and longer.

Helping Your Baby Nap

The periods of day sleep and night sleep do not develop at the same time (Mindell et al., 2016). Night sleep develops first, so you will notice longer sleeping periods at night before you notice longer naps. Between 12 and 16 weeks of age, day sleep organization develops. Getting the baby to take a nap long enough for you to accomplish something becomes challenging. He falls asleep on the breast but awakens when you transfer him to bed. Or, you successfully make the transfer, and the baby awakens before you have a chance to take a shower or complete a task. Daytime sleeping was not a problem when your baby was younger because he was not as social and was less interested in his environment. Now that the 3-to-4-month-old is more aware of his surroundings, outside stimulation like light, noise, or motion can affect his sleep. Also, for naps, there is a lack of darkness and quieting behaviors that adults do to prepare for bed—things that ordinarily support the baby's bedtime transition. To promote healthy naptime habits, follow these Baby Watching techniques: timing, soothing that is not overstimulating, and consistency.

Timing

Keep the intervals of wakefulness short. While you are still learning your baby's cues, peek at the clock when your baby wakes up. After about 1 hour, you can expect to see early fatigue cues. At this time, begin a soothing process before he appears grumpy, crabby, or drowsy. Usually, the total period of wakefulness, plus soothing, should be less than 2 hours. Avoid the mistake of keeping your baby awake for 2 hours or more before trying to soothe him to sleep. Some infants go to sleep after being awake for only 1 hour. Perfect timing produces little or no crying.

Motionless Sleep

For some parents, motion is a "go to" solution to get their baby to sleep. But infants need motionless sleep to get good sleep. A car ride, infant swing, or vibration of a stroller can force the brain to a lighter sleep state and reduce the restorative power of sleep. You may wish to use motion for a few minutes as a part of the soothing process but be sure to stop the motion once you see deep sleep cues. If the baby falls asleep on your breast and you try to put him down in light sleep, it may cause waking, so wait for the transition to deep sleep.

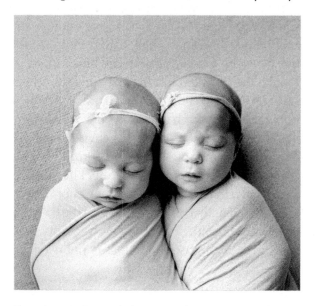

These identical twins help us see what two stages of sleep look like. The baby on the left is in deep sleep. Notice her relaxed eyes, head, and cheeks. The infant on the right is in light sleep. She shows more muscle tone, present by a furrowed brow, open mouth, strain within the swaddle, raised head, and tighter cheeks. You can tell there is movement behind the eyelids, showing this baby is in REM.

Consistency in Soothing Style

There is not a right or wrong way to soothe a baby to sleep. Falling asleep is simply a habit that your child will learn best if you are consistent.

CONSIDER FACTORS THAT AFFECT SLEEP

Illness and Sleep

When your baby is sick, everything "goes out the window." The days are long with erratic behaviors and sleep. Forget about routines, rules, and structure, and instead, do what you need to do to calm the baby. A sick infant may not have a big appetite for a while and lack energy to finish meals. This may leave the baby feeling hungry more often. A stuffy nose can also prevent the baby from completing a meal and lead to sleep disrupted by hunger and thirst more often than normal. A bit of patience will help you overcome this challenge.

How Temperament Affects Sleep

Your baby's individual personality traits, known as temperament, can impact the ease of falling asleep, length of sleep, and waking. Some babies are more organized than others. What we mean by that is they can get themselves to sleep faster and stay asleep longer. They also develop the ability to soothe themselves sooner, while others need more time. The latter babies take longer to fall asleep and are more sensitive to ambient sounds and sights, which makes them more likely to have their sleep disturbed. That sensitivity is genetic. Beware of those who tell you to expose the baby to your lifestyle so the baby learns to sleep through anything. On the contrary, it will likely result in an evening spent holding a very fussy baby.

Babies' activity level can also affect how easily they relax to sleep and how still they are during sleep. Mothers of the active child may find themselves perplexed by their sleeping gymnast. Babies also differ in their predictability. You can practically "set your clock" to the schedule of the predictable baby. Others, with little predictability, are so erratic that it makes it difficult to establish a bedtime, anticipate fatigue, and predict when the baby will wake up. For example, the irregular baby might be up at 4 am one day after "sleeping through the night," then 8 am the next after five night-wakings.

A baby's inherent adaptability is also relevant to sleep. Many expectant parents imagine how easy it will be taking their sleepy newborn on a road trip to see relatives, only to find that they are up all night shushing and pacing with a screaming baby in someone else's home. Some babies are extremely adaptable, making it easy for them to sleep anywhere. Others are more sensitive to change because it is disruptive to their rhythm and the organization that they feel. It might take several days in a new environment before they can adjust. Once you return home, it will require a few more days to get back to normal.

Mood affects how babies react when cycling in and out of sleep. Parents are shocked by the baby who wakes up with the primal scream. Others are surprised to find that their baby has been awake for several minutes, happily babbling and looking at the mobile. How loudly and strongly they communicate their mood to you is a matter of intensity. When the intense baby doesn't want to go to sleep, he will scream. You can't avoid it. A baby with low intensity may feel the same inside but may not express his discontentment as strongly.

Distractibility is another trait that impacts sleep. A mother may struggle to settle the distractible baby because every noise in the room causes him to pull off the breast. This can be a source of family tension where the mother is having to quiet the behaviors of her partner or other children, before she can get the baby to sleep. The opposite scenario is the baby who can get to sleep in any environment. One characteristic that many parents talk about is the persistent child who is trying to master a developmental task (i.e., rolling over, crawling). Practice extends to sleep time, challenging co-sleeping tremendously.

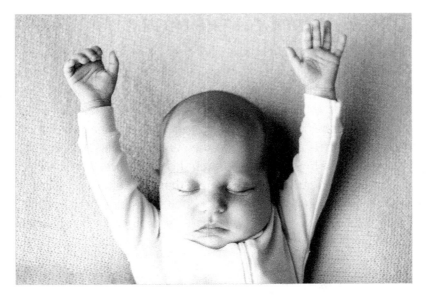

A baby that startles easily may need more external support to help protect her sleep.

The question is, how can you help when temperament affects sleep? First, be able to recognize if your baby is sensitive to his environment. You can tell if he startles easily to noise, makes jerky movements, easily reaches a crying state, and is not smooth with transitions between states of awareness. If you recognize your child is sensitive, you'll need to be like a mama bear and protect your baby by keeping the house quiet and preventing visitors from passing him around. This baby also needs careful, slow handling and swaddling, so jerky movements don't wake him up. In general, sensitive babies need a tranquil, less-stimulating environment. Look for early signs of fatigue and respond appropriately before the baby becomes overtired to prevent crying jags. When traveling with the routine baby (one that doesn't do change well), try to maintain the same schedule that you have at home, (i.e., nap and feeding times). Anything that you can bring from his normal environment, such as bedding, sleepwear, and soothing blankets, may help him adapt sooner (more on temperament in the next chapter).

NURSING THROUGH THE NIGHT

Research shows that nighttime breastfeeds make an important contribution to a baby's total milk intake (Kent et al., 2006). If you are worried about your milk supply, realize that night feeds are not only important for your baby's growth, but they help develop your milk supply. Mothers struggling with attachment sometimes find more success at night, when they are both relaxed and less distracted by the household. Research shows that breastfed babies wake more frequently during the night than non-breastfed babies (Galbally et al., 2013). Rather than being discouraged by this, avoid comparing your baby's habits to your friend's baby, who exclusively bottle-feeds.

Night Waking

Waking is a normal characteristic of nighttime sleep for babies in the first year of life. Researchers have revealed that night feeds are necessary to protect lactation and ensure a continuous milk supply for 6 months and beyond (Galbally et al., 2013). There is a correlation between night waking and age, although it occurs at every phase of infancy. In one study, waking was reported in 46% of 3-month-olds, 39% of 6-month-olds, 58% of 9-month-olds, and 55% of 12-month-olds (Scher, 1991). The research shows that night waking begins to decrease between 3 and 6 months of age, and then increases again at 9 months, coinciding with significant socioemotional advances (Scher, 1991). In other words, learning disrupts the baby's sleep. It certainly wakes us up when we are stressed by new responsibilities or tasks (i.e., tax season, demands of the holidays, a new job).

Research also shows that most infants usually require their parent's help at night to get back to sleep after waking (Goodlin-Jones et al., 2001). While older babies have more self-soothing abilities than the younger ones, even at 12 months, 50% still require assistance from their parents to fall back asleep (Goodlin-Jones et al., 2001). This is a short phase in your baby's life. It's a time when your baby is not developmentally ready to sleep for long periods, and his schedule is driven by frequent hunger. He may be sensitive to environmental stimulation that triggers crying, or shutting down and sleeping. So, expect at least 2 to 3 wakings a night, including one around 3 am. If you find that the baby has long crying episodes during the early evening hours combined with lots of night feeds, try taking him back to a dark, quiet room after 75 to 90 minutes of wakefulness during the day.

Nurture Effectively

During the beginning of your newborn's life, tending to the baby to breastfeed when he begins to stir is good practice to help him return to birthweight, reduce the risk of jaundice, and bring in an ample breastmilk supply. But once your baby is doing well, has past his birthweight, and is gaining about an ounce a day, you can start to extend night nursing intervals. When your baby begins to move during the night, wait a few minutes to see if he is transitioning into a state of light sleep, upon which he might settle and return to sleep, or is actually waking up. Mothers tend to bring their infant to the breast quickly the moment they stir, not realizing those little movements are cues that signify light sleep and not hunger. The baby suckles briefly before returning to sleep. This disrupts the sleep cycle and risks creating a habit that you don't intend to maintain—one that can lead to excessive night waking (up to every hour of the night).

Nurturing effectively can help you minimize excessive night feeds. Really try to understand your baby's cues and learn what his sleep states look like. This will help you avoid mistaking light sleep behaviors for waking (review States of Awareness in Chapter 5). If you wait until the baby is wide awake, he will more likely be able to finish a meal, and you two will have better rest. Waking cues include open eyes, hands to mouth, rooting, and grunting sounds. You'll see the baby's arms flexed upwards and held under his chin while he roots, looking for the breast. The exception to waiting for wakefulness is the fussy baby that has rapid state changes. You'll want to catch this baby in light sleep to nurse before he fully wakes up. During the breastfeed, make sure he has a good deep latch and is gulping with rhythmic little "ka" sounds.

At around 3 months of age, if your infant was born full-term and is eating well during the day, you can start to reduce the number of night feedings. The infant who is thriving in terms of growth and sleep organization may have an easier time giving up late-night snacks. However, many babies need help. If you want to limit night nursing, try gradually reducing how long you breastfeed and stretch out the time between feedings. Delay feedings by offering other forms of comfort, one at a time, starting with the least stimulating: your voice, shushing, a lullaby, a hand on the back, massage, picking up, holding, then rocking. It is important to pay attention to your body while extending intervals. Engorgement or painful breast fullness can lead to plugged ducts and mastitis. Some women have to always continue the night feedings because their breasts can't tolerate longer intervals due to smaller storage capacity. Between 8 to 12 weeks, when the baby starts to sleep longer stretches at night, some women find that they experience less discomfort if they pump their breasts well before their baby goes to sleep.

· · · · · · · · · · · · · · · · ·

CHAPTER NINE

Sleep Safety: Protecting Your Infant Day and Night

Chapter Goal: Learn how to make a sleep environment that protects against SIDS and other sleep hazards while being supportive of breastfeeding.

SLEEP SAFETY

Those first few nights with your newborn can be terrifying. You lay there listening closely as he takes each breath. Before you have the confidence in your mothering instincts, you also might wonder whether you will wake to his sounds amidst sleep deprivation. These feelings can go on for weeks and be amplified by postpartum depression or baby blues that might make you weepy, anxious, or fearful, particularly of sudden infant death syndrome (SIDS). One practical way to help stifle these fears is to create the safest sleep environment possible and follow the most up-to-date American Academy of Pediatrics (AAP) medical recommendations. It is also important to be flexible. That may mean ignoring public opinion, including the unrealistic expectations that promote the concept of the independent newborn who sleeps in his own bed in a separate room. Plenty of parents set up the perfect nursery modeled after designer catalogs. They intend for their baby to sleep there and be independent from the start. Then, motherhood alters the brain remarkably, making you more nurturing and protective. Try not to be disappointed if your reality changes prenatal plans.

Infant sleep environments have become a complex subject in the last two decades, strewn with widespread realities that contradict social norms and blanket recommendations against Western parents who are increasingly adopting co-sleeping habits (McKenna & McDade, 2005). The result is parents are left with a void of information on how to co-sleep safely. While co-sleeping is how much of the world population nurtures their babies at night, Western medical authorities cannot recommend it because mystery still surrounds SIDS, and co-sleeping is sometimes a factor when combined with other hazardous situations.

Bassinet or Crib

Baby merchandisers have long enticed consumers to adorn their baby's crib with lush linens, bumpers, plush blankets, and stuffed toys. Even though researchers have since stressed the safety of a bare crib, it has been a struggle to change. The AAP states that no bumper pads, positioners, wedges, toys, or pillows should be in the baby's sleep space. The mattress should be firm. Caution should be taken to be sure that there are no gaps between the sides of the bed and the mattress, where the baby could fall or become wedged. A bassinet is a safe way to keep your newborn close at night. In a study of nearly 900 infants, the most common age to transition the baby to a crib was between 3 and 4 months (Wooding et al., 1990). The latest AAP recommendation is to make sure that the crib or bassinet is in the same room as you (which is likely your bedroom) for the baby's first 6 months to 1 year, if possible (AAP, 2016).

To Swaddle or Not to Swaddle

Newborn care classes and hospitals across the nation prioritize teaching how (and how not) to swaddle a baby. This may give you the impression that it is essential. For most babies, swaddling is calming when there is an absence of a warm embrace. It makes them feel safe, like being inside the womb. In addition, many new babies have trouble controlling their arms and easily startle. For the baby with a sensitive Moro reflex, these movements can be very disruptive to sleep. Research shows that swaddling supports a baby's sleep, resulting in shorter arousal duration during REM sleep and more REM sleep overall (Gerard et al., 2002). Note that if your baby's Moro reflex is not sensitive (reactive), and he does not have trouble completing a sleep cycle, he may not need to be swaddled.

Safety Guidelines

There are various ways to swaddle. You can choose to leave the baby's arms free or secured. What matters most is that you follow safe swaddling guidelines, including the following:

» Never place a swaddled baby on his belly or side. Back is best.

» Be careful not to wrap the chest too tightly. Doing so can restrict the lungs' ability to expand and may increase the risk of respiratory infections.

» Take care to prevent overheating, especially if his head is covered, he has a fever, or is co-sleeping. When co-sleeping or in the case of fever, check your baby throughout the night to make sure the body isn't too warm (obvious with the presence of heat or perspiration). Be advised that when your body is nearby, there is heat transfer to the baby.

» The baby should be able to rotate his hips freely and flex his knees to prevent hip dysplasia.

» In a hospital nursery, cotton blankets are used to swaddle but should be discontinued quickly after discharge. They should be replaced with a Velcro or zipper swaddle.

» Be aware of swaddles that have loose parts (i.e., zippers, ribbons) that can break off or loosen. Parents often wonder if they should continue to swaddle their baby when they see that the infant seems to resist this care, or the swaddle comes undone during the night. If no swaddle stays in place, then stop using one. Once the baby makes attempts to roll over, it is no longer safe to swaddle. Many parents stop swaddling after 3 months or sooner but then find that the baby is waking more and sleeping for shorter periods. This is a transition time, as parents try to find new ways to settle their baby and lengthen sleep stretches. A transitional swaddle that keeps the arms out can help.

PREVENTING SUDDEN INFANT DEATH SYNDROME

SIDS is the sudden death of an otherwise healthy baby under 1-year-old, which remains unexplained after a thorough investigation, autopsy, and review of medical history (AAP, 2005). It usually happens during sleep and most commonly occurs between 2 and 3 months of age (AAP, 2005). According to the AAP, approximately 3,500 infants die every year from sleep-related deaths, including SIDS and accidental suffocation and strangulation (AAP, 2016). That number was even higher when it was commonplace to put young infants to sleep belly-down (the prone position). In 1992, the AAP released a recommendation that infants be placed on their back (supine position) to sleep (AAP, 2005). After a massive campaign to reverse infant sleep positioning to back-down, habits started to change. Mothers began to comply with the back-down recommendation. What followed was a notable decrease in infant sleep-related deaths (AAP, 2016). In fact, since the push began to stop putting babies to bed on their bellies, the number of deaths dropped by more than 50% (AAP, 2005). While SIDS is still not completely understood, the major decrease in the number of SIDS deaths is telling. The recommendation stands; babies should be put to bed in a supine (back-down) position.

Risk Factors

The AAP Task Force on SIDS said studies consistently identified independent risk factors for SIDS, including prone sleep position (belly-down), sleeping on a soft surface (such as a sofa, couch, soft mattress, or waterbed), a mother that smoked during her pregnancy, overheating, late or no prenatal care, a young mother, preterm birth and/or low birthweight, and being a male infant (AAP, 2016). Babies are at increased risk of SIDS if they bedshare with parents who have been smoking or consuming alcohol (Blair et al., 2014). Other risk factors include bedsharing with other children (AAP, 2005).

Prevention

Since the cause of SIDS is still somewhat of a mystery, prevention is focused on reducing risk factors. It is NOT safe to co-sleep with your baby in a hazardous environment that includes any of the above risk factors. The AAP's latest protocol recommends you (AAP, 2016):

» Put the baby down on the back to sleep for every sleep until the child reaches age 1.

» Make sure the baby is on a firm mattress with only a fitted sheet (no other bedding, bumpers, pillows, hanging strings/cords, or plush toys).

» Breastfeed exclusively for at least 6 months.

» Room-share but not bedshare for at least the first 6 months (ideally, the first year). It's the proximity of the parent that is protective.

» Consider offering a pacifier at nap and bedtime after 1 month of age.

» Dress the baby in no more than one layer more than you dress yourself to avoid overheating. Signs of overheating include sweating and a chest that is hot to touch. Avoid over-bundling or covering the baby's head.

» Follow the CDC and AAP immunization schedule because recent evidence shows vaccinations may have a protective effect against SIDS.

» Supervise awake tummy-time daily to help your baby develop upper body strength, motor skills, and reduce time putting pressure on the back of the head, which can cause flattening.

PREVENTING HEAD FLATTENING

The newborn's skull bones are soft and malleable to mold and safely pass through the birth canal. They are made to expand during the early period of rapid brain growth. This can make the head susceptible to abnormal shaping. Young infants that spend much of their time on their back for sleep, frequent long car rides, bouncy seats, and swings commonly develop an abnormally shaped skull that is somewhat flat in the back, known as flat-head syndrome or plagiocephaly. The incidence in 7-to-12-week-old infants observed in the first population-based study is estimated to be over 46% (Mawji et al., 2013). Other studies estimate the prevalence in infants overall is about 8% (Boere-Boonekamp, 2001). This is a relatively new phenomenon that began to grow in numbers since the 1992 AAP recommendation to place all infants "back-down" to sleep. While the practice drastically reduced infant deaths from SIDS, flattening skulls was a consequence. Contributing to this phenomenon is a cultural push to nest our infants in anything but the mothers' arms. Witness the number of accessories gifted at baby showers, all intended to cradle the baby in an artificial nest.

There are other less-common causes of head-flattening, such as torticollis where muscle tightness causes the baby to prefer turning and resting on one side of the head over the other. Lactation consultants are reporting an increase in the incidence of torticollis cases that lead to breastfeeding issues. They postulate that it may be caused by longer births where babies spend more time in the narrow birth canal. While wedged in a position too long with a mother who is immobilized by an epidural, it can cause abnormal pressure on the skull and/or muscle tightening (torticollis). In a study of nearly 10,000 babies diagnosed with skull deformation, more than half also had torticollis (Wood et al., 2013). Periodically look at your little one's head from various angles (top, sideways, back). If he has a thick head of hair, feel with your hands. Look at his face. Are the cheeks equal? Are the ears at the same level? Cranial Technologies offers an online assessment tool that you can try at home (www.cranialtech.com/online-assessment/).

If you notice that the head is misshaped, or the face is asymmetrical, see your baby's practitioner. It is critical to diagnose the reason for cranial asymmetry. Radiological imaging should be undertaken in extreme cases to rule out other conditions, such as lambdoid synostosis, which requires surgery (Kalra & Walker, 2012). This is a rare condition where skull bones fuse too early, putting the baby's brain at risk. Infants with severe cases of flattening may form asymmetrical facial features, which, if not treated and diagnosed early, can be permanent (Mawji et al., 2013). New research also points to possible abnormal developmental outcomes (Shipster et al., 2003). Head Shape Clinics specialize in correcting deformation caused by caregiver positioning by using custom helmets. This approach has been proved effective. There is some controversy, however, regarding whether intervention is always needed due to over-diagnosed cases and the profitable business of treating it.

Prevention

Try the following techniques to prevent flat-head syndrome:

» Wear or carry your baby as much as possible.

» Incorporate "tummy time" into your routine after every diaper change or when your baby is alert. Turn your infant on his belly, bringing the elbows under the chest. Then, gently press on the small of the baby's back to stabilize the hips and prevent him from arching his legs up in the air. This will make the baby more comfortable and encourage him to lift his head and strengthen the muscles in his neck and upper body. Do not leave your baby unsupervised. Many babies don't like tummy time at first and protest. You can encourage it by getting down on the ground with your infant and making sessions short, about 3 to 5 minutes each time.

» Try repositioning techniques by rotating the direction you place your baby in his bed. When sleeping near their mother, babies tend to turn their head in her direction, causing more time spent on one side and increased risk of developing a flat spot.

» Limit time in car seats, swings, and bouncy chairs. If you notice a flattening area, help prevent putting further pressure on that part of the skull by rolling a receiving blanket or small towel, and wedge it behind the shoulder to keep the baby from leaning in the direction of the flat spot. Always supervise when you place an object under your baby.

» Use laid-back breastfeeding positioning. If your infant has already formed a flat spot, be aware that holding him in the crook of your arm while nursing could put pressure on the flat spot.

SHARING THE PARENTS' BED: CO-SLEEPING

Many parents feel more at ease when their baby is within reach, especially at night. They want to hear those tiny breaths and be able to check on their baby in an instant. Research shows that nursing mothers are more responsive to their baby than non-nursing mothers at night (Baddock et al., 2007). Bedsharing supports the closeness mothers and babies need to sense each other and make frequent physical contact. It gives the mother a heightened sensitivity, increasing the chance that she will alert to a danger and intervene in a life-threatening event (Mosko & McKenna, 1997). The frequent arousals mean the baby spends less time in deep sleep, which has been identified as a possible risk factor for SIDS (Mosko et al., 1996). The latest research shows safe bedsharing (where there is an absence of hazardous conditions) beyond 3 months postpartum is protective against SIDS (Blair et al., 2014).

Numerous studies show that bedsharing also benefits breast-feeding. Mothers who sleep next to their baby breastfeed three more times than those who have their infant in a separate room (McKenna, 1994). In one study, bedsharing babies suckled more often at night and longer than babies who slept separately (McKenna et al., 1997). The frequent feedings and physical contact bedsharing facilitate plays an important role in the activation of milk-producing cells, increasing a mother's milk supply (McKenna & McDade, 2005). Co-sleeping also allows more total sleep for both mother and baby (Mckenna & McDade, 2005).

Divided Over Co-sleeping

Many health authorities discourage all forms of bedsharing, in part, because there are no consumer safety standards for infants in adult beds. More pointedly, they have concerns over accidental entrapment, overlain by a sleeping adult or child, and risk of SIDS (ABM, 2008). Investigations into SIDS deaths uncovered that in almost all the cases where bedsharing was involved, there was also formula-feeding, parental drug or tobacco use, and/or the sleep position and/or surface was unsafe, such as a couch or waterbed, and the infant sleeping belly-down (Gessner et al., 2001).

A lack of complete understanding about the cause of SIDS has created a stigma around co-sleeping. Following a review of studies and data looking at the co-sleeping controversy about SIDS, bedsharing, and breastfeeding, renown researchers James Mckenna and Thomas McDade fired back against a cultural norm, which has become taboo. Their review concluded that "co-sleeping at least in the form of room-sharing, especially with an actively breastfeeding mother saves lives, is a powerful reason why the simplistic scientifically inaccurate and misleading statement 'never sleep with your baby' needs to be rescinded, wherever and whenever it is published" (McKenna & McDade, 2005, p. 134).

Anthropologists can tell you that across the non-Westernized world, co-sleeping is normal in more than 100 cultures (Latz et al., 1999). Historically, it was recommended in North America until the start of the 20th century, when social norms began to change (Ball, 2014). Due to the stigma, many more people bedshare than they care to admit. In a review of 10 studies conducted by anthropologist Helen Ball, observing the prevalence among over 30,000 families with an infant age 3-to-6-months-old, 40 to 77% said they co-slept (Ball, 2014). Many parents that do not plan on bedsharing with their baby inevitably succumb to its benefits because cribs are not designed to support breastfeeding. In general, breastfeeding mothers are three times more likely to co-sleep than bottle-feeding ones (McCoy et al., 2004). Some parents are hard-pressed to carry on breastfeeding without co-sleeping at least some of the time. What matters is that you do what is best for your family and make an informed decision.

How to Bedshare Safer

The Academy of Breastfeeding Medicine has extensively examined evidence-based research on sleep safety. For safer co-sleeping, it recommends you (ABM, 2008):

» Follow SIDS-prevention tips for avoiding hazardous sleep conditions and risk factors.

» Wait until your baby is 3-months-old before starting to co-sleep. If you are in bed, breastfeeding your infant who is under 3 months of age and you drift off to sleep, transfer the baby back to his crib or bassinet when you awake.

» Ensure the baby's head cannot possibly become covered.

» Use an infant sleep sack if needed to maintain warmth, or swaddle rather than using blankets.

» Make sure there are no gaps between the mattress and head-board, walls, or other areas, which could entrap the baby and lead to suffocation.

» Never put your infant down to sleep on a pillow.

» Understand that adult beds are not designed for use by infants, so there are no federal consumer safety standards to protect you. Never leave the baby alone on an adult bed.

» Consider the use of an infant bed that attaches to the side of your bed, which allows proximity and access to the baby without the need to share the same sleep surface.

» Don't co-sleep with your baby if there is another child or an unrelated adult in the bed.

Co-sleeping can get complicated with the 3-month-old who can roll over or the 6-month-old who can crawl. Infants get injured falling off beds and inadvertently whack parents on their heads while thrashing around in sleep. You can make bedsharing safer by removing the springboard and base of the bed so that the mattress is flat on the ground. Be advised that when you no longer want to co-sleep, it can be difficult to change. You may need to slowly transition the baby by first moving him to a crib in your room. To limit stress on the family, avoid making the transition when there is a major change at home, such as a parent returning to work. You'll also need to take into consideration your baby's phase in development and personality.

Research shows that co-sleeping leads to less crying (McKenna & McDade, 2005). Without having to face the nightly stress of separation and crying to sleep, the baby learns to feel safe at night. This early dependence grows independence. When the child is developmentally ready and old enough to be an independent sleeper, the parents who met their baby's needs will likely have an easier time putting the child to sleep, keeping him in his bed all night, and less waking and night intrusions.

COPING WITH SLEEP DEPRIVATION

Sleep deprivation following a lack of continuous, uninterrupted sleep is taxing. The feeling combined with a dominant right brain over the cognitive left can make you feel a lot less like yourself. Research shows that the sleep deprivation new parents experience with their young infant limits physical and cognitive function and leads to increased stress (Lee, 2003). It affects our relationships with other adults and even how we interact with our babies (Lee, 2003). Inadequate sleep can also lead to postnatal depression (Armstrong et al., 1998). It is important that you prioritize rest whenever possible. Try side-lying breastfeeding and co-sleeping to lessen fatigue. The National Sleep Association recommends the following tips to adjust for the baby who wakes through the night and/or rises early (National Sleep Foundation, 2017):

» Make your bedtime no later than 10 pm to shoot for maximum cumulative hours of rest.

» Disconnect from social media, cellphones, tablets, etc. one hour before bedtime.

» Keep sleepiness at bay during the day by taking walks, getting fresh air and sunshine on your skin.

» Nap when your baby naps or ask a support person to take over care so you can take a nap.

» Use a white-noise machine. Relax the mind and drone out little sounds made in light sleep.

If you take anything from these sleep discussions, realize that new babies have irregular sleeping patterns, take short naps, take preference to falling asleep at the breast, frequently wake throughout the night, and sleep best when close to their mother's heart. If parents see these normal behaviors as problematic or expect that they can control or change them, they are more susceptible to feeling depressed (Muscat et al., 2014). Know that this is a short phase of your life, although it feels like forever. Sleep is in your destiny.

CHAPTER TEN

Personality Matters: Unveiling your Baby's Unique Temperament

Chapter Goal: Begin to identify your baby's individual characteristics that describe his temperament and any areas that may require sensitive support or care for successful breastfeeding, calming, sleeping, and learning.

WHO IS THIS PERSON?

Four-week-old Allie looks directly at her mother and smiles intently while onlookers gaze in amazement. In a neighboring town, Tina tries to make the same connection with her newborn, Grace, but instead, it seems to overwhelm the baby. Grace is not the cuddly social baby her parents expected her to be. In fact, Tina must protect her from visitors—their eye contact and touch. It can be the hardest thing for parents to face the reality that their new baby does not react like they expected. Matters become more complicated when parents either fail to recognize differences that may require a sensitive response or try to change the infant to fit their idea of an ideal baby. They must recognize that their baby is different from them, with his own personality, mood, and general approach to the world, known as temperament.

201

WHAT IS TEMPERAMENT?

When professors of psychiatry Stella Chess and Alexander Thomas first explained their temperament research findings to the world in the 1950s, they, too, shattered expectations. The prevailing ideas of the time theorized that babies were born "blank slates," their personalities shaped by their upbringing rather than genetic inheritance (Kurcinka, 1991). In groundbreaking research, they studied hundreds of babies looking at each one's reaction to routine activities, such as sleeping, eating, dressing, eliminating, and moving about. The babies differed in their reactions, from their general mood, activity level, sensitivity, adaptability to changes in routine, intensity of their responses, tendency to approach or withdraw in a new situation, persistence, and distractibility (Thomas & Chess, 1977). They also varied in regularity of sleep and eating cycles. Temperament is a baby's way of reacting in all nine categories and how they mesh. The various traits essentially describe how a person responds to the world—his natural disposition or personality style. A baby's temperament determines his general activity level, attention span, level of distractibility, and ability to adapt, self-regulate, and be soothed (Thomas & Chess, 1977). It also affects the quality and intensity of his emotional reaction in response to his environment and needs (Thomas & Chess, 1977).

The early temperament research has since been replicated, and ranges of the same nine categories continue to help define who we are as individuals. This chapter explains each of them and will show you how to make observations about your baby's budding temperament. Tuning in will help you tailor your response when your baby signals his needs. The objective is to help heighten your sensitivity to his individuality and adapt the environment to make caregiving go smoother and help the baby maximize his potential, rather than reinforce characteristics that would make his life more difficult. For example, the baby who is really sensitive to stimulation and either sleeps or cries all day, as a result, will learn to be calmer and interact more when the parent adjusts the environment. The baby's development is then enhanced because his experience is positive. Through the concept of "goodness of fit," you will learn what it means when you and your baby have opposite traits. The goal is to prevent parent/infant relationship strain caused by a mismatch to avoid potential long-term mental and emotional health issues.

When Temperament Is Revealed

A newborn's responses to stimulation and state control do not necessarily predict temperament because the baby may still be recovering from the effects of labor and delivery. The newborn may have a tender, swollen head. Maybe one shoulder hurts, which makes lying on one side to breastfeed uncomfortable. Because of this, he may be irritable and less cuddly, making it difficult to distinguish whether it is a matter of temperament or just a temporary condition that will change with time. So, be sure to give your baby at least 10 weeks to mature and adjust before making predictions or judgments about his temperament. By about 3 months and continuing through 6 months, your baby's temperament will begin to emerge. From waking to nursing, your little one will reveal his personality style and offer you clues as to who he is and how he needs to be treated.

WHY TEMPERAMENT MATTERS

Temperament matters for reasons that will continue to be seen throughout your son or daughter's lifetime. Discovering and under-standing your baby's unique traits in the nine temperament categories will help you to respect and adapt to his individual differences rather than try to change them. You will have more patience with your fidgeting toddler who you've recognized as active, rather than label him uncooperative. In the early days, parents are typically instructed to wake a sleepy baby to breastfeed by undressing him. But is that baby sleepy because he needs to be stripped naked, or is that baby sensitive to light, sound, and/or touch, and consequently needs a quieter, warmer, and darker environment so he can stay awake enough to focus on eating? Is that baby fussy because he needs a quieter environment to become calm? Perhaps he is responding by fussing and screaming because he needs to be swaddled and calmed down. While these situations are different, they equally affect feeding and how that child adjusts to different experiences.

Temperament Affects Your Baby's Behavior

How a new baby behaves and expresses his needs and feelings is influenced by the child's temperament, the ability to self-regulate, and states of awareness, such as (Brazelton & Nugent, 2011, March of Dimes, 2003):

> » **Alertness:** The level to which the baby can focus his attention by looking, listening, or sucking.

> » **Visual Response:** The degree to which he reacts to who and what he sees.

> » **Auditory Response:** How your infant responds to voices and noise in his environment.

> » **Habituation:** Whether the baby can shut down (decrease his response to repeated stimuli) to protect himself from too much noise, light, sound, and/or motion.

> » **Cuddliness:** How the baby responds to being held, whether he snuggles into the contours of your body or seems to resist.

> » **Consolability:** How quickly and easily the newborn can calm down into a quieter state.

> » **Motor Behavior:** How active the baby moves in response to touching and other stimulation.

It Can Affect Breastfeeding Duration

One important finding in a Norwegian study of over 30,000 infants, babies who were perceived as difficult by their mothers were less likely to be breastfed exclusively for the recommended 6 months (Niegel et al., 2008). In other research, the Cambridge Baby Growth Study, breastfeeding mothers rated their babies during their first 3 months as having more challenging temperaments and less control over their feelings compared to formula-feeding ones (de

Lauzon-Guillain, 2012). Because of the natural dynamics, breastfed babies control their intake and learn to signal their hunger. They learn to ask for what they need instead of waiting passively, which long-term, makes them more confident and assertive. This active interaction is commonly misperceived because it does not fit in with our cultural expectations that the parents should be in charge. This is normal, not temperament, but note the more active and intense baby will signal even louder.

It Can Lead to Misdiagnosis

It is also common for mothers to misinterpret their baby's responses and behaviors, when so often it is just a matter of finding a way to modify the environment so that the infant can stay alert long enough to interact and feed. For example, sometimes mothers think their baby is fussy due to reflux or an allergy to their milk, when the behavior may be caused by an unrecognized sensitivity. Normal developmental growth that causes crying, fussiness, and more frequent than normal feedings could also be confused with difficult temperament.

Cambridge researchers conclude that parents must increase their awareness of the behavioral dynamics of breastfeeding, gain a better expectation of normal infant temperament, and find support to cope with difficult infant phases, so that caregivers can prevent the misdiagnosis of problems that might otherwise lead to premature weaning.

UNVEILING A BABY'S TEMPERAMENT TRAITS

Now that you have had experience Baby Watching, you've taken the time to understand your infant's unique language. This same approach (stop, look, listen, feel, evaluate) will help you observe individualistic qualities about his nine temperament traits. Observing your baby's responses during interactions will help you discover the depths of this little person.

Activity Level

Babies vary in their degree of activity level, which in the newborn period, is revealed by how much they move their arms, legs, head, and body. A highly active infant seems to wiggle and squirm a lot on the changing table and while resting on your lap, while a baby who is less active is good at staying relatively still during routine activities. Highly active babies may become very difficult to diaper change as they get bigger and stronger.

Nursing Notes

ACTIVITY LEVEL

How much does your baby move during diaper changes, dressing, and times resting on your lap?

_____

Does your baby complete his meals quickly or slowly?

_____

Your newborn's feeding style will provide early clues as to his activity level and intensity, as you begin to investigate his overall temperament, such as the length of his meals. Active, intense babies tend to wake up, scream, and gulp down their milk quickly. Less active infants are slower, steadier feeders. They wake up slowly and quietly reveal their hunger. They may take an hour or more to drink the same amount of milk an active baby takes in 20 minutes. They pause frequently and lose interest if not helped to stay on task.

Intensity of Response

Whether positive or negative, each baby responds to their feelings, sensations, and caregivers with different intensity. This trait is understood by the amount of energy the baby puts into his expression. Highly intense infants have responses that are strong, urgent, and energetic. They noisily let parents know when they are hungry with loud and piercing cries. They tend to react with pleasure or drama to even minor events. Those with a high intensity of reaction seem to experience emotions at an altered level, whether it's with great pleasure or discontentment, and they are sure to express it. This can be exhausting. Yet, lusty infants are more likely to have their needs met compared to the placid baby with a low intensity of reaction.

Babies with low intensity may react quietly when upset and cry softly. They may wake and stir a bit, or move about restlessly. They don't start crying unless these signals go unnoticed or are ignored. They may shut down or tune out when bothered. They are less likely to express their feelings of pleasure or displeasure, and are consequently difficult to read and understand.

One way you can observe your baby's intensity trait is by noting his feeding behavior. Lusty, intense infants scream for food and drain the breast quickly. They usually make it just as clear when they are full. Some of these babies will clamp their lips tightly when they finish, and some will kick and scream. Milder babies, however, might just doze off, letting the nipple slip from their lips. Also, look at how demanding your baby is when he is ready to eat. An intense infant might show less patience and distractibility when hunger calls.

Nursing Notes

INTENSITY

How does your baby usually let you know that he's hungry?

_____

How does your baby let you know when he is full?

_____

When your baby has a need, how intense is his reaction to discomfort? Does he give you a sense of urgency or signal in an easy-going way?

_____

Not recognizing these temperament traits can cause parents to misinterpret their baby. For example, the baby with a mild intensity that wakes up quietly and contently sometimes doesn't get fed often enough because he's not demanding. This can decrease the mother's milk supply. However, the super intense baby that cries often and loudly may make his mother feel less confident about breastfeeding. It can cause her to worry about the quality or quantity of her milk, resulting in a switch to formula or change in her diet, as she suspects allergies. She will likely make more trips to the pediatrician. Parents must take care to meet the needs of the baby with low intensity. These infants tend to appear easygoing and may not signal hunger strongly enough. It is not uncommon for parents of the easy baby to find themselves surprised at a visit to the pediatrician when they learn that their baby is underweight.

Distractibility

Distractibility is measured by how well a baby maintains attention. Naturally, when a person loses interest, they begin to look around and tune in to their immediate surroundings. Non-distractible babies will usually nurse without interruption until they are full, no matter what is going on around them. Highly distractible babies have a hard time maintaining focus when there is a lot of activity in the room and stop nursing to check out every noise or movement they sense.

Distractibility is viewed as positive or negative, depending on the age and agenda of the parents. For example, if the baby suddenly wants to nurse and Mom is in the shower, Dad may be able to distract the baby with a toy, or by picking him up and talking to him. In this case, the child's distractibility is positive because the mother can buy time to finish taking care of her personal needs. Hence, very distractible babies can easily be soothed by an alternate activity. A hungry baby who scores low on the distractibility scale is more focused. He might set out to cry and continue to cry until he tastes milk, defying his father's efforts to distract him. No amount of jiggling, cooing, or cuddling can divert his attention, even momentarily.

Nursing Notes

DISTRACTIBILITY

In a quiet alert state, can your baby focus on your face when there are other people nearby?

_____

When your baby is hungry and you need to stall the feed for a few minutes, are you able to distract your baby while you prepare?

_____

Can your baby continue nursing if there is activity going on around him? What does he do while he's nursing when the phone rings?

_____

If you have a baby who is not easily distracted, once he is on the move at around 7 months, detailed babyproofing will be essential because these focused, non-distractible babies can be very persistent and difficult to redirect. A simple "No, don't touch," is not going to keep this child from going back to power outlets, cords, stairs, drawers, etc. Of course, all babies need good childproofing and a safe environment. Set your baby up for success by blocking the things that you don't want him to touch. Otherwise, if you continue to punish him for his persistence, he may not feel good about himself owning this special trait, which later in life, could bring him great success. For example, for the schoolage child, low distractibility is the quality of a good student, which amounts to focus and attention for completing classwork.

Regularity

While the newborn does not have a regular sleep and feeding schedule, over time, you'll notice your baby may have a sort of regularity to his biological functions like appetite, excreting, sleeping, and waking. Regularity is essentially how predictable your baby is. If you have a predictable baby, you'll be able to tell, in each developmental phase, how long he can stay awake before getting tired and needing to go back to sleep. The length of naps can be consistent. How often and when they have bowel movements can be expected. A predictable baby makes it easy for the mother to know when the next meal will need to begin. She'll be able to plan her day and errands around her baby's routine. Daniel's mother revealed that from the moment he was born, she could predict exactly what time he would want to eat next. Paul was less predictable. His pattern changed daily. Daniel's mother developed her parenting confidence quicker than Paul's.

A regular baby is born regular. Highly regular babies need consistency to feel right with the world and may feel all out-of-sorts or stressed when things are out of place. If you miss their nap, they are miserable. If you are traveling, you need to make sure your baby sleeps on schedule. The higher the regularity, the less flexible the baby is going to be. In this way, the irregular baby is easier to manage. You can't change these traits but understanding them can help you adapt. If you are irregular and the baby is regular, you will find it easier if you get the baby's meals and sleep on a regular schedule. It also helps the regular baby feel more secure by changing diapers in the same place each time and going to the same place to nurse.

Some babies have so little regularity about their routine that it makes it very confusing for the mother to know what's next. If this is the case for you, be flexible in the beginning and feed your newborn on-cue. As the baby grows, you can start offering food at more regular times. Rest when that baby rests. Watch for signs of fatigue (yawning, red skin around the eyebrows, fussing, slowed motor movements, suckling on hands and fingers) and start putting the baby to sleep as soon as you see early cues. Try to introduce a schedule by putting your baby down for naps and bed at the same time every day. This will establish a sleep routine that your baby will be able to anticipate and eventually learn to follow.

Nursing Notes

REGULARITY

Does your baby last about the same amount of time between most meals?

_____

Does your baby seem to have a consistent "awake window" before needing to go back to sleep?

_____

Is your baby flexible or easily bothered when his routine is disrupted?

_____

The parents of an irregular baby are often able to go about their lives as before, traveling and going out to dinner with their infant in tow. Babies with little regularity often become grownups who travel well, adjust to change easily, and have no problem working a job with erratic working hours. If you find yourself having a hard time observing this temperament trait, try keeping a sleep/wake log for a few days to see if you notice any patterns.

Approachability/Withdrawal

The approachability trait describes how one initially reacts to new experiences, new tastes, people, and places. Some children seem fearless and don't hesitate to jump right in to try something new. Others are slow-to-warm-up and behave cautiously, thinking before they act. They just need a little bit of time observing before approaching the new experience. The baby with little approachability will withdraw and shut down when faced with something new, appearing fearful and shy when introduced to new faces and strangers.

To test for this trait, offer a sip of water or a textured toy to his mouth, and observe his reaction. When given a different food, babies who happily approach new experiences smile and smack their lips. They might even lean toward it to try again. Others will withdraw from the new experience and will show you by turning their head, arching, gagging, or twisting away. Some babies fall in between and have mildly negative reactions to new tastes. When it comes time to introduce solids, understanding the characteristic of your baby's personality trait for approachability is important so you don't wind up creating a list of foods your baby dislikes. When he spits out his first taste of mashed peas, is it because it's something new and he tends to withdraw to new experiences, or is it because he'll never like peas? The answer is most likely the first. You may need to introduce a food many times and give the baby time to make it his idea. Never force it, just offer it again. To avoid creating food issues, meal times should be free of all forms of pressure, including positive (for example, "One more bite for Mommy. Yeah, you did it!") or negative (for example, "If you don't eat your veggies, you can't have dessert").

Nursing Notes

APPROACH OR WITHDRAW

How does your baby react to new tastes?

_____

Does your baby brighten to new faces or tend to hide?

_____

Adaptability

The adaptability trait explains how easily your infant adjusts to transitions and new experiences, activities, people, and changes. When one activity ends and the next one begins, like breastfeeding to diapering, does this seem to bother him or is he happy to roll with it? Babies with little adaptability find transitions uncomfortable. They have a hard time readjusting and act out-of-sorts until they adapt. The baby may not take a bottle or pacifier if he is not regularly using them. Generally, new experiences tend to be difficult. The opposite is the baby who never knows a stranger. This trait also affects new experiences, such as moving from two naps to one, or accepting a new person or experience.

Nursing Notes

ADAPTABILITY

How does your baby respond to changes in his routine?

_____

How easily does your baby adapt to new places and people?

_____

A baby that does not adapt well cannot be handed to Grandma right away. If he doesn't see her often, he will need time to adjust. The baby with low adaptability usually leans toward the shy type. He won't jump into new situations eagerly. Be patient, flexible, and help your little one adjust. For example, you may need to arrive early to an event. Sit next to his grandparent for a while prior to handing him over so he can take his time to warm up. Prepare the toddler to make him more comfortable, perhaps by showing him pictures of what to expect. For example, Dan's parents recognized that he had trouble adapting to new situations. When he was old enough for a Disneyland trip, they showed him a video about it. A highly adaptable child wouldn't need this extra support and would be joyful to dive right in without any preparation. Take careful steps and try not to force the slow-to-warm-up or difficult child to do things; it can hurt them in the long run in terms of their mental/emotional health. You can't make these individuals more adaptable, but you can give them the skills to work with who they are. Shifting your approach can help them explore and make stronger relationships long-term.

Sensitivity Threshold

Each baby has their own sensory threshold or level of sensitivity. Sensory threshold describes how much stimulation in terms of light, sounds, smell, touch, and temperature changes elicits a response from the baby. It's essentially the, "I've had enough" moment. This is a very important trait to identify early on, when your newborn is learning to self-regulate to be able to accomplish the task of eating and sleeping for healthy growth and development. You'll want to identify the things (sensitivities) that disrupt this ability. The baby who is trying to nurse after his sensory threshold is overwhelmed may shut down before he's full. When you are feeding a baby, you are stimulating five senses: vision, taste, touch, hearing, and smell.

Frequently, women coming in for lactation help suspect that they lack a sufficient milk supply. What Andrea often discovers is that there is nothing insufficient about her milk, but rather, the feeding environment and the baby's response to it. An infant hypersensitive to noise may struggle to put on weight if a loud home shuts him down and prevents him from drinking enough milk to gain weight. Too much noise impedes his concentration to maintain suckling. As parents, we typically expect our babies to adapt to our lifestyle (an idea our society projects), but for some children, it is harder than for others. It can be an unrealistic expectation. Instead, we must strengthen our awareness of the baby's responsiveness and how it affects his eating. If your baby often cries or falls asleep before he is full, you can help by experimenting with one or more of the following to see what makes him concentrate on eating:

» Hold him close, but do not rub or pat him while he is eating.

» Have as much skin-to-skin contact as possible but always keep his back covered. If the baby gets cold, he may spend more time trying to stay warm than eating and, consequently, wind up habituating (shutting down).

» Feed him in a quiet, dark area if he is too sleepy or too fussy.

» Introduce a white noise (dull background sound) if he is a baby who cries a lot.

» Keep lights turned down while breastfeeding.

» Swaddle the arms if they are flailing so much that they interfere with staying on the breast. This may be more of a problem if sitting upright to nurse, so try laid-back nursing first.

Sensitivities also play a role in sleep interferences. For example, if a baby is napping in the living room, he may wake up from a sleep state due to noise or too much light if he has a sensitivity to either or both. This baby may be hardpressed to complete his natural sleep cycle. One sign of this sensitivity is a baby that startles easily. The startles wake him up. Swaddling safely will benefit this baby and promote sleep.

The infant that has a sensitivity to touch may not be as cuddly. If this is the case for your newborn, try not to be offended by it. These babies tend to be bothered by the feel of material against their skin, particularly clothing tags. It helps to remove tags and avoid rough synthetic fabrics. He may need to wear loose, light cotton clothing to feel more comfortable. It's tough to be a highly sensitive baby.

Since the infant has a low threshold for stimulation, he must work very hard to avoid becoming overloaded. If he is sensitive to sound, he may be easily startled, as noted by the Moro reflex. Loud and unpleasant sounds could also cause him to react by shutting down, habituating, or going to sleep. Uncomfortable sensations could cause the sensitive baby to stiffen his body. For example, 8-week-old Gianmarco consistently showed hypersensitivity to motion. He screamed uncontrollably in a rocker, swing, or car seat. His parents stopped using rockers and swings and avoided long trips in the car as much as possible. It took the baby 5 months to adapt to the motion in the car and more than a year to enjoy a swing.

Nursing Notes

SENSORY THRESHOLD

Does your baby respond intrigued or startled by certain sounds?

_____

Does your baby have a hard time staying awake when there is a lot of light or activity in the home?

_____

How smoothly or challenging are diaper changes?

_____

With time and care, a hypersensitive baby can learn how to process his experiences without needing to shut out the world. Be aware, however, that one's instinctive eagerness to calm a hypersensitive baby could be the very thing that sets him off. Attempts to calm must be made in slow and gradual steps. Dr. Brazelton's literature recommends approaching the baby in only one manner at a time. For example, when you gaze into his eyes, do it without speaking or rocking. After the baby has responded to your gaze, you can gradually add speaking softly or rocking gently—but only one. Finally, all three activities can be combined once the baby is paying attention and is responsive. If you increase your interaction and the baby stiffens, wait until he relaxes before making any more attempts. Realize that handling sights, sounds, and movements all at the same time is a big accomplishment for a hypersensitive baby (Brazelton, 2006). These babies need a firm, slow touch. Light tickles will be uncomfortable. When you begin feeding solid foods around 6 months, note that the sensitive baby may be challenged to enjoy new foods.

Persistence

As the baby's motor skills improve, parents can recognize specific characteristics that represent their infant's level of persistence or attention span. You can observe this trait by watching your baby as he faces a personal challenge, like stretching for a toy out of reach. Does he accept defeat quickly in the face of an obstacle or does he continue to try until he succeeds? Persistency is time dedicated to difficult tasks. A persistent baby will continue to reach for the toy without interruption, while a less persistent child easily moves on to try something else.

This personality trait can affect an infant's success in having his needs met. For example, a persistent hungry baby will elevate the intensity of communication cues from rooting to crying until he is brought to the breast, while an infant with little persistency might give up after early cues go unnoticed, missing a meal. The less persistent baby may even adapt to minor hunger sensations and become accustomed to ignoring them. "Failure to thrive" may be seen in infants who are often underfed because they don't persistently demand milk. Like other personality traits, persistence is sometimes viewed positively and other times negatively. In the future, a persistent baby who continues to play in a kitchen drawer, despite his mother's request to stop, may be perceived as stubborn, while the persistent 8-month-old is admired for continuing to pull himself up, despite his wobbly legs that make him fall every time.

Mood

Mood is another trait that becomes more apparent with the older, settled baby. Mood explains whether a person tends to respond to the world in an enthusiastic, happy, or serious way. Once your baby becomes more alert and responsive, you can assess whether he is generally quiet or happy. For the young infant, you can tell early on whether the baby is a quiet looker who gazes peacefully and calmly, the bubbly type who smiles easily, or the very irritable baby. People with good mood tend to see the patch of blue sky among the rainclouds. They approach the world through a positive lens. The opposite is the serious child who is more observant and quietly thoughtful about new situations. You might feel that it's harder to connect with the quiet baby who is fussier and more irritable.

Seven-day-old Ethan would lie on the changing table, look at his mom, and smile. There are other babies, that if you look at their face, they can't handle it. They don't seem to want to cuddle. You may have had this dream that you would have a cuddly baby that would just mold into your body—one that you couldn't put down. Then you get the baby who does not like to cuddle, that turns away from you, that is sometimes happier being on his changing table kicking his legs than being on your body. It can be a real adjustment for some parents.

TEMPERAMENT TYPES

Doctors Chess and Thomas discovered that most babies seem to have one of three basic styles: easy, slow-to-warm-up, or difficult. Easy babies take things pretty much as they come and seem comfortable most of the time. Slow-to-warm-up babies usually need a little time before they feel at ease in new situations. Difficult babies tend to have a harder time getting comfortable and staying comfortable. You might find that you have the best baby in the world or an infant that seems very challenging. If your newborn is content and easy, take credit. If he is difficult and fussy, rest assured that it is not your fault. While the causes of these personality differences are up for debate, it is believed that heredity, as well as experiences in the womb and throughout birth, influence temperament (Barnard & Thomas, 2014).

While it may seem unsavory to place such labels on innocent children who have yet to express themselves, it is important to recognize your baby's general personality traits early on because the cues, adaptability, transition from one state to another, and maternal response required for an easy baby are different than what is needed for a difficult baby. If you recognize your baby's style, you can work out a mutually satisfactory compromise between his own needs and your perception of the baby's needs. Watch your infant and ask yourself, "how does my baby respond to his environment? Is he easy, slow-to-warm-up, or difficult?"

Easy Babies

Easy babies appear to be born more organized than other types and have excellent self-consoling skills. For example, the easy baby wakes up, and if her hands are free, she brings them up to her mouth, looks around, and maybe goes back to sleep. The easy one fusses infrequently and is easily soothed. Easy babies seem to handle anything and have a long attention span. They can shut out stimulation, perhaps by sleeping more rather than crying, and adapt well to new experiences. The easy baby can handle lots of activity and visitors in the home. About 3 months from now, you might hear from another mom who has a baby sleeping through the night (lucky lady). You can bet she has an easy baby.

Sometimes a baby can be so good, parents will say, "We hardly know he's around." This can be a mixed blessing for the whole family. Easy newborns are subtle and will give you very mild signals—cues that they have a need. If you fail to notice what they are communicating, they will probably go to sleep. These babies are sometimes so easy that parents fail to feed them frequently enough, resulting in slow weight gain. They assume that if the baby doesn't fuss, he must not be hungry. Other mothers interpret the easy baby's calm and quiet approach to life as a rejection. They expected to be needed more, and without these demands, they may feel less valuable as a mother. When a baby is so undemanding, the mother may spend less time bonding and relating to the baby as she should. The busy parent is particularly at risk for under-stimulating the easy baby. If you have an easy baby, don't let his politeness cause you to ignore his real need for interaction, attention, and love.

Slow-to-Warm-Up Babies

Slow-to-warm-up babies gradually adapt to new situations if they are handled sensitively. Unrealistic social expectations and inappropriate environments can be harmful to the shy child with this trait. He isn't going to feel good about himself if he is forced to do every event the family wants to do. If, instead, the baby is given time to adjust to things and is introduced to new experiences slowly and at his own pace, he may be more confident and adventurous long-term with better self-esteem. This baby can possibly overcome his shyness and slowness-to-warm-up.

Andrea experienced this with her son. She said, "He was very shy and attached to me. He lacked interest in getting out and having new experiences. I recognized very quickly his temperament traits. So, rather than forcing him, I gave him time to adapt, brought in a familiar friend to ease transitions to new experiences, and let him make it his idea. If I had pushed him, it might have hurt him long-term. Instead, I had the shyest baby who later turned into the social chairman of his college fraternity." If you identify your child as slow-to-warm-up, it is best not to be too concerned about how long it takes him to change his schedule or begin eating solid foods. And when he gets older, don't pressure him to go into the water at a beach or pool. At the playground, the child may be content to sit and watch.

Difficult/High-Needs Babies

Difficult infants are very clear and fast to react. They communicate with potent cues and quickly start loud crying when in need. For example, the fussy baby wakes up and immediately screams. Difficult babies are not easily soothed. They can be intense, impatient, and highly irritable. They seem to have a short attention span. These little personalities cannot shut out the bothersome and normal lights and sounds of daily activities. Consequently, they may respond by getting stuck in a crying state. Difficult babies are often the ones who experience colic. If your baby appears this way, before deciding that he is just difficult, inform your baby's health provider so that any physical or health reasons can be ruled out. You must realize that you are not responsible for your baby's temperament and you are not alone. Many babies are difficult. Be prepared for endless crying and unpredictable meal and nap times. Keeping a sleep/wake scale is very helpful with this type of baby. Keep track of his schedule and then see if you can anticipate his feeding time and try to help him sleep before he is so tired that he can't sleep.

Difficult babies require extra care and attentiveness. A mother may have to adjust her plans to manage the demands with less frustration. For example, if you see that when you undress your baby, he goes ballistic, you may need to postpone the bath. But if you must bathe him, clean one limb at a time or give him a sponge bath until he is ready to be submerged in water. Avoid forcing activities. Realize that your high-needs child is particularly vulnerable and requires protection from the minor stresses of daily life. Restrict visitors or introduce them one at a time. If you see that when the baby goes from the arms of one relative to another, he sleeps all day long but then he is awake all night and fussing, it should tell you that your baby cannot handle being passed around. The difficult baby should not be kept in the living room all day, where there are all sorts of bright lights and loud sounds. Instead, this infant should be taken into a dark, quiet room for naps. A white noise machine that amplifies the soothing sounds of static, ocean waves, or running water can help relax the disorganization he may feel.

The best way you can help your difficult baby is to be flexible in your responses to his needs and to keep the stress he feels to the lowest levels possible. By the end of the first year, he will probably respond more consistently and predictably. Also, it's very important to elicit the help of relatives, friends, and trusted babysitters so you can have breaks from this labor-intensive baby. Many a mother have confessed that if only they had help during this difficult, early time, they would have coped better.

GOODNESS OF FIT

Temperament matters because of the concept of "goodness of fit," which is the compatibility between the baby's temperament and environment (Thomas & Chess, 1977). When there is goodness of fit, children are more likely to reach their potential and feel good about themselves. A poor fit happens when the child's temperament is not respected, and parents try to change it rather than adapt the environment. Difficult infants can influence their mother's psychological state, causing depressed mood and post-partum anxiety to emerge early on (Britton, 2011). Interventions to improve the goodness of fit, beginning with understanding temperament, can help you reduce stress on your relationship (Britton, 2011). This method can also help you with your partner, siblings, parents, colleagues, and other children.

There are effects for babies that do not have goodness of fit with their caretakers. If the parents' idea of how the baby should be differs from how the baby is, this can lead to poor expectations and non-acceptance that can set the baby up for long-term self-esteem issues, which can impact his success. Parents must recognize that these temperament traits are not purposeful and cannot be changed in the short-term. What can happen, however, is you can adapt to each other. This adjustment may require some time.

First, you, as parents, need to analyze and identify what your own temperament is like. Do a little assessment using the Infant Toddler Temperament Tool (IT3) found online at the Center for Early Childhood Mental Health Consultation, funded by the government Office of Head Start (https://www.ecmhc.org/temperament/). There, you can conduct the short survey, which will help you recognize your traits and similarities to your baby. Most importantly, you might recognize how you are different. These are the areas that may prove to be challenging.

You may need to consider making adaptations to how you parent this baby based on what you have learned. For example, if you have an active baby and your temperament puts you at the low activity level, you'll need to find activities that suit your need to be sedentary and his need to be stimulated. Sitting on the sofa with your baby on your lap while you wiggle his arms and legs would make a suitable and satisfactory activity for the both of you at playtime. You could also lay on the floor with your baby while he gets activity doing tummy time.

TAILORING YOUR CARE: SENSIBILITIES FOR SENSITIVITIES

Each of your baby's activities, everything from eating to sleeping, are affected by the stimuli in his environment. Stimuli is what helps babies maintain their level of awareness (state). Take the time to get to know your baby. Ask yourself, how does my baby respond to the stimuli in his surroundings, including visitors, activities, touch, noise, and light. The answers will help you determine how the environment affects your new baby. The results may also tell you that perhaps you need to make changes, so you can better meet your infant's needs.

For example, nurses noted that newborn Jack went from "0 to 60 in 3 seconds" as he wailed during every diaper change. They immediately labeled him an active, difficult baby. But his mother, Lindsey, realized that her baby was just not yet mature enough to have his arms and legs free and his body exposed to air. She tuned into his need and began swaddling him much of the time during his first 2 weeks. She used a white noise machine to help soothe him during diaper changes, when his limbs were free, and used warm wipes to ease the skin sensitivity. Also, unconventionally keeping his arms swaddled during nursing helped breastfeeding get off on the right start. Since all babies are unique, a different baby might like to have himself free and prefer to kick or use his hands to reach a state of calm.

Now that you are beginning to recognize your baby's characteristics, you can understand how his temperament affects the dynamics of your daily experiences with breastfeeding, sleeping, and interacting. You can begin to tailor your care so you can accomplish the first major step in supporting your baby's emotional development. According to research of the human emotional experience by Dr. Greenspan, by tailoring your care, you can help develop the baby's capacity for self-regulation and interest in the world to lengthen and increase the frequency of alert periods. It also creates an emotionally supportive environment that is needed for this growth. Through these positive experiences, you can essentially teach babies what it is like to be calm or engaged so that they can eventually begin developing ways to get there on their own through associations they learn through you. The more parents understand what their infant needs to help him stay awake, and not cry or sleep too much, the sooner he will become the settled baby that can communicate and trust that "my mom and dad are trying to figure out what I need." After all, the baby is trying to figure it out too.

In *What Babies Want*, Debby Takikawa, D.C. and Carrie Contey, PhD explain how babies rely on their caregivers to give them cues about their surrounding environment, including the way in which they should form relationships with other members of the family. They write, "The effect of the environment and the care your baby receives is the nurture aspect of life. This part of her development helps her formulate her ability to express her inner nature" (Takikawa & Contey, 2010, p. 45). We hope you've gained a few ideas and a greater understanding of who your baby is and how he needs to be nurtured so that you can support his rapid development and blossoming personality.

PART IV

Dazed and Confused: Preventing Premature Weaning

. . . .

CHAPTER ELEVEN

The Need to Supplement: Determining When, What, and How

Chapter Goal: Be able to weigh whether supplementation is absolutely necessary or a matter of choice to fulfill a temporary need. Learn what steps to take.

WHEN THE NEED ARISES

Erika was devastated when she was told she needed to feed her baby something other than her breastmilk. Before birth, she was determined to breastfeed and believed nothing would stand in her way. But once she had baby Dublin in her arms, the mother found herself wondering how she could possibly deny medical advice that would deprive her newborn of getting the nourishment she needed.

"I felt like I failed as a mom," Erika said. "Nobody prepared me for this—the fact that I might not be able to breastfeed. As a mother, your instinct is that you just want to provide." Erika experienced postpartum hemorrhage, following a long labor. This delayed her milk coming in. She was physically exhausted and mentally fatigued. She said, "I remember telling the nurse I just don't feel like myself. The nurse said, 'you just lost over a third of your blood. You are not going to feel normal for a while.'"

From the start, Erika and Dublin had challenges breastfeeding. They tried numerous supplementation methods, including spoon and dropper-feeding colostrum, formula supplementation at the breast with a feeding tube (SNS), and bottle-feeding. Erika didn't give up. Instead, she put Dublin to the breast every time the baby signaled her hunger, then followed by supplementing and pumping. After about 2 weeks of this routine, every 2 hours around the clock with very little milk expressed, Erika went in for blood tests. The clinician looked at the results and informed Erika that "her milk was just not going to come in." Family members advised her to stop trying, fearing that she would exhaust herself to the point of no recovery.

Considering her risk factors for insufficient milk supply, the stats were not in her favor. But Erika didn't want to be a textbook case of failed lactation due to severe anemia from postpartum hemorrhage. She wanted a story of perseverance, and with Dublin, they would win their first mother/daughter challenge together. They went to Growing with Baby and concurrently worked with an acupuncturist. For several days, Erika sipped an organic chicken bone broth with lemon, garlic, and ginger prescribed by the acupuncturist to help replenish her body, following major blood loss. She had acupuncture and saw Andrea for lactation consults to monitor her progress. Erika continued to stimulate the breasts every 2 hours with breastfeeding and pumping, even if the milk wasn't there. Meanwhile, she made sure Dublin received the nutrition that she needed. "I felt defeated and discouraged, but I didn't give up," Erika said. "I knew I was going to take on the job of trying to get my milk to come in."

With skilled lactation help, family support, and determination, Erika overcame what seemed impossible. About 3 weeks after giving birth, her milk did come in—late but not never. Because she breastfed regularly, Dublin knew what to do when the milk finally arrived. "I always started with Dublin at the breast, and she would get frustrated, and I would get frustrated, but we just kept trying," Erika said. "I told her, we are a team. We are in this together. And we did it together." She went on supplementing her nursing until, with regular test weights, she grew confident that Dublin's needs were being met through breastfeeding. "I would not want to look back and have it any other way," Erika said. "Even the struggle in the beginning—that's all a part of our story—Dublin and I, building our bond, and my start with motherhood."

THE LEARNING CURVE

Ideally, every breastfed baby would start out obtaining all his nourishment from his mother's breast. Once breastfeeding is well-established, and both mother and baby are confident with nursing, the parents could then willingly choose to give an occasional bottle of expressed breastmilk. Unfortunately, reality happens. When life is not picture perfect, the first rule is to feed the baby. That may mean supplementation. Supplementation seems to be a part of the breastfeeding experience for countless mothers, who use it to fill a temporary need. When the hospital's lactation consultant rolls in a mechanical breast pump and suggests you get to pumping, it is not the end-all. Even if you feel discouraged by it, don't be derailed. Plenty of mothers have taken this short detour before getting back on track with breastfeeding and ultimately meeting their long-term goals. Even in normal cases, activation of milk making cells and development of the milk supply continues for several weeks until it settles between 40 and 60 days (Allen et al., 1991). So, there is a grace period.

There are few new jobs that anybody takes on that require less than 6 weeks to master. This is called a learning curve. In the workplace, you realize you are past it when you suddenly have a sense of confidence as you go about your duties faster and with ease. Recognize that you are learning under very stressful circumstances: no sleep, new roles, and new boundaries in your home. Meanwhile, you are worried about your baby's well-being. This, combined with feedback from relatives and friends who project an attitude like "it worked fine for me so why are you struggling?" can make it even more challenging. Give yourself these first 10 weeks to figure it out while your milk supply develops and your baby settles.

WHEN TO SUPPLEMENT: DETERMINING NECESSITY

Be aware that there are certain times when you will be told to supplement and it may not be necessary. Sometimes, busy medical professionals who are worried about time and the safety of the baby may be biased toward giving a bottle because it is easier than troubleshooting breastfeeding mechanics. This is magnified by a knowledge deficit among health professionals about breastfeeding and how to resolve attachment challenges. Research shows that medical personnel often interfere with breastfeeding and supplement healthy breastfed babies with formula as common practice when mothers are tired after childbirth (Gagnon et al., 2005).

While formula might be the easy way out, if it is not necessary, it can do more harm than good (see Formula: The Great Debate ahead). For one, mothers who supplement their newborn with formula are less likely to stimulate a full milk supply and meet minimum breastfeeding recommendations (Perrine et al., 2012). The culture of where you birth will affect many of the practices that either support or hinder breastfeeding. For example, if you give birth at a hospital where breastfeeding rates are low, and formula-feeding is high, the staff is more likely to encourage you to supplement when your baby records even a normal weight loss. If your medical facility has a Baby-Friendly designation, have peace of mind that the staff is trained to give breastfeeding the benefit of the doubt before considering supplementation.

Poor Reasons to Supplement

Many new mothers lose confidence right off the bat with breastfeeding when they learn that their baby has lost weight. Understand that weight loss is the result of a normal physiological process after birth when the baby starts excreting and shedding the extra fluid absorbed from the placenta (Zangen et al., 2001). Breastfed babies lose more weight at first compared to formula-fed newborns and sometimes take longer to regain their weight (MacDonald et al., 2003). According to the Academy of Breastfeeding Medicine, most breastfed newborns should not require supplementation for normal weight loss (Kellams et al., 2017). Normal weight loss for exclusively breastfed babies is 5.5 to 6.6% of their birthweight (ABM, 2009). They typically return to their birth weight by the 8th day (MacDonald et al., 2003). If the baby is approaching the 5th day of life, has not started to gain weight, and is still showing a weight loss of 7% or more compared to the birthweight, he needs to be closely monitored until weight gain is well-established (Evans et al., 2014). Although some healthy babies do take longer to get back to birthweight, be aware that if your infant has reached the 10th day of life and hasn't returned to birthweight, it is an indication that medical and breastfeeding evaluations should be initiated along with a feeding plan.

During the first few days of your baby's life, insufficient breast-milk is not a valid reason to supplement. The breasts typically contain only small amounts of colostrum—just enough for the newborn's tiny stomach. At first, breastfeeding is less about fulfilling nutritional needs than it is about immunity-building through colostrum transfer, infant state regulation, and learning to coordinate the suck, swallow, and breathe rhythm. Early frequent feeds are essentially placing the order for milk, which, when it comes in, is usually more than the baby needs.

The most common time a baby is supplemented for the first time is at night, when the mother is exhausted (Gagnon et al., 2005). New parents often become nervous when they are unable to settle their newborn and start thinking that the free formula sample in the cupboard will rescue them. Fussiness often means that the infant needs more time skin-to-skin with his mother to regulate to a calm state. The baby may need to be swaddled while you try other calming techniques. Young infants also have periods where they "cluster feed," needing back-to-back breastfeeds several times an hour. Keeping your baby on your bare chest and allowing him to suckle as needed can help satisfy this need until he falls asleep. If the fussiness does not improve after this course of care, have the baby evaluated. Some infants are born with injuries and have pain from being wedged in the birth canal too long during difficult deliveries.

If you are told to supplement with formula, realize that you have options. If your baby is term, not sick, without risk factors, looking active, waking up and trying to feed, and having an adequate output (see diaper output on page 269), then you may be able to wait. In general, healthy babies should be allowed the first 24 hours to get themselves together. Even poor feeding is not a valid reason to supplement the healthy baby during the first 48 hours of life (Powers & Slusser, 1997). If your newborn fits the criteria for a healthy baby and the hospital recommends supplementation, the first thing you do is request to see a skilled consultant to assess you and the infant before, during, and after a breastfeed. The consultant should be able to evaluate adequate milk transfer (swallowing). She may be able to help the baby drink more colostrum by improving your technique. The following checks will help you ascertain the necessity when hospital personnel tells you that you need to supplement:

1.   Have you had a complete assessment by a lactation professional to see whether your baby is nursing well? If not, seek skilled lactation help before supplementing.

2.   Have you been given a hospital-grade pump and told to express your milk without instructions? Some mothers report that the pump is just wheeled in and left at the bedside. Ask for sufficient instructions to use the pump.

3.   Have you been taught how to hand-express your breasts and spoon, dropper, or cup-feed your baby colostrum? If not, request assistance from a lactation consultant.

Are you being told you need to supplement because your baby had a drastic weight loss during his first 24 hours? If so, did you have more than two bags of IV infusion during labor and delivery? Did your baby make many wet diapers the first day of life? Three "yes" answers are reason to dispute the need to supplement (see excessive infant weight loss on page 270).

Valid Reasons for Supplementation

There are valid reasons to supplement using alternative feeding methods that will be discussed ahead, in conjunction with breastfeeding or, in some cases, in lieu of nursing with milk expression. In fact, sometimes pumping and supplementing is the course to building or maintaining a milk supply when the baby is having trouble nursing or still learning how to do his job, particularly for the mother who has risk factors for insufficient milk, or a sick or premature baby. If you think your milk supply is low, be aware that supplementing a bottle of formula without pumping will further decrease your milk supply. In the following cases where supplementation may be necessary, plan to express remaining milk from both breasts after most feedings to build and protect your milk supply.

The Well Baby

A healthy full-term newborn without risk factors may require supplementation of expressed colostrum or breastmilk following breastfeeds because of:

» **Latch Issues:** If after 24 hours, the baby is not successfully nursing.

» **Sleepiness:** If after 24 hours, the baby does not wake up regularly to nurse (see sleepy baby on page 318).

» **Difficulty Calming:** If after 24 hours, the baby cannot calm down enough to organize himself to feed (see difficult to calm on page 317).

» **Severe Weight Loss:** If the baby has lost more than 8 to 10%of his body weight 120 hours after birth or 5 days old (Kellams et al., 2017) (see excessive infant weight loss on page 270).

» **Jaundice:** If you have been informed that the baby has a high bilirubin count and is not actively feeding at the breast (see jaundice on page 323).

» **Not Passing Stool:** If the baby is still having black, tarry (meconium) stools by day five (120 hours old), the baby may not be getting enough to eat if he has fewer than four stools on day four of life (Kellams et al., 2017). This is a strong indication that it will help to pump your breasts after breastfeeding and give the baby the additional expressed milk. Breastmilk is what helps the baby pass the dark stool and changes it to a yellow color and seedy consistency.

The Sick or Premature Baby

Babies who go to special care units, such as the neonatal intensive care, are held to different standards when it comes to supplementation. Their feeding plan is carefully decided by the neonatologist in charge, based on each individual baby's health, needs, and weight-gain goals. Mothers are encouraged to express their milk for the sick or premature baby who requires supplemental feeds. Donor human milk from a designated milk bank is often the next protocol. Supplementation is valid and may be essential for:

» **Prematurity:** The baby who is born premature or late preterm (34 to 36 weeks gestation) may not yet be strong enough to breastfeed. The preemie should be supplemented after an evaluation shows that he is not swallowing at the breast or transferring sufficient milk.

» **Sick Infants:** Babies that are too ill to breastfeed, such as those born with heart disease or metabolism errors (Walker, 2014).

» **Baby with a Congenital Anomaly:** Babies born with congenital anomalies, such as cleft palate, cleft lip, or other physical characteristics that mechanically interfere with the infant's ability to milk the breast.

» **Hypoglycemia:** A baby with low blood sugar may be too lethargic to breastfeed (see Hypoglycemia on page 327). It is appropriate to supplement if hypoglycemia is validated by blood tests conducted before and after feeding, and a skilled professional can document that the baby is not transferring milk at the breast. Hypoglycemia commonly occurs in infants of diabetic mothers who are on insulin.

» **Dehydration:** A baby with dehydration will feed poorly and be very sleepy. Babies who are losing weight and have laboratory evidence of high sodium chloride levels indicated by a blood test need to be supplemented. Meanwhile, a complete breastfeeding assessment should be given, including a test weight to determine milk intake.

Maternal Reasons for Supplementation

You may not be able to breastfeed and may need to supplement due to:

» **Sickness:** You are too sick due to severe illness, such as chickenpox, Lyme disease, sepsis, psychosis, eclampsia, postpartum hemorrhage, Sheehan syndrome, retained placenta, or shock (Walker, 2014). In the United States, if the mother has active chickenpox at birth, it is recommended that she and the baby are separated until she is not contagious anymore.

» **Serious Disease:** If you are infected with HIV (U.S. protocol), untreated Tuberculosis, or herpes simplex virus type 1, where there are lesions on the breast (Walker, 2014).

» **Weakness:** You are too weakened by circumstances that put you in the ICU, such as severe postpartum hemorrhage, postpartum infection, sepsis, pulmonary hypertension, or HELLP syndrome.

» **Drugs or Medications:** Supplement if you have certain medications or street drugs in your system that would make breastfeeding dangerous for the baby.

» **Separation:** For example, if the baby is transferred to a neo- natal intensive care unit at another hospital. Express your milk regularly during separation.

» **Delayed Onset of Copious Milk Supply:** Supplement if your milk has not come in after 3 to 5 days since birth and there are signs that your baby is not getting enough to eat. Pump after each nursing to stimulate the breasts and create demand for the milk to come in.

» **Pain:** If anything causes you pain so severe that you need time to recover, such as bleeding nipples, you may need to temporarily stop breastfeeding until pain subsides. With a clinical-grade double-electric pump, express both breasts for every feed you replace.

» **Breast Surgery:** Supplementation may be necessary if prior breast surgery or procedures have interfered with the normal production of milk. Breast reduction surgery could result in low milk production if a large volume of glandular tissue was removed and milk ducts were severed. Nerve damage from surgery could inhibit the milk-ejection reflex (Geddes, 2007).

» **Hypoplastic Breasts:** If you have a lack of breast development indicated by no breast growth during pregnancy and no breast growth after 3 days postpartum, you may need to supplement.

» **Adoptive Nursing:** Supplementation with at-the-breast tube-feeding while the mother is trying to induce lactation may be a long-term way of breastfeeding.

» **Re-lactation:** Women who wean and decide to re-lactate may need to supplement.

Once you have confirmed medical necessity to supplement any of your infant's feeds, know that you have options so you can make an informed decision as to what is right for you.

WHAT TO SUPPLEMENT

Ideally, every baby that needs to be supplemented on day one would receive the mother's hand-expressed colostrum. After that, the mother who is separated from her baby would start pumping 8 to 10 times a day and supplement with her breastmilk. If this is not possible, the second-best case scenario is to give donor human milk by a doctor's prescription and safely supplied by the hospital. The last resort would be to offer a formula that you and your health provider agree upon. Hospital personnel sometimes supplement newborns with water or glucose water. This should be avoided because it can put the baby at risk of increased bilirubin (jaundice), excess weight loss, and possible water intoxication (ABM, 2009).

Breastmilk

Human milk is the gold standard for human babies. It is a living food, special for its many nutrients, antioxidant, antibacterial, prebiotic, probiotic, and immune-boosting properties (Eglash et al., 2017). The amount of milk you give your baby will depend upon how many days old he is and your baby's hunger/feeding cues. The jury is still out on how much the newborn should be fed at each supplemented breastfeed. Note that infants who are fed formula take in larger volumes than breastfed babies, but the consensus is they are often overfed (Owen et al., 2005). The nearby chart from the Academy of Breastfeeding Medicine shows the average reported intakes of colostrum for healthy breastfed babies.

TABLE 11.1: Average Reported Colostrum Intakes. Source: The Academy of Breastfeeding Medicine (Kellams et al., 2017).

Time Since Birth	Volume per Feed
1 to 24 hours	2 - 10 ml
24 to 48 hours	5 - 15 ml
48 to 72 hours	15 - 30 ml
72 to 96 hours	30 - 60 ml

Donor Milk

The next best thing to your own milk is another woman's breastmilk. In terms of the main contents and nutritional benefits, human milk does not vary too much from mother to mother. What matters most is that the milk is safe. Only feed donor milk from a qualified milk bank under the direction of your hospital or practitioner. Milk banks treat donor breastmilk and screen for serious infections, such as HIV and hepatitis, to make sure it is safe for babies. There is a growing trend to obtain donor milk through online communities, such as Craigslist. This can be dangerous and we don't recommend it. There is no guarantee that the milk was stored or handled properly. It can have unsafe levels of bacteria. Even if the donor woman does not have an infectious disease, alcohol, drugs, and certain medications can jeopardize the safety of it. Recipients of donor milk received through informal communities have reported that the milk they were given was watered down, presumably to top off or reach a desired amount.

Formula: The Great Debate

When breastmilk is not an option, formula is likely the easiest solution for parents who plan to bottle-feed long-term. For those who want their baby breastfed, however, the decision to supplement with formula should not be taken lightly because even one bottle dissolves some of the health benefits that an exclusively breastfed baby receives. Renowned author Marsha Walker, RN, IBCLC, presents what formula supplementation does to the gut of the breastfed baby. She summarizes that just one supplemented bottle of formula every 24 hours can raise the infant's gut pH and change the flora so much that it no longer resembles that of a breastfed baby (Bullen et al., 1977; Walker, 2014). It takes 2 to 4 weeks of exclusive breast-feeding for the intestinal environment to return to a "normal" state (Brown et al., 1922). Because the gut is more open and penetrable, it can allow big proteins in. The exposure to formula early on puts the baby at risk of forming allergies (Saarinen et al., 1999). Infant intake of formula changes the balance of friendly bacteria (see the infant microbiome on page 37), potentially increasing the risk of inflammation and lifelong disease (Di Mauro et al., 2013). When possible, formula should not be given before gut closure occurs around 6 months past birth (Walker, 2014).

Formulas differ in their macronutrients and micronutrients, such as long-chain polyunsaturated fatty acids, nucleotides, and oligosaccharides (Eshach et al., 2004). Because formula does affect infant health, consult your doctor for a recommendation. The Academy of Breastfeeding Medicine recommends a protein hydrolysate formula, such as Enfamil Nutramigen or Similac Alimentum, instead of a standard artificial milk for the newborn to avoid early exposure to cow's milk proteins. Early introduction to cow's milk protein can damage the baby's gut mucosal barrier and lead to inflammation (Savilahti et al., 1993). Cow's milk-based formulas given to the young infant can also increase the child's risk of developing type 1 diabetes during the first 5 years of life (Holmberg et al., 2007).

Most parents are unaware that formula is basically modified cow's milk with the contents specific for the growth of very large animals. Protein hydrolysate formula, such as Nutramigen, contains proteins that have been broken down (hydrolyzed) into smaller particles than those in cow's milk and soy-based formulas. For the baby who is being supplemented due to jaundice, a protein hydrolysate formula is known to reduce bilirubin levels effectively (ABM, 2009). Soy milk-based formulas pose risks and nutritional disadvantages to young infants, so they are not recommended during the first 6 months of life (Nevo et al., 2007).

Confusing infant fussiness and unsettled behaviors commonly lead to a formula switch. In one study, 47% of the babies had their formula changed (Nevo et al., 2007). The most common reasons for switching were regurgitation, vomiting, and restlessness. These are some of the same confusing behaviors that lead nursing mothers to give up breastfeeding. Researchers conclude that parents perceive common infantile symptoms and behavior patterns as formula intolerance. In other words, parents switch because they believe the formula does not agree with the baby's digestive system. Researchers were surprised that most parents switched to another cow's milk-based product (Nevo et al., 2007). This showed a lack of understanding.

Formula-Feeding Safety

If you choose to give your newborn formula, avoid the powdered form during the first 2 months because it is not sterile and can put the baby at risk of getting a bacterial sickness called Cronobacter infection (CDC, 2011). According to the Centers for Disease Control and Prevention, the illness is rare, but it can cause severe blood infections or meningitis, and may result in death (CDC, 2011). Cronobacter is a group of bacteria that are naturally found in the environment, so it is very difficult to prevent contamination. Symptoms of the disease are fever, poor feeding, crying, and listlessness.

Offer ready-made formula, sold in the liquid form, until the baby is older than 2 months, when the risk of developing infection is less likely. If your baby is premature or has a weakened immune system, continue to use only the ready-made liquid form. When using powdered formula for the older baby, close formula containers as soon as possible after opening and take care about being sanitary when setting down scoops and lids. Don't put the scoop back in the can. Mix the powder with water that is at least 158 degrees F. To mix the formula, shake rather than stir. After heating formula, you'll need to cool it in an ice bath. Don't let the nipple touch the ice water. To make sure the temperature is suitable for the baby, squirt a few drops onto your wrist. The formula is fresh for 2 hours. The unused amount should be disposed of after the feed. If you prepare formula and immediately refrigerate it for later use, it is good for 24 hours.

HOW: YOU'VE GOT OPTIONS

Since the quantity of milk needed the first few days is relatively small, you have many options for feeding your newborn, including a supplemental nursing device at the breast (if the baby can nurse), finger-feeding, and bottle, cup, spoon, or dropper-feeding. Each has its benefits and disadvantages. The method most protective of breastfeeding is a supplementer-at-the-breast. Your final decision will have to do with your individual situation, your infant's health, and the anticipated duration for supplemental feeds. Don't be afraid to try more than one option.

Supplementer-at-the-Breast

For the baby who can attach to the breast but suckles weakly, a tube feeding device may be beneficial. It prevents nipple confusion and provides the mother and baby with some of the benefits of breast-feeding, including state regulation through skin-to-skin contact. The baby receives milk from a small tube attached to the nipple while simultaneously stimulating the mother's milk producing system. For a woman with delayed milk, this is an ideal choice.

Erika, introduced earlier, described the use of the Medela Supplemental Nutritional System (SNS) as a pivotal moment for her and her baby girl: "I was able to feel what it was like for her to get what she needed nutrient wise," Erika said. "I felt like I was providing it for her. Mentally, I needed that."

A lactation consultant can help you obtain a commercial supplementer-at-the-breast, such as Lact-Aid Nursing Trainer, Medela SNS, or a Supply Line. There are different types of tubing that vary in firmness and negative pressure, required to drain the milk. There are also many other at-the-breast feeding devices, such as a syringe attached to a small feeding tube, or a bottle with a feeding tube where a hole is made in the nipple to access the feeding tube. It takes time to get accustomed to using an at-the-breast device—to feel comfortable with it and be good at it. Like any new skill, the motor skills needed are different. Give yourself a few trials to learn how to use this valuable tool while keeping your long-term goals in mind.

How to Use a Tube Supplementer at the Breast:

1. To keep the supplementer tube from rolling, attach tape along the length of the tube. Experiment with the placement of the tube, either on top of the breast or by the baby's lower lip. Either way, it should extend slightly past the tip of the nipple. Some women prefer to use an adhesive bandage. Regular paper tape is good for sensitive skin.

2. Run the tubing under your bra or top, keeping the milk container at the side of your breast or high enough so the

baby cannot grab it or become entangled. Gravity will affect flow, raising the pouch of milk will increase speed while lowering it will decrease flow.

3. Be sure that the baby does not suck on the tube like a straw by checking that the attachment at the breast is deep enough. If he is not able to drink the milk within 30 minutes, or leaves the breast full, you may need to consider a different method (Genna, 2009). Babies who are not effective in removing milk can become overtired and burn too many calories.

Unfortunately, these at-the-breast supplementation devices can be costly when parts break and are cumbersome to clean (Walker, 2014). Mothers still need to pump after feeds to build and protect their milk supply. Many mothers get very adept at just holding the tube in place until the baby starts nursing. It is easier if the supplementer is cleaned and filled, then refrigerated immediately after use. If you put it on a few minutes before nursing, your body will warm the milk. YouTube has examples of mothers using supplementers. Take the time to learn. It is a valuable tool to reach breastfeeding goals.

Finger-Feeding

For the newborn who requires supplemental feeds and cannot nurse, finger-feeding can help him learn to open his mouth wide and keep the tongue down, forward, and cupped, mimicking oral movements needed to breastfeed (Walker, 2014). For premature babies, finger-feeding is sometimes used to assist the newborn to develop rooting, latching, and sucking patterns, including the coordination of the suck-swallow-breathe rhythm needed to breastfeed. A supplementer-at-the-breast is a better alternative, but finger-feeding may also be used with formula occasionally if you are not able to breastfeed temporarily due to a medication that makes your milk unsafe, cracked nipples, or a health/safety reason, such as testing positive for hepatitis C.

How to Finger-Feed:

1. You'll need a baby bottle, artificial nipple, 36-inch #5 French feeding tubing, a small syringe to clean the feeding tube after each feed, scissors, and tape.

2. Trim and clean the nail of the index finger you plan to use. Wash your hands with soap and water, and dry with a clean towel.

3. Working on a clean surface, prepare the supplementer. With sterile scissors, widen the hole of the bottle nipple. Thread the narrower part of the tube through the hole.

4. Add your breastmilk, close the bottle, then push the tube until the wide end rests at the bottom.

5. Hold the baby in a cross-cradle position.

6. Tuck the bottle into a shirt pocket or rest it nearby in a place that is level with the baby's head. The position of the bottle affects flow. If too high, the flow may be too fast and cause the baby to choke. A level too low could tire the baby before he finishes the feed.

7. Line up the feeding tube so that it ends at the tip of your index finger. Tape it to the bottom of the finger around the second joint so that the baby does not suck on tape.

8. Place your tube wrapped finger on the baby's lips, nail facing down. Allow your baby to open up and draw it into his mouth, just past the gumline. Keep your finger flat and straight to promote natural breastfeeding positioning (tongue down and jaw forward).

9. The infant will draw milk from the tube. Avoid letting your baby suck on the tube alone.

10. The tube must be cleaned and air-dried after each feed. Fill the syringe with cold water first to flush any residual milk from the tube to prevent milk from curdling and clogging. Then, flush hot water into the larger end of the tube. Do this about five times, followed by two plunges of air to clear remaining water.

Hang dry the tube in a clean space away from the kitchen. A clothespin on a hanger works well.

Finger-feeding allows the baby to be in control and still feel human skin in his mouth. The baby can pace himself, which is better for him. Both Mom and Dad can do it, ideally being cuddled against the parent's bare chest. There are some disadvantages to this feeding method, however. For one, it is only ideal for small amounts. Trying to get 3 ounces into a baby who is finger-feeding can be laborious and time-consuming. It can be mechanically difficult and not very hygienic because it's hard to clean well under the fingernail. The other downside—a finger is not a breast. The finger is firm and does not mold into the baby's mouth like the mother's nipple. Because the finger is inserted into the baby's mouth, he does not develop the skill to draw the nipple in. Consider your baby's ability and weigh the benefits vs. disadvantages.

Bottle-Feeding

When a baby requires supplementation, a bottle may seem like the obvious choice for its fast flow and place as a cultural standard. However, if you are determined to meet your breastfeeding goals, consider the evidence carefully because supplementation with a bottle can interfere with exclusive breastfeeding. Some babies can transition easily from the breast to the bottle and back, but others have difficulty with it. It's unclear why. What we do know is there is not one bottle on the market that makes the newborn's mouth work the same way as it does on the breast. As a result, bottle-feeding changes the muscle function in the mouth, tongue, and jaw, which can lead to trouble transitioning back to the breast (Ferrante et al., 2006). Many babies are not able to develop the skills and strength needed to breastfeed when they get accustomed to the bottle, including the suck-swallow-breathe cycle (Goldfield et al., 2006). With bottle-feeding, there is the risk of obstructed breathing, apnea, bradycardia, and lower vagal tone (Walker, 2014). Babies who are not used to the fast flow risk aspiration (Wilson-Clay & Hoover, 2008). Overall, bottle-feeding results in higher heart rate and lower blood-oxygen levels (Marinelli et al., 2001).

Bottle-fed babies become accustomed to a firmer object in their mouth, making them reject the soft breast. Artificial nipples can cause the infant to become nipple-confused. When switching back to the breast, he might also expect a fast and immediate flow. He may become frustrated, sucking with no milk, and find it difficult to wait for a let-down. Artificial nipples can cause gagging, and the fast flow of the bottle can lead to choking. Newborns who are bottle-fed formula often take in more milk than they need, causing overfeeding, which has led to an increased risk of obesity (Owen et al., 2005). Most bottles do not allow the baby to set the pace, so they tend to overeat to meet their sucking needs. This stretches the stomach. A mother whose milk supply is still developing may be challenged to meet her baby's exaggerated milk demand.

When feed volumes are small, you can avoid the adverse effects of early bottle-feeding by supplementing with an alternate feeding device. If supplementation is long-term for your baby, the benefits of using a bottle likely outweigh the risks. Mothers may find other supplementation devices cumbersome and time consuming for feeding the older baby, who takes larger amounts of milk. Although there is no bottle comparable to a breast, a wide-based bottle, such as Lansinoh, Munchin, Latch, Advent, or Playtex Natural Nipples, in conjunction with paced-feeding, may be less interfering with later breastfeeding.

The Centers for Disease Control and Prevention stresses care-givers take certain steps to bottle-feed safely and protect the baby from infections and dangerous germs. It recommends bottles be prepared with clean hands on clean surfaces. Sterilize bottles in a dishwasher or in boiling water for 5 minutes after washing with hot soapy water. If your baby is full-term, healthy, and your water supply is known to be safe and your plumbing is relatively new (built within the last 10 years), sterilization may not be necessary. Hot water and dish soap, combined with good rinsing and air drying, may be enough, depending on the country you live in.

Pace Bottle-Feeding

Pace bottle-feeding is a technique that can help your baby transition back and forth from breast to bottle because it slows down the flow of milk into the nipple and the mouth, allowing the baby to eat more slowly and take breaks. Paced-feeding reduces the risk of overfeeding. The goal is to mimic your baby's milk flow pattern where there are breaks between sucking bursts. Figuring out your baby's pattern requires a little tracking, which you can do during a normal breastfeed. While your infant nurses, count the number of times you hear him swallow before he takes a pause. Jot down the number of swallows in the nearby chart. This is the first cycle. After the rest, start counting swallows again, beginning at one. Record cycle number two. Continue to count and record until the baby has completed the feed. You'll notice that the number of swallows decreases as you get closer to the end of the feed. You can now bottle-feed at the baby's familiar breastfeeding pace. This teaches him to be an active eater, rather than a passive one, who gets to decide how much milk he needs and how fast (just like breastfeeding).

TABLE 11.2: Let-Down Tracker

Let-Down Cycle	Number of Swallows
1	_____ / Rest
2	_____ / Rest
3	_____ / Rest
4	_____ / Rest
5	_____ / Rest
6	_____ / Rest
7	_____ / Rest
8	_____ / Rest
Continue if there are more	

How to Pace Bottle-Feed:

1. Start with a bottle that has a wide base and slow flow, unless your lactation consultant has determined that another one is better for your baby.

2. Hold your baby in the cradle hold, positioned so that he is semi-reclined and slightly upright with his chin tilted down.

3. With the bottle in your free hand, hold it horizontally and touch the nipple to your baby's lips. Wait for him to open his mouth and draw the nipple in by himself.

4. Once he begins sucking, tip the bottle up slightly, just enough to allow the milk to flow.

5. Listen closely. Once the number of sucks reaches the number of swallows in the first cycle, tilt the bottle down and sit the baby up so that the milk leaves the nipple.

6. Just like breastfeeding where the baby stays latched on, keep the bottle nipple in his mouth while he takes a moment of rest. Soon, he will begin suckling for more.

7. Once he begins again, elevate the bottle so that milk flow returns. Use your cycle record as a guide while you roughly follow your let-down pattern (tilting the milk from the nipple and raising the baby during breaks) until the feed is complete.

If the baby sputters, chokes, or looks overwhelmed, the flow may be too fast. Switch to a slower-flow nipple. You may need a faster-flow nipple if he has to suck more than three times between swallows or pulls on the nipple. Tightening the ring that attaches the nipple to the bottle too tightly will slow the flow. If the baby hasn't breastfed, the feeder sets the pace. Let him suck for 10 continuous swallows, then tip the bottle down to give him a break. When he starts sucking again, repeat the same number of sucks and pauses. As he slows down, try not to push him to finish unless you are worried about poor weight gain. Look for satiation cues.

Cup, Bowl, Spoon, Dropper

If you are worried about nipple preference, consider supplementation by cup, bowl, spoon, or dropper. They are effective and inexpensive tools for feeding breastmilk to the newborn baby who takes only tea-spoons of breastmilk at each feed. These alternative feeding methods are also good tools for occasional supplementation of the preterm infant, and in the case of older baby bottle refusal. Cup feeding may interfere less with learning to breastfeed compared to bottle-feeding (Howard et al., 2003) because it moves the tongue down and forward without altering the function of the mouth and jaw muscles (Walker, 2014). This great way to feed colostrum allows the newborn to pace himself and have successful feeding experiences.

How to Cup or Spoon-Feed:

1. The baby should be awake and alert, hungry but calm.
2. Start with a clean or sterilized plastic medicine cup, shot glass, or small spoon. Fill it three-quarters of the way full of breastmilk.
3. Cradle your baby upright in one arm or on your lap. Support the upper back and neck. Place a cloth under his chin to manage any spillage.
4. Put the cup or spoon up to his mouth, tilted slightly, and just let him lap it like a kitty. Never pour milk because it can cause him to choke and possibly inhale the milk into his lungs.
5. Keep the supplementer held up to his lips throughout the feed because babies who root to the smell of milk or the feeling of hunger might knock the milk and cause spillage.
6. After each feeding, wash the cup or spoon with hot soapy water and dry it completely.

A syringe or eye dropper may be used instead with the same baby-led approach. Cup, spoon, or dropper feedings are useful when the feeds are small (5 to 10 ml) but are not the most efficient to feed larger volumes of milk. These devices do not stimulate the breasts and hamper the development of the mother's milk when feeds are not replaced with milk expression.

· · · · · · · · · · · · · · · ·

CHAPTER TWELVE

Milk Expression: Learning How to Pump and Store Your Milk

*Chapter Goal: Learn a valuable skill
that supports lactation and, at times,
helps overcome breastfeeding difficulties.
Find guidelines for handling and
storing breastmilk safely.*

EXPRESSING BREASTMILK

Learning to express your milk is useful for multiple reasons besides supplementation. For instance, in the case of flat or inverted nipples, a breast pump can evert the nipple enough so the baby has an easier time taking the breast into his mouth. If the breasts are too full when you set out to feed, hand expressing some milk before nursing can make it easier for the baby to latch-on, while hand expressing or pumping afterwards makes the breast softer and relieves discomfort.

If you plan to return to work or school, pumping and storing some milk in the freezer ahead of time will give you confidence and a sense of security in anticipation of the upcoming separation. If your baby only takes one breast at a feed, pumping the other breast several times daily is one way to collect milk. If the baby always requires both breasts at a feed, pumping after nursing during your most productive times of the day is one way to collect extra milk. If you are not planning to return to work, take care not to pump too often, as it can lead to overproduction. Limit pumping to after feeds, when your breasts feel the fullest or after any long intervals when the baby finishes nursing. Once you return to work or school, you'll need to pump for every breastfeed that you miss or any time that you feel too full or engorged. For some mothers, pumping takes longer because they let down less milk compared to when they breastfeed. Mothers and babies who don't do well with this arrangement (i.e., bottle refusal), but have no choice, tend to breastfeed a lot more when they reunite, to make up for the separation and missed feeds. They nourish and comfort each other on an alternate schedule and seem to adapt to their circumstances.

In the past, there was a pediatrician who wrote a book on how to nurse at night and skip day feeds. She didn't want her baby to bottle-feed while she was away at work, so they found a way to compensate. Even if you do not plan to return to work or school, having expressed milk in the freezer can give you peace of mind in case of unanticipated separation from your baby or a need to temporarily stop breastfeeding.

Be aware that the amount of milk you occasionally express with a pump is not always a representation of how much milk your body is producing. The intimate connection between you and your baby is largely responsible for stimulating oxytocin, which then targets your milk cells to empty the milk. The rhythm of your baby's sucking elicits multiple milk releases. At first, you may only collect a small amount of milk. Your body needs time to adjust to a "mechanical baby."

If you are pumping without separation, keep your baby close or even skin-to-skin. Pumping one breast while breastfeeding on the other is likely to yield a good amount of milk. When your baby isn't close, some ways to promote milk flow are darkening the lights, finding a private place, looking at a photograph or video of your baby, massaging the breasts, starting with hand expression, applying warm washcloths to the breasts, sipping a cup of hot tea, and/or smelling your baby's blanket. Making pumping less mechanical and more right-brained (emotional) will help you relax and stimulate the hormones that help release the milk.

There are many options available for milk expression from the lowest tech (hand expression) to electrical pumps. You may wind up using hand expression sometimes, but if you are separated from your baby for illness or special care (i.e., NICU stays), most lactation consultants find a clinical electric pump that pumps both breasts simultaneously is optimal to bring in milk and maintain the supply. Familiarizing yourself with some basic techniques can help you get over the awkwardness you might feel when expressing milk for the first time.

Hand Expression

Hand expression is a good skill to learn and is always available. You don't have to wash a bunch of parts and it can also help stimulate a let-down quicker. For the babies struggling to take the breast, the rapid reward of a quick milk flow often entices them to breastfeed. If you are hand-expressing to treat a plugged duct, placing your thumb above the affected area and gently pressing can help loosen the blockage. If you are not needing to save and store the milk, but merely seeking to relieve discomfort or prepare the breasts for a feed, you can hand express in the shower or while leaning over a sink. If you plan to feed the milk to your baby, wash your hands first and use a clean collection container. The breasts and nipples do not require cleaning prior to milk expression (Pittard, 1991). Find a container with a wide mouth. For colostrum collection, a tablespoon works well.

Steps for Hand Expression

1. Start by preparing your breasts and let-down reflex with a gentle massage. Express one breast at a time. Place a hand at your chest and gently rub toward the nipple. Then, make little circles with three fingers as you work your way around the breast, getting closer to the nipple. Some mothers find it helpful to shake the breast or brush it with their fingertips.

2. Now it's time to attempt to milk the breast in a way that mimics how a newborn stimulates the ducts. Work with one breast

at a time, using your right hand for your right breast or your left hand for your left breast. Cup the breast with your hand and fingers resting under the areola and your thumb above it. The forefinger and thumb should make a C-shape, each placed about an inch from the nipple.

3. Push back toward your chest wall. Do this several times while looking for drops of milk to appear at the nipple tip. If you don't see milk after several attempts, move your hand further back, repeating the compression until you find the right spot on the breast that releases milk. Once you find your milk release spot, you can begin the following: (1) push into the chest wall; (2) pinch the fingers together without sliding; (3) gently pull forward. When you are in the right spot, milk will spray.

4. Find your rhythm: push, pinch, pull. Once you know how far you need to be away from the nipple, you can rotate your hand and repeat the press/release pattern, compressing ducts around the breast. Be gentle. It should not be painful. Signs of incorrect technique are bruising and skin irritation.

5. If you need to express a predetermined amount to supplement your baby (rather than merely trying to relieve engorgement or prime the breasts for a feed), switch breasts as soon as the sprays slow. Switch side-to-side each time the milk slows until both breasts are softened.

Electrical Pump

There are three main parts to any breast pump: the breast shield (flange) that covers the nipple and areola during expression, a component that creates suction, and one or two containers to collect the milk. There are many brands and types of pumps on the market. The most effective way to extract milk in lieu of a vigorous, hungry newborn is with a double-electric breast pump. Mothers report higher milk yields from clinical-grade pumps than consumer pumps sold at retail stores (Hill et al., 1999; Hopkinson et al., 1988). A baby sucks at 240 mm Hg negative of pressure. Many consumer-grade pumps put out only about 200 mm Hg negative of pressure. Mothers generally need about 200 to 230 mm Hg negative pressure from a pump that cycles about 40 to 60 times per minute (Alekseev et al., 2000) to mimic how a newborn feeds. Models like the Ameda SMB or Medela Classic have some of the highest pressures.

If you are not able to rely on your baby to bring in your milk, a multiuser clinical grade pump is highly recommended to help you establish a generous supply. A lactation consultant will be able to help you decide which pump is best for you, fit the flange to your breast, and may even offer a rental service or suggest a nearby hospital or WIC clinic (see appendix). If possible, pump both breasts at the same time. This stimulation often produces numerous let-downs and saves time. For some mothers, it may be easier to pump one breast at a time. In this case, switch breasts when the milk flow stops. After the second breast stops releasing milk, you can switch back to the first for potentially more let-downs.

Research shows that when expressing milk at the maximum comfortable vacuum, there is a higher rate of milk flow with the first let-down. But after about 15 minutes of pumping, the cream content of the milk is at its highest (Kent et al., 2008). Note: Some mothers need the highest vacuum, while others do better with less pressure. Some mothers report their milk stops after 10 to 15 minutes. Others need 45 to 60 minutes to complete an adequate milk expression. Read your instructions thoroughly to find out how your pump operates. A good pump has different vacuum settings and speeds that mimic the newborn's feeding pattern. Some have a button to push, and others have a dial. Be aware that some pumps will shut off after 30 minutes to prevent overheating.

Adjust the speed in a way that mimics your baby's nursing rhythm. When the milk flows, slow down. A baby's non-nutritive sucking is about two sucks per second (Medela, 2015).

Using an Electric Breast Pump

1. First, turn your suction up to the highest you can tolerate until you see milk start to spray. If your breast pump has a let-down or initiation mode, start there.

2. As soon as the milk flow speeds up or sprays, turn the let-down mode off or slow the speed.

3. When the milk slows down, hit the let-down (initiation) button again or turn up the speed. Keep repeating the cycle until you see just drops of milk for at least 5 minutes.

4. If you don't have a let-down mode, stop and hand express for a minute each time the milk flow slows.

5. Try to relax as your pump does its job. When you no longer see milk flowing, stop the pump. You can either switch breasts or take a break if your goal is quantity. Often, a mother can trigger another stream of milk flow after a few minutes of rest, just like how babies often take a break, then start again.

6. Once you are done using your pump, follow the manufacturer's guidelines for dissembling and sterilizing the parts. Take care that you don't miss a piece that requires separation and cleaning before reusing, or it could lead to bacterial growth. Most rubber membranes need to be taken off and cleaned.

Troubleshooting Discomfort

Female nipples differ in size and elasticity. It's important that your flange fits correctly in order to drain the breasts and prevent discomfort or injury. The breast shield (flange) fits over your nipple and seals to the breast under vacuum pressure. Fortunately, most pumps can accommodate different-sized shields. Start by centering the flange. There should be enough room for the nipple to pull through without touching the sides of the tunnel. If the flange is too small, it will cause friction and lead to sore nipples. A tight flange can also block milk flow, limiting your ability to express milk, increasing the risk of mastitis, plugged ducts, and low milk supply. If your skin is turning blue or white, it means the suction is probably too high.

If you experience burning and stinging after pumping, the diameter of the flange and pressure may not be right for you. Note: Your breasts may change throughout lactation, especially after your milk supply settles. You might need to update your flange.

Some women have nipples that greatly expand as they pump. This can cause pain and irritation. Be sure to turn the pressure way down if you see your nipple start to expand. Stopping and starting the machine will also help. One very important note: the flange should push into your breast enough to seal but not cause pressure, or else the milk flow will stop. It will also cause nipple tenderness. Many women decrease their milk supply by pressing into their body too hard. Lubricating the areolar area with a small amount of nipple cream, olive oil, or coconut oil will decrease friction.

Hand-Operated Pump

If you don't own a pump and find yourself needing one late at night or weekend hours, you can purchase a hand-operated manual pump at a pharmacy. They are typically priced under $50. Most hand pumps rely on your hand strength and energy to squeeze, pump, or compress a handle. There are a few battery versions available. Once you get comfortable, it can be quite effective in expressing breastmilk, especially if you are using it to treat painful plugged ducts or to soften the breasts prior to a feed. Take care not to strain yourself using a hand-operated pump and follow manufacturer instructions.

EXCLUSIVE PUMPING

Some mothers initially rely on exclusive pumping to bring in their milk supply if the baby is not well or mature enough to breastfeed effectively. It does require some discipline, but the benefits are priceless. Keep in mind that this situation is usually temporary. Many new mothers who are faced with exclusive pumping to bring in their milk experience feelings of grief or anger that they are using the "mechanical baby," not their precious newborn. These feelings are normal. If this is your experience, talk to someone who can help you get through it. Before you get started, be sure to have the breast flange fitted.

Breastfeeding authority, Nancy Mohrbacher, IBCLC, FILCA, discusses three stages of milk production and strategies for bringing in a maximum milk supply with exclusive pumping: Stage 1) birth until the milk comes in; Stage 2) a period of milk increasing until full production; and Stage 3) a full production of the milk supply. See the accompanying chart for techniques and goals to achieve a full milk supply without an actively nursing baby.

TABLE 12.1: Strategies for Expressing Milk at Each Stage of Milk Production. Source: Adapted from Mohrbacher, 2016.

Milk Production Stage 1: Birth Until Milk Comes In

Expression Techniques:	Goal:
- Massage the breasts before you pump. - Pump both breasts at the same time until milk-flow stops. - Hand-express at least 6 times a day after the mechanical pump. - Pump 8 to 10 times in 24 hours (schedule the longest stretch of 6 hours from 9 pm to 3 am).	- Express colostrum until you see transitional milk, which is higher in volume and beginning to look like breast milk.

Milk Production Stage 2: Through Day 10 Until Full Production

Expression Techniques:	Goal:
- Massage the breasts before you pump. - Pump both breasts at the same time until milk flow stops. - Add hands on expression, switching from breast to breast until milk ceases to spray. - Pump 8 to 10 times in 24 hours.	- By day 10 postpartum, express 750 mL (25 oz) in 24 hours. - Seek help if you express less than 500 ml (17 oz) in a day.

Milk Production Stage 3: Full Production

Expression Techniques:	Goal:
- Pump 7 times in 24 hours. - Develop a routine for the best times. - Be sure to pump right before bed and then first thing in the morning. If you become engorged during the night, you must pump. - After 1 week, record your 24-hour milk yield.	- By day 10 postpartum, express - 750 ml (25 oz) in 24 hours. - Seek help if you express less than 500 ml (17 oz) in a day.

If after stage 3, you followed the 8 to 10 times a day protocol, and achieved less than 350 ml (11 oz) in 24 hours at 7 to 10 days postpartum, intervention from a skilled lactation professional to increase the milk supply is recommended (Riordan & Wambach, 2016). Once a mother is at her goal milk yield, she can usually decrease the number of pumping sessions to about seven per day, dependent upon how much milk her breasts can hold. Some mothers at this point can sleep 8 hours, then pump 16 ounces in the morning. Others, unfortunately, can never go longer than 4 hours without engorgement that impacts the milk supply. Continue to keep a record of how often you are pumping and your daily yield, aiming for at least 750 ml (24 ounces). Depending on your breastmilk storage capacity, the number of pumping sessions can vary from 5 to 7.

How long you need to pump per session will vary. Some mothers have a very quick let-down and fill two 4-ounce bottles. Others need 45 minutes to fill two 2-ounce bottles. For at least three pumping sessions, pump until your milk barely drips. This will tell you about how many minutes your body needs to fully release the most milk. Mothers who have breasts that can hold larger volumes of milk may be able to pump less often. If you easily feel engorged and, at most, collect 2 ounces per breast when you pump, then you will need to pump more often.

You don't need to space out the pumping sessions evenly, but rather, notice when your breasts start to feel full. Contrary to most practices, fuller breasts (uncomfortably full) make less milk. Be sure to wake to express milk at least once a night (ideally, when you wake up naturally after completing a sleep cycle or need to use the bathroom). Unless you know your breasts can comfortably hold 16 ounces, never go longer than 5 to 6 hours without pumping. Discomfort from fullness or engorgement can lead to breast infections and decreased milk supply, telling you you've waited too long.

Breast massage and stimulation are essential for mothers to bring in a full milk supply without the help of their infant. Dr. Jane Morton studied this technique and found that the mothers who massaged during pumping, then hand expressed when finished, had a milk yield increase of more than 48% compared to the women who didn't (Morton et al., 2009).

When using a hands-free bra or when holding flanges against the breasts, make sure they are not too tight. Pressure against the milk ducts in the areola inhibit milk flow. Many mothers find a commercial pumping bra or an old bra adapted by cutting, then reinforcing holes large enough to fit the shaft of the flange, allows hands-free pumping. You can also make your own hands-free device by intertwining two hair bands, then put one around the shaft of the flange and attach the other to your bra cup hook. While the pump is expressing your milk, using your hands to press any firm areas of the breasts towards the flange will release more milk. Don't forget the bottom and sides. Note: Stress inhibits milk ejection, so seek ways to reduce it as much as possible. Other strategies to increase milk output prior to pumping include applying warm compresses to the breasts and warming the breast shields.

STORING BREASTMILK

Supplementing with milk expressed within the last 24 hours is the ideal choice because it contains the most active antibodies and nutrients. The second-best choice is breastmilk that has been refrigerated for up to 8 days. Before you set out to pump or handle breastmilk, be sure that your hands have been cleaned with soap and water, or hand sanitizer to prevent milk contamination. Breastmilk is a living food. Like all food, it is susceptible to be exposed to viruses and bacteria transmitted through poor hygiene and handling.

In terms of storage containers, glass, steel, and plastic have been studied to determine any changes to the milk during storage. Glass and plastic containers are ideal. They should be strong enough that they do not chip, break, or become punctured. The Academy of Breastfeeding Medicine (Eglash et al., 2017) recommends the following: avoid storage products made with bisphenol A (BPA), which is found in some plastic containers, including baby bottles. Plastic containers should be food grade and not hospital specimen storage containers. Before use, any bottle, nipple, or container you use should be washed in a dishwasher, or with soap and water, and dried completely. When soap is not available, boiling is sufficient.

Do not use chemical disinfectants. Rather than fill up a storage container, prepare small bags or containers of milk with about 15 to 60 ml (1/2 to 2 ounces) each. This will help you prevent waste. If you plan to freeze the milk, leave space at the top (about 1/4 of the container) because the contents will expand during freezing.

Shelf Life: Fresh, Frozen, Refrigerated

Freshly expressed breastmilk can be kept at room temperature (60 to 85°F or 16 to 29°C) and fed within 4 to 6 hours (Eglash et al., 2017). The warmer the temperature, the sooner the milk should be refrigerated. If you have not served the milk by then, it must be stored in the refrigerator or freezer to maintain freshness. Once the milk is refrigerated, it is still safe to serve for 4 days at a maximum temperature of 39.2°F (4°C). If you have a refrigerator that maintains a temperature below 39°F (4°C), the milk will keep for up to 8 days in very clean conditions. Purchase a refrigerator thermometer if you are unsure. If you are expressing milk away from home, such as the workplace, the milk can be kept under ice or ice packs in a cooler at 59°F (15°C) or less for up to 24 hours (Hamosh et al., 1996). Avoid combining fresh warm milk with older cold or frozen milk.

Table 12.2 Guidelines for Storing Milk Safely

Storage Location	Temperature	Maximum Storage Time
Room Temperature	60 - 85 F. (16-29 C.)	4 to 6 hours
Refrigerator	39.2 F. (4 C.) / Less than 39.2 F (4 C.)	4 days / 8 days
Cooler with Ice	59 F. (15 C.) or less	24 hours
Freezer	24.8 F. (-4 C.) or less	6-12 months

Breastmilk can be stored in a freezer at 24.8°F (-4°C) or less for up to 6 months optimal, 12 months acceptable (Eglash et al., 2017). Fresh milk is certainly better than frozen milk because, after 3 months in the freezer, it loses some fat, protein, and caloric value (Garcia-Lara et al., 2012). It's good practice to label the milk storage container with the baby's name, and the date and time the milk was expressed. Store it in the back of the freezer, where the temperature is more stable, as opposed to the interior of the door. Seal the container to prevent contamination. Store the milk in proportions less than 4 ounces (120 ml). Mothers find it helpful to have a few single ounce portions. Please note that there are different storage and handling requirements for babies who are staying in the NICU.

Serving

How much to supplement depends on the baby's age, weight, and number of feeds per day. Weight is less of a factor after the first month. After the first week, most babies take 1 to 2 ounces (30 to 60 ml) at each feed. During week two, they increase their intake to 2 to 3 ounces (60 to 90 ml). Then at one month, the average breastfed baby drinks between 3 to 5 ounces per feeding, which is consistent for the first 6 months (Mohrbacher, 2010).

There is conflicting information regarding the amounts of formula to supplement. New feeding guidelines to prevent obesity recommend that babies work up to no more than 2 ounces of formula per feed by one month of age (Perez-Escamilla et al., 2017). It is best to prevent over or underfeeding by paying attention to the baby's cues. Look for a cluster of feeding cues (arms flexed under the baby's chin, mouth searching, chin bobbing on your chest, and desperate cries for when you've waited too long). Feed the baby until the arms and body become totally relaxed. If bottle-feeding, be sure to follow the paced method. When babies eat too fast, they overeat and then act unsatisfied.

Once the baby has reached the "back to birthweight milestone" and until age 3 months, you can calculate precisely how much milk to feed with the following equation; multiply the baby's weight in pounds by 2.5. This gets you the total number of ounces needed for 24 hours. Divide the total number by the number of times you feed in 24 hours to get the amount to supplement for a feed. For example, a 10-pound (4.5 kg) baby needs 25 ounces (750 ml) during a 24-hour period. If the baby is doing about 8 feeds a day, he needs about 3.2 ounces (90 ml) at each feed.

If you would like to supplement with frozen breastmilk, thawing it overnight in the fridge is the ideal way because it causes less fat loss than warming methods (Thatrimontrichai et al., 2012). If you choose to thaw the milk slowly at room temperature, refrigerate it as soon as it becomes a liquid with remaining ice crystals to prevent bacteria growth (Jones & Tully, 2006). Placing the container of milk in a warm water bath for about 20 minutes or holding it under warm, running water are also safe preparation practices. A bottle warmer is okay to use. Microwaving can cause hot spots in the milk and reduce the quality. Milk that was previously frozen can be at room temperature for up to 2 hours (Handa et al., 2014), but should be discarded after the feed is over.

Once the milk is stored, you'll notice a normal separation of the milk fat. Fat freezes at a different rate than protein and water (Jones & Tully, 2006). As you prepare the milk that had been frozen or refrigerated, there may also be an odor. This is believed to be caused by oxidation of fatty acids released during a lipase triglyceride breakdown (Spitzer et al., 2013). Previously, mothers were told to scald the milk before storage to deactivate the lipase, but this is no longer advised because it can destroy immunological properties (Eglash et al., 2017).

If you find that your defrosted milk does smell soapy and your baby consistently rejects it, experiment. Does he take the milk immediately after it is expressed? If so, that means it's not the bottle causing the rejection, but rather, the milk. For some mothers, it takes up to 24 hours to change the odor of their milk. You can express one ounce and then check it hourly to see how long it takes to change. That length of time is how long you have before needing to scald and freeze the milk. Although it may change some of the immunologic properties of your milk, expressed breastmilk that is scalded is better than using formula. To prevent this change, heat the milk until you barely see bubbles, then cool and store it.

CHAPTER THIRTEEN

When It's Complicated: Solving Initial Breastfeeding Challenges

Chapter Goal: Overcome any initial discomforts with breastfeeding and difficulties that interfere with your newborn's ability to nurse effectively.

THE HOMECOMING

As Jenny prepared to be discharged from the hospital two days after giving birth, she felt ready to go home with her newborn, Kaden. After all, her plan for an all-natural childbirth had been disrupted by a series of complications, including gestational diabetes and preeclampsia, a serious condition that required an immediate induction at 37 weeks. Jenny was hospitalized, and it was four days of labor and treatment before Kaden finally arrived. After the difficult hospital experience, returning home proved to be just as overwhelming. "That night, we took him home and I thought, 'I know babies cry but this baby is crying non-stop,'" Jenny said.

After a long and difficult night, the new mother felt that something was wrong and rushed Kaden to his pediatrician the following day. "They said he's starving, basically. 'Give him some formula.' We gave him some formula and he just sucked that down," Jenny said.

Both the mother and baby were struggling with breastfeeding. Kaden was very sleepy after a highly medicated birth and Jenny's health obstacles interfered with her milk coming in. "This breastfeeding thing is not easy," Jenny said. "It made me feel like a failure because the way they were portraying it was, 'it is so simple, so pleasant, and wonderful.' I was thinking, what is wrong with me? Because it's not pleasant and wonderful, and I want it to be."

Research shows that breastfeeding challenges during the first week are common (Dewey et al., 2003). The top problems are sleepy baby, sore nipples, leaky breasts, newborn spitting-up, and maternal weepiness (Kearney et al., 1990). A fussy baby that isn't getting enough to eat and maternal engorgement are also common concerns. Unfortunately, most postpartum women are in the moment and fail to recognize that these challenges are usually temporary. Some give up. Reasons for weaning from the start include latch difficulties, the perception that the baby is eating too frequently, maternal fatigue, feeling isolated, and finding time for oneself (Dennis, 2002). When initial discomfort is seen as insurmountable, it is likely to cripple a mother's confidence. However, with the right support and motivation to continue breastfeeding, these are all challenges that can be overcome.

Try not to be traumatized by breastfeeding difficulties. Stress activates an inflammatory response in the body, which increases the risk of depression (Kendall-Tackett, 2007). Seek help immediately if you find yourself crying more than usual, feel too tired to care for yourself or the baby, feel more anxious than usual, or have thoughts of harming yourself or the baby (see postpartum depression on page 338).

Consider Your History

When you face an early breastfeeding challenge, always take into consideration your medical history as a couplet, including your pregnancy, birth experience, and any medical interventions you might have had. This information will help you determine what steps to take and whether you can try self-help or need to seek skilled assistance. Solutions to each breastfeeding difficulty could depend on whether you had a high- or low-risk pregnancy, or a birth procedure that could potentially lead to further complications.

When there are no risk factors, you might be able to resolve the difficulty on your own. However, when there are risk factors, a professional breastfeeding consultation is recommended. Conduct a review of your medical history in the adjacent boxes to see whether you or your newborn have any risk factors that might interfere with effective breastfeeding. Take into consideration any possible risk factors that could delay your milk coming in. All mother and baby couplets should be evaluated 3 to 4 days postpartum, as recommended by the American Academy of Pediatrics (Dewey et al., 2003).

Nursing Notes

Sometimes we don't know that we need help until it is too late. Seek support from a lactation professional if any of the following scenarios resonate with you. Check all that apply.

[_] My baby is more than 3 days old and he has orangish-red specs in his diaper.

[_] At 4 days old, my baby has less than four wet diapers every 24 hours.

[_] My newborn has lost more than 10% of his birthweight.

[_] My baby is older than 5 days and his stool has not turned yellow.

[_] It seems my baby cries excessively.

[_] My baby does not wake up to nurse, or is very sleepy and hard to wake for feeds.

[_] My baby seems to want to eat every hour and is never satisfied.

[_] It's been 10 days since he was born and he has not returned to his birthweight.

[_] My baby is older than 10 days and is not gaining at least 3/4 to 1 ounce daily.

[_] More than 24 hours passes before my newborn makes a poopy diaper.

[_] I am experiencing unrelieved engorgement.

[_] I never felt engorgement.

[_] My nipple pain is beyond discomfort.

[_] I have damaged nipples.

[_] I feel unusually worried, anxious, and, or depressed. (Call your doctor and notify the baby's medical professional.)

Other Concerns:

_____

Work Through It

This chapter will help you assess how to deal with many common initial breastfeeding challenges. We will give you a way to evaluate your body and your baby to determine whether physical characteristics are contributing factors. A plan to overcome will follow. When you face a true breastfeeding obstacle, three priorities are paramount in maintaining your milk supply and your baby's health. Number One: Feed the baby, even if it means supplementation. Number Two: Preserve your milk supply by bringing your baby to the breast on-cue and often, and/or emptying with a clinical-grade multiuser breast pump. Meanwhile, the third step is to work with a lactation professional, or other members of

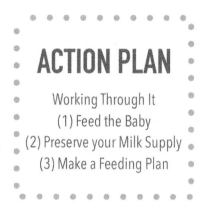

ACTION PLAN

Working Through It
(1) Feed the Baby
(2) Preserve your Milk Supply
(3) Make a Feeding Plan

your healthcare team, to develop a feeding plan that you feel you can accomplish. Children are resilient. You can have a plan with an A, B, and C before eventually getting back to plan A and going on to meet your goals with this baby.

Common Concerns

Breastfeeding problems are often associated with the newborn being sleepy after birth and less vigorous, combined with decreased feeding reflexes, including a less-active rooting reflex. The baby may have trouble locating the breast. The biggest job seems to be waking the infant up to nurse, then keeping him alert long enough to stimulate the breast and drink sufficient milk.

"My Milk Has Not Come In"

During the first 2 days after birth, a mother produces very small amounts of milk in the form of colostrum. By the second day, her body responds to the drop in her hormone (progesterone) levels, triggered by removal of the placenta, and her milk production increases. On average, mothers experience their milk coming in (secretory activation) 2 to 3 days postpartum (Dewey et al., 2003).

If your breasts are not noticeably fuller by 72 hours postpartum, you may be experiencing a delayed onset of milk production. Other signs include a fussy, cranky baby that wants to be held all the time, a baby whose diaper output is less than normal, and/or has yellowing of the skin, which is a sign of jaundice. If you experience any of these symptoms, seek medical assistance. In one study, 22% of mothers were tasked with overcoming a delayed onset of lactation (Dewey et al., 2003). Research shows several associated variables, including medical management of labor, like overhydration with intravenous fluids (Noel-Weiss et al., 2011). There might be inherent maternal physical reasons for delayed milk production, which is why a medical evaluation is needed (see Risk Factors for Delayed or Insufficient Milk Supply on page 352). Know that with the right help, nearly all mothers with delayed milk can eventually establish an adequate milk supply for their baby (Dewey et al., 2003).

Feeding Plan for Delayed Milk

1. See your medical professional as soon as possible for an evaluation.

2. Make an appointment to see a lactation consultant for an evaluation of both you and the baby. The specialist will be able to tell you how much milk your infant is drinking during a feed and give you a feeding plan based on your milk supply and baby's weight.

3. Make your home environment as private as possible.

4. Keep your newborn skin-to-skin as much as you can. Breastfeed every time he nuzzles up to the breast or shows feeding cues (at least 8 to 12 times in 24 hours).

5. Avoid pacifiers. Newborns need to do all their suckling at the breast.

6. Listen for swallows and when they become infrequent, or you see the baby pause, press on the breast, holding your

hand in place until he stops swallowing. Move around the sections of the breast that feel firm (alternate breast compressions). When pressing fails to make the baby swallow, switch breasts until he is uninterested. If there are concerns about your baby's weight or your milk supply, do not spend too much time on this intervention. Stop as soon as the baby appears sleepy.

7. Hand express after every nursing, then feed the baby through an alternate method (see chart for amounts).

8. Once colostrum turns to milk, start pumping after every feed.

9. Consider taking a galactagogue, which is a drug or herb that can potentially increase your milk production (see galactagogues on page 362). A knowledgeable medical professional can help you find the correct medicinal choice and dosage, depending on your history and physical issues.

Feed the Baby Adequate Amounts

TABLE 13.3: Feed the Baby Adequate Amounts. Source: Adapted from the Academy of Breastfeeding Medicine Protocols.

#Hours Since Birth	Amount the Newborn Needs Every 2 to 3 hours (factoring 8 feeds per 24 hours)
Less than 24	2 to 10 cc (about a teaspoon)
Less than 48	5 to 15 cc (1/2 oz or less)
Less than 72	15 to 30 cc (1/2 to 1 oz)
Less than 96	30 to 60 cc (1 to 2 oz). Feed less if the baby is under 7 pounds.
More than 96	Take the baby's weight and multiply it by 2.5, and divide by the number of feeds. For example, an 8 pound baby would be fed 2.5 oz per feed. The equation is 8 x 2.5 = 20 / 8 = 2.5 oz.

DIAPER OUTPUT

Keeping track of the baby's output can give you a good indication of whether he is having enough to eat (see nearby chart). You should see the baby's stools change in color from black and tarry to yellow between day 4 and 7. The stools will be loose and seedy or appear to have curds. By age 6 to 10 days, the average newborn is stooling almost every time they nurse (Wambach & Riordan, 2016). At least four of the stools should be larger than a quarter. Wet diapers are just as important. They increase in number with each day. Call your medical practitioner if you see red crystals and/or scanty urine by day 4 to 5. Little girls may have vaginal mucus, and possibly a small amount of bloody smear. This is normal.

TABLE 13.4: Diaper Output Parameters with Normal Milk Intake.

Day of Life	Urine	Stool
First 24 Hours	1 or more, pale color	1 or more, black sticky
Day 2	2 or more, pale color	1 to 2, greenish black, less sticky
Day 3	3 to 4 or more, pale color	3 to 4, green-yellow, looser
Day 4	4 to 6 or more, pale color	4 to 10, yellow-seedy, liquid
CALL THE DOCTOR	dark yellow, reddish color, crystals present	less than 4 stools on day 4

How to Tell a Diaper is Wet

It helps to be able to tell if a diaper is truly wet. Try this little experiment. First, feel a dry, disposable diaper. Notice that when you squeeze it with your fingers, it feels firm and does not dent. Next, pour an ounce or two of water on the dry diaper. Then, pinch it between your fingers and notice how different it feels. Once the gel inside becomes absorbed with liquid, it's squishy. This observation will help you detect when your baby's diapers are wet.

Excessive Infant Weight Loss

Most nursing newborns lose some weight the first 3 days after birth, during the colostrum phase, when the mother's milk volume is minimal. On average, they lose 5 to 7% of their birthweight (Manganaro et al., 2001). After the copious milk production begins, newborns show a typical pattern of weight gain after day 5 and beyond. When all is well, a baby should regain the lost weight and return to birthweight by age 7-to-10-days-old. According to the World Health Organization weight standards, normal weight gain is 5.5 to 8.5 ounces per week during the first 3 to 4 months (www.who.int/childgrowth/ed/). Many factors are involved in weight gain, including stomach size, breastfeeding frequency, and how well the baby drains the breast.

Be sure your baby is weighed by day 5. Health providers become concerned when the baby loses more than 10% of his weight. This is an indication that the baby may be dehydrated, and also susceptible to higher levels of jaundice. Some causes of excessive weight loss are delayed milk production, ineffective nursing position, and a sleepy baby with depressed feeding cues, caused by medications administered during labor (Dewey et al., 2003). Research further shows that excess infant weight loss can be associated with maternal obesity, cesarean delivery, long labor (greater than 14 hours), and flat or inverted nipples (Dewey et al., 2003). An online calculator, known as Newt, can help you see how your newborn's weight loss compares with a large sample of newborns. Go to www.newbornweight.org.

If your baby appears vigorous and is feeding well, but on paper, looks like he has lost too much weight, take into consideration how much IV fluid was administered to you during labor. Babies can have an inflated initial weight because they absorb the IV fluids through the placenta (Chantry et al., 2011). A drastic weight loss in the first 24 hours, with 4 to 6 wet diapers, but little-known intake of colostrum at the breast may indicate that the baby is passing those excess fluids (Noel-Weiss et al., 2011). If this is the case, try to work through it without supplementation. Of course, both mother and baby should be monitored for progress.

Feeding Plan for Excessive Weight Loss

1. You can be assured that your milk has arrived if your breasts feel fuller, and even lumpy and hard in some spots. Feel your breasts before and after nursing. They should soften.

2. Get an assessment from a lactation professional to confirm that the baby is drinking milk at the breast.

3. Be sure to express (pump) your milk if you miss a breastfeed.

4. Avoid pacifier use. It's the baby's strong sucking drive that helps bring milk in.

5. Breastfeed on-cue and frequently, every 2 to 3 hours or sooner.

6. Be sure to relieve any engorgement by breastfeeding or pumping.

NIPPLE PAIN AND SORENESS

Nipple pain is one of the most common reasons new mothers stop breastfeeding (Tait, 2000). There are varying degrees of nipple pain, soreness, and injury, which we will discuss and assist you to diagnose so you can begin treatments to relieve and heal this discomfort. First, it is important to understand that it is normal in the beginning to experience mild soreness and feel a strong pull of the baby's mouth, even when the latch is correct. Welcome this feeling that you are not used to because research shows that a lack of nipple discomfort during the first few days of breastfeeding may indicate a weak infant suckle, which is less simulating to the breast and may lead to a delay or decrease in the milk supply (Nommsen-Rivers et al., 2010).

Events leading to nipple soreness or injury vary. They can be very complex or as simple as the way the mother holds the baby when nursing (Tait, 2000). Because you and your baby are a couplet, the cause of your pain can be related to the way the baby's mouth, face, and head are shaped, or your unique breast and nipple anatomy. Nipple trauma can also result if the baby experienced a breech delivery, has a tight neck, bruised head and face, and/or shoulder injury. Lastly, the effects of labor medications can influence how well the baby nurses (Smith, 2007).

Treatments for nipple pain focus on detecting the cause, promoting healing, and preventing further trauma. Emphasis is focused on learning how to hold the baby in a manner that accommodates a deeper hold of the nipple, which usually results in a more comfortable and effective breastfeed. Often, the mother and infant just need practice, and time for the baby to grow and the mother to heal. If you follow the breastfeeding checklist on page 25, and you continue to have pain and damage, it's time to see a professional for help. If you are dealing with sore nipples,

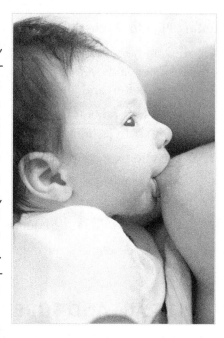

A bad latch causes pulling, nipple soreness, and possibly injury.

observe the appearance of your nipples and areola to assess the severity so you can determine what treatment plan will give you the best results until you see a consultant. See the Breastfeeding Challenges: Symptom Checker in the back of the book for direction to the relevant chapter topic that will help you further assess, treat, and resolve the problem.

Mild Nipple Pain

During the first 2 weeks, most mothers experience mild nipple irritation. It should feel like when the weather changes and your lips suddenly need more lubrication. When the baby pulls the nipple deep into his mouth, stretching it to twice its size, it can be quite uncomfortable. It takes time for the nipples to adapt and for the skin to stretch and build elasticity. With mild nipple pain, your nipples shouldn't hurt between feeds, although clothing rubbing against them could feel irritating. When you examine your nipples, they may look slightly red and irritated. For most, that will abate after a short time once the nipples acclimate. Research shows that for the majority of breastfeeding mothers, nipple pain decreases to minor discomfort at about 7 to 10 days postpartum (Dennis et al., 2014). Many mothers report that this early latch-on pain goes away after the baby starts swallowing milk. Mothers seem to handle it better with the second baby because they know it is normal and only lasts about 10 days.

In the beginning, some women have very sensitive nipples due to the extra blood flow to the breasts. Other mothers who have had breast surgery may have increased or decreased nipple sensitivity. This puts them at risk for injury because they may not feel the pain, or they feel so much pain that it deters them. These sensations will also diminish with time.

Tips to Manage Nipple Pain

» Continue breastfeeding but verify that you are holding the baby correctly so he can take the breast deep into his mouth.

» Try to trigger your let-down sooner with skin-to-skin time, privacy, relaxation techniques, and gentle massage.

» Breastfeed on the less sore nipple first until the baby starts gulping. Switch as needed so you release milk from both breasts.

» Mothers report the usefulness of pure and natural products, such as purified anhydrous lanolin, coconut oil, and olive oil. Research the product prior to use to understand if any risks are involved (i.e., allergic reaction, recalls). Do not use lanolin if you are allergic to wool. So far, researchers have not found evidence to support any one treatment over the other (Dennis et al., 2014). In fact, they found applying expressed breastmilk or nothing at all can be just as effective in resolving minor nipple pain.

» Hydrogel pads may help with nipple pain. Read instructions before using to prevent infections.

» Wash your breasts once a day with mild soap and water during your typical bathing ritual.

» Use nursing pads without plastic lining and change them regularly to avoid irritation.

» Breastfeed on-cue and often to avoid engorgement, plugged ducts, or pain caused by an intense, hungry baby.

» Soften the breasts before the baby nurses if you are engorged. Otherwise, the infant will not be deep enough on the breast and may cause damage (see reverse-pressure softening on page 299).

» Be sure to break suction before removing your baby from the breast.

When nipples continue to be injured and tender beyond week two, the cause may be more complicated. The hardest thing is you will have to continue nursing to prevent complications and avoid reducing your milk supply. Since poor positioning and attachment at the breast are the two most common causes of nipple pain, check that you are holding the baby correctly (Tait, 2000). If the initial pain does not abate after several sucks and swallows, break suction and start over. Timing matters; wait for the baby to be wide awake and showing active feeding cues. Be sure that your hands and clothing are positioned out of the infant's chin space so he can get deep on the breast (see breast attachment on page 293).

Cracked and Bleeding Nipples

When mothers have cracked and bleeding nipples, they often dread breastfeeding. It's amazing to see how many soldier on. Look at your nipple when the baby lets go. It should appear slightly elongated, perhaps even a bit creased, but not white edged, lipstick shaped, or unusually shaped. Correct positioning and breast attachment are the most important factors in preventing nipple damage and pain. It also matters because poor positioning can impact the milk supply. Since the ducts that transport breastmilk are tiny and close to the surface, getting smaller toward the tip, a baby who is not positioned or attached correctly takes a superficial hold, which can easily compress the ducts, blocking milk flow (Gooding et al., 2010).

Ineffective hand positioning can lead to nipple injury. Are your fingers in the baby's chin space? If so, he will have no choice but to hold the nipple superficially. You will usually know it's wrong if you feel pain, followed by notably injured skin below the nipple. Are you pressing on the breast to make an airway above the baby's nose? This tends to lead to an abraded raw tip (face) of the nipple. Instead, tuck your baby's hips against your belly. This will lift the baby's nose off the breast. If the area above your nipple is injured, make sure the baby is not tucking his upper lip. To untuck, gently press into his cheekbone and lift. Avoid flipping the lip with the tip of your finger because this will break suction and require you to start again.

If you know you are positioning your baby correctly and your anatomy is normal, then it may be the way your baby suckles the breast. Signs include poor or slow weight gain, combined with nipple pain and damage. There are certain physical characteristics that are consistent in infants that are found to have suckling problems. Check your baby and see if you notice any of the following: Does he have any lumps or bumps on his head? At birth, did they say he had a cephalohematoma (a raised, spongy collection of blood on the head)? Did your birth attendant use a forceps or vacuum to assist the newborn out of the birth canal? Look at his face and head—does it look even on both sides? Babies typically have a small chin, but some have an overbite and a dramatic receding jaw, caused by genetics or positioning inside the womb. Does the infant keep his head turned to one side? If so, does one nipple hurt more? Is it damaged more than the other side? Does your baby have a thin or thick fold of skin anchoring the tip of his tongue to the base of his mouth behind his lower gum (tongue-tie)? Look at your baby's palate when his mouth is open wide. It should be smooth and gently sloped. The baby's palate can trap your nipple if it is too shallow or too high. Tense, strong babies tend to have a stronger suckle. Affirmative responses to many of these factors may increase a mother's nipple pain and damage.

If you see any of the preceding, skilled help is essential to take you through healing. The following can be started right away.

Plan to Promote Nipple Healing and Help Prevent Infection

1. Clean the nipples three times daily with saline soaks. Mix 1/2 teaspoon of table salt in 1 cup of warm water. Either soak the nipples with a washcloth or soak in a wide-mouth cup (a shot glass works well) until the water cools. Following the soak, rinse the breast with plain water so too much salt does not transfer to the baby.

2. See your medical practitioner and ask if an antibiotic ointment can help. Topical mupirocin will treat a superficial infection and a low-strength steroid cream may be recommended for inflammation (Walker, 2010). Be sure to gently wipe any excess medication off prior to nursing. A sterile, wet cotton ball works.

3. Look for signs of infection, such as fever, "flu" symptoms, and skin redness. Cracked nipples can be a precurser to mastitis (see breast infection).

4. Try the following comfort measures for sore nipples:

   » Take Ibuprofen or Tylenol. Ask your health provider for recommendations.

   » Start nursing on the least sore side first while the baby is most hungry.

   » Consider hand-expressing until the milk starts spraying before nursing.

   » Try hydrogel pads for comfort. Cooling the pads prior to a feed will make them ready to relieve pain after nursing.

   » To protect your tender nipples from rough clothing, consider wearing breast shells between breastfeeds.

Be aware that nursing with a sore nipple may make you involuntarily flinch and distance your body from the baby when bringing him to the breast. Some mothers with sore nipples have a fear response to the anticipated nipple pain. Since babies need to start their pull of the areola from below the nipple, flinching sabotages good positioning, making the sore nipples worse (Thorley, 2015). To prevent this from being a problem:

» Be mindful of your posture and what your arms are doing.

» Lower your shoulders and press them against the backrest.

» Hold the baby close.

» Be aware of not bending your elbows up and jerking. This action lifts the breast, and the baby ends up on the nipple rather than with a deep hold of breast tissue.

» Try laid-back positioning, which is more relaxing and can help prevent this issue.

YEAST INFECTION (CANDIDA)

There are some conditions that make a mother and baby suscep-tible to a yeast infection after breastfeeding is well established. Rarely, it happens early on if the newborn has thrush. Normally, we have candida on our skin and mucus membranes as part of our healthy skin flora. Under some circumstances (i.e., broken skin from nipple trauma, antibiotic use, or a baby's mouth infected with candida), the balance becomes upset, allowing the yeast spores to overgrow and penetrate the skin, causing infection. The mother will suddenly notice very red, shiny, even peeling skin on her nipples. The nipples may appear swollen and bumpy. Women complain that their nipples itch, burn, and throb. Mothers say they can't even stand to wear their bra and dread feeding the baby.

If this occurs, check your baby's mouth, looking for white fluffy patches in the inner cheeks and inside the lips. Also, look for a thick white coating on the baby's tongue that doesn't wipe off. Finally, check your baby for a bright red shiny diaper rash that isn't getting better, despite good diaper hygiene. Be aware of risk factors that could potentially make you vulnerable to developing this type of infection.

Maternal Risk Factors

» Just having a pregnancy lowers a mother's resistance to vaginal candidiasis

» A current vaginal yeast infection

» Taking antibiotics during labor and delivery, or anytime afterward

» Experiencing skin breakdown from nipple trauma

» Thrush infection exposes nipples and areola to the yeast spores

» Mothers with diabetes or other medical illness that lowers their resistance (Walker, 2017)

» Not changing your breast pads frequently enough (yeast thrives in a dark, wet environment).

Infant Risk Factors

» Pacifier use can be a carrier of yeast in the baby's mouth, making it more difficult to heal

» The use of bottles in the first 2 weeks of breastfeeding (Francis-Morrill et al., 2004)

» Exposure to maternal antibiotics during labor

If you suspect you or your baby have a yeast infection, it is best to be examined by your medical provider. It is usually diagnosed by symptoms and can be difficult to treat. The most common treatment is oral nystatin for the baby and a nystatin cream for the mother's breasts. These medications are commonly prescribed four times daily. For improved effectiveness, ask your health provider if you can divide the medication into a dosing after every feed.

Infant Treatment Tips for Thrush

See the baby's healthcare provider to discuss treatment and follow the directions carefully, including these tips:

1. Treat your nipples and the baby's mouth after every nursing session. Start by wiping his mouth with a clean, wet washcloth.

2. Pour the scheduled medication dose into a small medication cup.

3. Dip a Q-tip into the medication and apply it to the baby's entire mouth.

4. At the next feed, repeat the mouth cleaning, followed by the medication. Then have the baby drink the rest. Wash the cup thoroughly.

5. Wash the baby's hands with every diaper change.

6. Boil all the bottle nipples and pacifiers you use, daily.

Maternal Treatment Tips for Candida

1. Purchase over-the-counter Monistat/miconazole 7 (not the 3 because it is too concentrated), Lotrimin AF, or Micatin.

2. Gently wipe the nipples with plain water, then apply the medication. Unless you nurse immediately after application, there is no need to wash it off before breastfeeding.

3. Make sure that the baby is positioned correctly to avoid further trauma.

4. Wash your hands frequently, especially before handling the baby or touching your breasts.

5. Make sure to change your breast pads between feeds so that they are mostly dry.

6. Change your bra daily and wash it in hot water with a bleach solution.

7. Sterilize any pumping equipment you use.

8. Consider probiotics for yourself and the baby.

9. If you are too sore, express your milk with a double electric pump or hand express at least seven times in 24 hours for a day or two while you start treatment.

Candida is a stubborn fungus to treat. If the standard treatment doesn't make you and your baby feel better, ask for a referral to a dermatologist for a definitive diagnosis. For years, nipple pain and damage was largely treated with candida medications. Mothers and babies were treated repeatedly, and when improvement wasn't seen, they were started on a strong drug called fluconazole. There are many other possibilities that explain these symptoms. Suckling issues from breast and infant anatomical variations may also leave a nipple looking red, swollen, and cracked. More commonly, red cracked nipples may have a bacterial cause and may need an antibiotic (Livingstone et al., 1996). Remember that chronic trauma from poor infant positioning at the breast is the leading cause of nipple pain (Thompson et al., 2016).

STRONG VACUUM: ANOTHER CAUSE OF SORE NIPPLES

In most instances, early nipple pain resolves in a few weeks but some women are never totally comfortable when feeding, no matter how perfect the positioning and anatomy of the mother and baby are. There are not many studies that look at chronic pain, but in 2015, a study revealed new findings. It found that some babies produce a stronger suction than others, which can lead to nipple pain that doesn't resolve (McClellan et al., 2015). The study showed that these babies also express less milk from their mother, even when the latch appears correct. Using ultrasound imaging of mothers with persistent nipple pain, researchers found that these infants didn't lower their tongue as far when filling their mouth with milk compared to the no-pain control couplets, which increased vacuum levels. It was surprising when they learned that the mothers complaining of pain had babies with suction levels (tested by using a pressure sensor taped to the nipple) twice as strong as the mothers without nipple pain.

Unfortunately, the tools used in research aren't available in day-to-day practice. Lactation consultants don't have a gauge to tell them if a baby's suck is too strong. An experienced mother can tell you if her new baby has a stronger suck than what she was accustomed to with a prior baby. While there is not a treatment plan for this condition, hopefully it helps to know that it's not something you are doing wrong—you can be sure of this once you've ruled out all other possible causes. Time will improve this condition.

VASOSPASM OF THE NIPPLES: RAYNAUD'S PHENOMENON

If you feel intermittent throbbing pain in your nipples, it is important to quickly examine your breasts because you may be experiencing vasospasm. You will see that your nipple first appears white, then turns blue, before returning to pink or your normal color. This is a painful condition that results from the spasm of the blood vessels in the nipples. Exposure to cold temperatures increase episodes. In the past, we believed vasospasm of the nipples was rare but with better diagnosis, it is noticed more often. Research shows that the condition may affect 20% of women in the childbearing age (Anderson et al., 2004).

Women with the following conditions are more susceptible to vasospasm: cold sensitivity (hands and feet turn white when cold); an autoimmune condition, such as systemic lupus, rheumatoid arthritis, or hypothyroidism; Raynaud's nipple trauma; history of breast surgery; or extreme stress. Some medications can also be factors, such as caffeine and estrogen in birth control (Anderson et al., 2004). The increased hormones of pregnancy can also be a trigger. When vasospasm is caused by nipple trauma, the nipple or a part of the nipple will be white when coming out of the baby's mouth. Anytime the nipple gets cold (such as turning the warm shower off), Raynaud's can trigger the painful nipple spasm. If you suspect that you have this condition, see a lactation consultant.

Treatment Plan to Overcome Vasospasm of the Nipples

1. Be sure that the baby has a deep hold of the nipple. Your nipple should appear slightly elongated, round, and normal when the baby comes off the breast.

2. Avoid exposure to cold. To keep the nipple as warm as possible, store your nursing pad under your breast while nursing. Once your baby finishes the feed, quickly slide it up.

When showering, make the room warm and cover yourself immediately after turning off the water.

3. Apply dry heat to the breast when symptomatic, like a warmed rice sock.

4. Massage the nipples three times daily with warm olive oil.

5. Avoid nicotine and eliminate caffeine.

6. Some medications and supplements are helpful, such as 500 mg of calcium/magnesium three times daily, fish oil supplements (Lawrence & Lawrence, 2011), or vitamin B complex. If you get no relief, ask your health provider if a low dose oral Nifedipine (a blood pressure medication) will help (Lawrence & Lawrence, 2011).

ENGORGED BREASTS

It is normal to feel increased fullness of breasts when colostrum shifts to mature milk. This is due to increased blood and lymph flow to the breasts. Active babies that nurse well relieve the fullness. But when babies are separated from their mother, are sleepy, and/or ineffective when nursing, the fluids build up, allowing the proteins to seep into surrounding tissues (Mohrbacher, 2010). The breasts become so full of milk that they feel hard and heavy. The skin appears so stretched that the skin looks shiny and the veins become visible. The breasts may feel hot and tender with painful throbbing and/or lumpiness that can extend into the armpits. Some women experience breasts so full that the areolae become swollen and their nipples flatten (see areolar engorgement). This can cause breast-attachment problems. The hungry infant cannot grasp this firm unyielding breast. The baby just bobs and cries at the breast in frustration.

Sometimes the way we breastfeed or manage feeding can unknowingly cause engorgement. Examples include restricting the number of breastfeeds by timing or limiting nursing to a schedule, unnecessarily supplementing the baby with formula, missing the newborn's early hunger cues, pumping without clinical reason, which causes an oversupply of milk, and not holding the baby correctly on the breast. Breast implants can also exacerbate engorgement. Previous breast surgery may result in certain segments of the breast becoming engorged. Unfortunately, some women are just more prone to engorgement, no matter how well they try to follow best practices. Many women fear that treating engorgement with milk expressions will make it worse. Engorgement must be relieved because pressure on the milk ducts caused by being overfilled signals your body to make less milk. Repeated or habitual engorgement can lower your milk production overall.

Feeding Plan for Engorgement

1. To relieve discomfort, apply cold cloths for up to 20 minutes before nursing. Avoid heat because it increases swelling (Walker, 2017).

2. Gently massage each breast from the armpit to the nipple before nursing.

3. Following cold therapy, hand express or pump, using low pressure until the areola is soft. Or, do reverse-pressure softening (see areola edema) immediately before each attempt to latch.

4. Feed the baby frequently, aiming for every 2 hours or when your breasts start to feel full.

5. If the baby is too sleepy to nurse frequently, hand express or pump the breasts often.

6. While the baby is nursing, gently press on the full breast spots during pauses. Use a laid-back nursing position while doing this to protect the baby from your vigorous milk flow.

7. If the breasts still feel engorged after nursing, pump or hand express to achieve comfort.

8. After breastfeeding, cover your engorged breasts with a light cloth and apply ice packs (or bags of frozen veggies) for at least 15-20 minutes.

9. If your engorgement appears to be caused by inadequate milk transfer, work with your baby to help his mouth achieve a deeper hold of your breast.

10. Ibuprofen can help relieve pain and reduce inflammation while you work through engorgement (Mohrbacher, 2010). Check with your provider before taking any medication.

If you are not able to relieve the fullness, it may be necessary to rent a clinical-grade breast pump for several days. Seek breastfeeding help for unresolved engorgement that lasts more than 2 days. Engorgement can sometimes lead to plugged ducts. Along with engorgement, you may concurrently have areolar engorgement. If so, you will notice that your areola is bulging, and your nipple appears to have flattened. You often will not be able to relieve breast engorgement without first relieving the swelling around your nipple (see areolar engorgement).

PLUGGED MILK DUCTS

Commonly, nursing has been going well and suddenly, a woman notices a hard, painful area on her breast. Her first thoughts may be fears of cancer. Most likely, the cause is a blockage of a milk duct. This condition is more common in women with too much milk. It can be caused by pressure on the outside of the breast from sleeping on the stomach or anything that puts pressure on the milk glands (i.e., a backpack with straps across the breast, an underwire bra). Returning to work or a social schedule that doesn't allow adequate time to express breastmilk is another culprit.

Women nursing multiples are more susceptible to plugged ducts. Often, it occurs after a frequent-feeding day, followed by a sleepy, less demanding day, or after the baby has his first long stretch of sleep. During the night, the mother wakes up because she feels uncomfortable but is so tired, she just goes back to sleep. The next morning, she discovers the plugged duct. The area behind the plug will swell and feel very hard and painful. It can be differentiated from mastitis because you would otherwise feel well.

Treatment Plan for Plugged Ducts

1. Look for preceding causes (e.g., bra too tight). Underwire bras that are not fitted properly are known to block milk ducts. Are you wearing a bra or a tank top you pull up across the top of your breast? Did the baby have a growth spurt, then a sleepy day? Anything that obstructs the breast or gets the milk supply out of balance is the possible cause.

2. Apply heat to the affected area for 10 to 15 minutes prior to nursing.

3. Nurse frequently, starting on the affected side.

4. Apply gentle pressure behind the area when the baby's sucking pauses.

5. Lean over a container of hot water and submerge the affected breast. Massage from the chest wall toward the nipple, then hand express.

6. If there is no relief after several days or you start to feel ill, you may be developing a breast infection. See your health provider or a lactation consultant.

7. If the lump reoccurs, see your health provider. It is important to determine the source.

BLEBS OR MILK BLISTERS

Sometimes a plug may be caused by a white spot (bleb) over a nipple pore that blocks the milk flow. It can occur when a tiny bit of skin grows over a milk duct opening, causing milk to back up behind it. It can also be caused by inflammation. Blebs can be very tender or just present without pain. The blisters can be stubborn and reoccur for weeks or months if the cause isn't determined. Treatment is centered around opening the blister, releasing the milk, and healing the area.

Treatment for Blebs

1. First determine the cause. Does the baby have a superficial hold of the nipple? Get a deeper attachment. Is your flow so fast that the baby pulls back? Lean way back.

2. The bleb must be opened or removed to relieve the obstruction. Do not poke or pop the blister because inserting an object can lead to infection. Start salt water soaks (see cracked/bleeding nipples treatment), followed by rubbing with a soft cloth to peel the softened skin away. Warm olive oil massages to the nipple may help soften the area.

3. Hand express the nipple after treatment and after every nursing until you are sure the area is healed. A steroid cream to decrease the inflammation and a topical antibiotic are often prescribed. Apply three times daily, wiping off any excess medicine before nursing.

4. Examine your nipple after feeds for at least a week past healing in case the bleb returns.

OTHER LACTATION RELATED CONCERNS

Overabundant Milk Supply

While mothers are often concerned about having enough milk, having too much can also wreak havoc. These mothers often feel like they have not emptied their breasts after nursing. The breasts feel full and tender between feeds, leaking continuously. The baby may act distressed while feeding. (Note that this symptom can be confused with a suckling problem.) The baby will pull off the breast, choke, and sputter. He may appear gassy and irritable from an overfull stomach. Often, the baby spits-up after meals, and has frequent loose stools. The baby puts on weight rapidly, gaining 3 to 4 ounces per day as opposed to the expected 3/4 to an ounce. As a result of having overfull breasts, a mother may develop plugged ducts and mastitis. If you suspect that you have an overabundant milk supply, get an assessment before making changes to your nursing routine. It should be differentiated from possible overactive let-down and a foremilk-hindmilk imbalance.

How to Overcome an Overabundant Milk Supply Following Professional Diagnosis

1. Offer one breast per nursing session for a period of 3 hours. Make that breast available on demand before switching to the other breast. For example, at noon, the baby would nurse on your right breast. If the baby wants to nurse anytime within the next 3 hours, you continue to offer the same breast. At 3 pm, when your infant cues his hunger, you would switch to the left breast. For the next 3 hours, only the left breast is offered when the baby wants to nurse.

2. While doing this, you would only express milk from the other breast for comfort prior to feeds and not to empty the breasts. Be cautious—some women develop plugged ducts while attempting to decrease their milk. If 3 hours feels too long (uncomfortable), try 2 hours.

3. These tactics can help stabilize the milk production to a supply that is more suitable to your baby. Be aware that some mothers have a very sensitive milk supply, which quickly decreases. Notice how your baby responds. If he starts to be more fussy or restless when nursing, have him weighed and your milk supply evaluated again.

Overactive Let-Down

Overabundant milk supply is sometimes associated with an overactive let-down, meaning the milk suddenly flows too fast and forcefully. It may feel painful beyond normal tingling. The flow may be faster than the baby can swallow. In response, he coughs and appears to gasp or choke. Loud gulps can be heard when the milk flows. Sometimes the baby lets go of the breast with let-down, making the milk spray across the room. Over time, the hungry baby may become fearful while breastfeeding, pulling off the breast and sucking his fingers instead. In addition, mothers with overactive let-down often experience frequent plugged ducts and breast infections.

An Overactive Let-down Can Be Managed with Various Methods

» Try using relaxation techniques like deep breathing and thinking of your favorite calm place.

» Use a laid-back nursing position. The infant will handle the flow better, being above the breast.

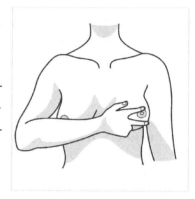

ILLUSTRATION 13.1: Scissors Hold. Illustration by Ken Tackett

» Listen for the baby's sucks and swallows. When he starts looking restless or you hear loud gulps, lean further back or take the baby off for a minute.

» You can hold back the flow of milk by crossing your index and middle fingers together like a pair of scissors and clamping behind the nipple. Be sure to rotate positions of your fingers. Practice this technique when hand-expressing or pumping your milk to see what slows the flow. Avoid pressing against the breast because it makes the sprays more forceful.

» To stop the flow of milk when the baby pulls off the breast, press hard on the nipple.

» To further help with this problem, burp the baby often.

Foremilk/Hindmilk Imbalance

Occasionally, a mother with a full milk supply notices that her baby acts unsettled after eating, expelling gas and fussily pulling up his legs before passing a diaper full of greenish, liquid stool. A Dr. Google search is bound to follow. The results of the search may yield a diagnosis of foremilk/hindmilk imbalance and a recommendation for block-feeding. Note that foremilk/hindmilk imbalance is a very rare condition but has become one of the most popular self-diagnoses around. Unfortunately, the recommendation for block-feeding often does more harm than good, jeopardizing milk supply in many mothers who don't have this condition. Mothers who block-feed without professional guidance are at higher risk of reducing their milk supply, developing painful blocked ducts, mastitis, and engorgement. Since milk supply concerns are so prevalent, any self-help efforts that can harm or reduce the milk supply should be done under the guidance of a lactation consultant.

So, how did we get to a point where mothers are overly concerned about foremilk and hindmilk? In the 1980s, researchers Chloe Fisher and Michael Woolridge discovered that breastmilk composition changes throughout a feed, becoming higher in fat the longer the baby feeds with later let-downs. Before that time, it was recommended that a young infant nursed 10 minutes on one breast and then 10 minutes on the other. Because babies were not being allowed to regulate their own balanced meal and were instead pushed to reach a time goal, the ones nursing on a mother with overabundant milk were getting too much low-fat milk that was high in sugar. As a result, the babies were gassy, miserable, and having diarrhea from sugar overload (Woolridge & Fisher, 1988). Many babies had colic and insufficient weight gain.

Fisher and Woolridge's discovery has led to new management of breastfeeding. Now, mothers are encouraged to let the baby finish the first breast and come off on their own, regardless of how long the feed is. If the infant is interested in more after a burp and a little break, then mothers are advised to offer the second breast until the baby is satisfied. Change is slow, and many mothers are still feeding by the clock.

One influencing factor begins with the first feeds in the hospital. Feeds are timed so staff can record data in the computer along with vital signs to track the newborn's progress and health. This hospital practice of timing feeds can give mothers the idea that *this is how it's done*. Be aware that there is no correlation between the timing, length of your baby's feed, and milk intake.

Many mothers are overly concerned about reaching the goal of hindmilk, which is higher in fat and calories than foremilk. Know that the total milk consumed each day determines weight gain, not the hindmilk (Mohrbacher, 2010). Research shows that infants regulate their fat intake and, over a 24-hour day, get roughly the same net fat intake, whether the mother is nursing one breast or two during a feed (Woolridge et al., 1990), along with the right amount of foremilk, hindmilk, carbohydrates, and proteins, among other essential nutrients and hormones needed for growth. So, use your Baby Watching techniques to look for those wonderful signs of satiety.

True foremilk/hindmilk imbalance can happen after a mother develops her full supply, due to a number of scenarios (Rapley & Murkett, 2012): 1) The baby is not spending enough time at the breast because the feed is cut short; 2) The baby is not feeding effectively; or 3) The mother is producing far too much milk (hyperlactation) for her baby. This can occasionally make digestion a miserable experience. In these cases, if the baby sets out for a long period of crying soon after nursing, he may have discomfort due to an imbalanced meal or overeating. Babies with this problem want to suckle more for comfort and pain relief, but it results in more overeating and further discomfort. The baby will be difficult to soothe and show abdominal pain by arching his torso and drawing his knees up to his chest. Relief may eventually follow an explosive release of greenish, watery, or frothy poop. If your baby has these behaviors, first see your health professional because the same symptoms can relate to other illnesses. In the short-term, you can help in several ways:

» See calming techniques in the crying chapter.

» Position the baby upright, massage his lower back, and offer a white-noise distraction.

» Check your baby's attachment and make sure he is feeding effectively.

» Avoid taking the baby off the breast when milk is flowing. Switch breasts following a short rest and diaper change, rather than make the move in the middle of a breastfeed.

» The most important action is to watch the baby—not the clock. As long as he is happily swallowing with a regular rhythm, let him come off the breast on his own.

If you suspect your baby is getting a foremilk/hindmilk imbalance, see a lactation consultant to assess whether you have an overabundant milk supply or a feeding issue. A possible fix may be as simple as correcting attachment, keeping the baby on the breast longer, or nursing one breast only at each feeding time with careful follow-up of the baby's weight gain.

CHAPTER FOURTEEN

Breast Attachment: Difficulty Taking the Breast

Chapter Goal: Find the right intervention to overcome any early attachment challenges.

HELPING YOUR BABY TAKE THE BREAST

There are times when a baby has difficulty taking the breast and holding it in his mouth, often referred to as latching-on. Challenges are associated with the use of labor pain medications, cesarean delivery, flat or inverted nipples, low breastfeeding confidence, supplementation of non-breastmilk alternatives, and pacifier use (Dewey et al., 2003). When it's seen on day 7, it can be associated with maternal obesity, stage II labor greater than one hour, and low birthweight (Dewey et al., 2003). In addition, adequate breast-hold issues are sometimes caused by the anatomy of the mother's nipple or the baby's mouth. Most of these breast attachment frustrations can be resolved with a bit of patience and time as the infant's mouth grows larger and he becomes accustomed to his mother's breasts. When a baby has trouble taking the breast, you may notice the following:

> » He starts to suckle, then suddenly arches away or appears to sleep (shut down).

> » Superficial sucking, causing nipple distortion, pain, and insufficient milk intake.

» As soon as you take what appears to be a satisfied, sleepy baby away from the breast, he wakes up and screams frantically.

Risk Factors for a Feeding Issue

Check all that apply:

[_] Fetal positions that interfere with breastfeeding, such as breech, and extension rather than tucked-infant posture (tight neck, known as Torticollis).

[_] A baby who was pushed out quickly and forcefully in what is known as a precipitous delivery.

[_] Infant head trauma due to extreme molding, following a long labor and/or extended pushing.

[_] Bruises, lumps, and bumps on the baby's head and/or face following forceps or vacuum delivery. Asymmetry of the face is also a risk factor.

[_] A baby born with a shoulder injury after being stuck in the birth canal (dystocia).

[_] A baby who weighs less than 7 pounds and does not have developed sucking pads in the cheeks that are strong enough to maintain suction.

[_] A baby who cannot organize himself (state organization) due to exposure to certain labor and delivery medications so he cries or sleeps excessively.

[_] A baby with a receding chin—a sign of micronathia.

[_] A baby with a short tongue, possible tongue-tie.

[_] A tongue that protrudes excessively.

[_] A baby who spits-up frequently and may have swallowed amniotic fluid.

[_] A baby that had deep suctioning may have an exaggerated gag reflex.

[_] A baby exposed to artificial nipples, such as pacifiers or bottles.

[_] A baby with a stuffy nose. Infants are obligate nose breathers. They have to let go of the breast to breathe.

[_] A baby who loses more than 4 ounces a day during the first 2 to 4 days.

[_] A baby that has medical issues: illness, jaundice, congenital heart defects, prematurity, neurologic or structural issues (high-arched palate or cleft palate).

[_] A baby born between 36 to 39 weeks, who is sleepy and weighing less than 7 pounds. He may not have the ability to empty the breast.

The nearby box describes several reasons why a baby may have difficultly seeking the breast and holding it in his mouth. Some may impact his ability to thrive. Having a step-by-step plan will guide you through difficult feeds. The goal is to help your baby learn to breastfeed, while at the same time, he gains weight and stimulates your milk production.

General Feeding Plan for the Baby Having Trouble Taking the Breast

1. Before you begin, make sure that your body is comfortable and well supported.

2. Work with your infant for short periods.

3. Undress the baby to his diaper but keep his back covered with a blanket. The exception to undressing is the late preterm infant (born between 35 and 38 weeks) due to increased risk of harmful cold stress (Wambach & Riordan, 2016). Maximize skin-to-skin contact by removing your top and bra. Spend time snuggling with no attempt to latch-on. This will help your baby become alert and stay awake once the feeding begins.

4. When the baby demonstrates feeding cues by putting his hands to his mouth and sucking on them, bring him to the breast. Lean back with the baby on top. If using a more traditional hold, express a bit of breastmilk to the tip of the nipple to entice him. Bring him up to the breast by letting his upper lip brush your nipple. Hold the baby so his chin plants below the nipple on the areola. When you feel his tongue, pull his body to your breast to tuck him close, rather than hold the back of his head.

5. If your baby cries, arches away, or pulls back, stop and calm him. A baby that is forced onto the breast while crying may have difficulty breathing because the tongue is up and back.

6. While he calms, you can allow him to suck on a clean finger. Then, try different positions and both breasts. Some babies are more successful on one breast over the other.

7. Work with your baby only if he is calm and willing to go to the breast. Do not push past his tolerance level or make him latch while he is crying. Working too hard without reward becomes aversive for the baby and that will interfere with success.

8. When he latches-on or makes good attempts, whisper positive reinforcing remarks but try not to distract him with loud cheers.

9. If he does not find success for that feeding, pump and feed the expressed breastmilk.

10. See interest? Try again. Attempt feeds before he is fully awake or crying, whenever possible. Babies commonly achieve the successful latch at night, when you are sleepy and relaxed.

11. Develop and protect your supply. Attempt to breastfeed at least seven times every 24-hours.

12. Until the latch issue is resolved, continue to pump your breasts 8 to 10 times a day until the milk flow stops. To maintain a milk supply, a mother must pump at least twice during the night. Once your milk is fully in and you no longer feel engorged, you can pump less.

13. Keeping a diary of feedings, diaper output, and any supplements will help you assess improvements. Of course, concurrently seek skilled lactation help as soon as possible.

FEEDING CHALLENGES DUE TO NIPPLE SHAPE

The anatomy of the mother's nipple area may challenge a newborn's ability to nurse efficiently. Often, a little work on tailored positioning can help you overcome this challenge. The nearby chart describes some tips for unique nipple anatomy.

TABLE 14.2: Aid for Your Anatomy.

Nipple Type	Mindful Tip
Flat Nipples Do not protrude in a normal state. Appear to blend into the areola. Stand out when stimulated.	If the nipple appears to blend into the areola and does not raise and become firmer with stimulation, it is a flat nipple. If the nipple is soft and stretches easily, flat nipples are not problematic. To make the nipple protrude, pinch the areola with your index and middle fingers while pulling back (see scissors hold). See areolar engorgement for other ideas.
Short, Inelastic Nipples Do not stretch to double their size (less than 7 mm).	Soften the areola with reverse pressure softening. Keep flow going with alternate breast compression. Change nursing positions frequently. Apply a good layer of organic virgin coconut oil on the nipple after nursing. If it hurts you more then the first 10 to 15 seconds of nursing or lesions appear (blisters, cracks, bleeding), seek help from an IBCLC.
Inverted Nipples Have a dimpled look, folding into the areola. They appear concave. A pinch test makes it flatten or bury itself.	If the areola is soft and pliable, an inversion may not be a problem. Otherwise, try pumping before nursing to evert the nipple or use a device that everts the nipple. Help the baby latch by pinching the areola with your index and middle fingers while pulling back (see scissors hold). See an IBCLC for tools to help.
Dimpled Nipples A type of inverted nipple with a partial inversion	The nipple is only partially inverted and usually can be pulled out. Take care to make sure the nipple is dry before putting a pad or your bra back over to cover up.
Double Nipples The nipple appears to have several canal-like separations.	Sandwich the breast in a way that gets the nipples and areola in the baby's mouth. You may need to pump after breastfeeding until the infant's mouth is bigger and able to relieve much of the milk on his own.
Large Nipples Larger than the size of a quarter. Average is 12-15 mm (1/2 inch); large is 16-23 mm (3/4 inch); extra large > 23 mm (Wilson-Clay & Hoover, 2017).	Make sure the baby opens wide before taking the breast. Tilt the nipple towards the baby's upper lip. Lift the breast away from the baby's chin and check that you see his lower lip curled down onto his chin with a part of the areola in his mouth. Listen for audible gulps and swallows to confirm milk transfer. Track that the baby has frequent stools. Try the football hold. You may need to express your milk for a while until the baby grows big enough to efficiently nurse.
Long Nipples Greater than 16-23 mm (3/4 to 1 inch).	The baby may fool you and look like he is nursing. Be sure that you see active feeding, hear the swallows, and notice your breast softens. The baby should have frequent stools (at least four yellow daily).

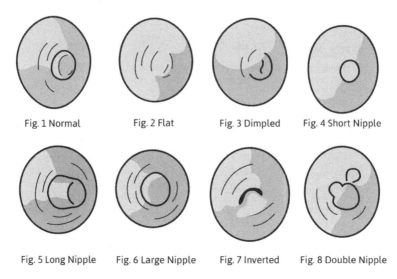

Fig. 1 Normal   Fig. 2 Flat   Fig. 3 Dimpled   Fig. 4 Short Nipple

Fig. 5 Long Nipple   Fig. 6 Large Nipple   Fig. 7 Inverted   Fig. 8 Double Nipple

ILLUSTRATION 14.1 - Nipple Types. Illustration by Ken Tackett.

Flat Nipples

Mothers who have nipples that appear flat do not necessarily have problems if they have an alert, unmedicated baby and the areola is easy to grasp. A recipe for breastfeeding difficulties is a flat-appearing nipple, combined with a thick and firm areola that doesn't stretch, and a sleepy baby, following a labor with complications (Walker, 2014). Newborns nursing on flat nipples can struggle to pull enough breast to form a teat that fills the mouth and stimulates them to suck. This can lead to damaged nipples and inadequate milk intake, so the baby's output should be monitored. Flat nipples can be caused by obesity, genetics, or be a side-effect of breast surgery. In the case of obesity, excessive weight in the breast makes the areola expand, pulling the nipple in. After the onset of lactation, the swollen areola may cause the nipple to appear flattened. Another cause is areolar edema (swelling).

Areolar Engorgement/Edema

To the surprise of many mothers, they notice that their nipples and areolae appear different shortly after delivery. Nipples that protruded have become flat and the areolae appear fuller, as if bulging. This phenomenon is called areolar engorgement or edema. Swelling from absorption of excess fluid given through intravenous administration during delivery is a cause (Mohrbacher, 2010). The swollen areola makes it difficult for the baby to draw it deep into his mouth. Usually, after a few days, the kidneys do their work and get rid of the extra fluid.

So, how do you know you have areolar edema? If you press into your breast with the pads of your fingers, it will leave indentations that don't immediately bounce back. When a baby is unable to nurse during the first or second day due to the breasts or areolae being too full and tight, you might see that he seems more frustrated or restless when trying to nurse. Typically, the baby will bob and bounce his head back and forth because he can't get a good grip of the nipple and areola to pull it into his mouth. Reverse-pressure softening can help move the excess fluid out of the baby's way by relieving over distention (bulging) of the milk ducts. This technique, developed by K. Jean Cotterman, can reduce nipple pain and facilitate breast attachment. Reverse-pressure softening pushes the fluid away from the areola and often triggers the milk to flow. Do not use a breast pump before reverse-pressure softening or hand expression because the pressure is often too much for this tender, swollen skin, and may even draw more fluids to the area, worsening the condition, blocking milk flow, and further damaging your nipples.

How to Perform Reverse-Pressure Softening

1. Lay flat on your back. Starting with one breast, place your fingers at the base of your nipple. Apply gentle but firm pressure on the entire areola, using the pads of your fingers while you press toward the chest wall. Use both hands if your finger nails are too long, placing the pads of your fingers on both sides of the nipple. Press in until it softens, rotating around the entire nipple. Keep the pressure constant for up to 60 seconds each time you press. The fluid will feel like it is shifting backwards, and the skin will start to give under your fingers.

2. Apply pressure again to the softened area. Move your fingers back slowly and continue to apply pressure as you feel softening.

Rotate your pressure around the areola until it is soft and the nipple is pliable. Usually colostrum or milk will start to release.

3. As soon as you feel the areolar area soften, try to nurse or pump. If there is not improvement, try reverse-pressure softening again, this time with more pressure.

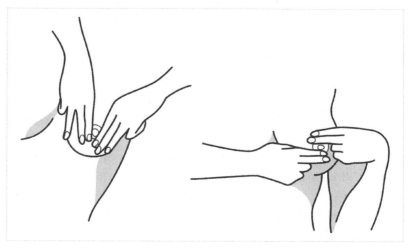

ILLUSTRATION 14.2 - Reverse-Pressure Softening. Illustration by Ken Tackett. Source: Jean and Kyle Cotterman

How to Position the Baby during Areola Edema

Good positioning is key. Mothers often find success with laidback positioning.

1. Try shaping the breast. Pinch the breast between your widely placed index and middle finger, positioned way below the areola.

2. Position the baby so that his chin can plant slightly below your nipple. When you feel his mouth, tuck his body close. The arm cradling the baby should be across his shoulders.

3. Once he starts nursing, you should see gulping. After the first few sucks, it should feel comfortable. If you feel pain, repeat reverse-pressure softening.

Short, Inelastic Nipples

Short nipples that extend less than 7 mm (about 1/4 in) can challenge mothers (Puapornpong et al., 2013). Nipples that lack elasticity can become very sore and traumatized, even when it appears that the baby is positioned correctly. To transfer milk effectively, the infant needs to form a teat from the nipple and the areola, then extend it deep into his mouth. When the nipple does not stretch easily, the baby often abrades the nipple tip with his tongue, causing pain and injury.

Feeding Plan for Short, Inelastic Nipples

1. To help the baby get a deep hold of the areola, lay way back so that he is above the breast. Nursing positions where the baby is under the breast can cause pulling.

2. Make sure the baby's mouth appears wide open on the areola. Pull the breast tissue away and look. The lower lip should be curled down on his chin. You shouldn't feel pain.

3. The baby should be vigorously swallowing. If he starts doing flutter sucks, see if you can increase gulping by gently pushing down along the side of his jaw bone until you feel less pressure on your nipple. Meanwhile, compress different parts of the breast when the baby pauses until softening.

4. If the baby starts looking tired, switch sides.

5. Work with a lactation consultant to see if using a breast shield would be right for you.

Inverted Nipples

Having a flat or inverted nipple is not necessarily a deterrent to successful nursing. Some nipples appear to be inverted but evert with stimulation. The baby should be able to stretch the nipple deep into his mouth and transfer milk. The mother may still be at risk for sore nipples because when the nipple inverts after the baby lets go, it stays wet. The moisture sets up the skin for irritation and infection.

If the nipple does not come out with a pinch test (place your thumb and index finger around the areola at about an inch behind the base of the nipple, then gently pinch the areola), the nipple will bury itself or retract. This is a true inverted nipple. There are degrees of inversion. If the nipple is flexible and easily pulls out, most can nurse. When the nipple is buried, and the surrounding areola is thick and not pliable, it can challenge breastfeeding.

Tips to Overcome Inverted Nipples

» Try Supple Cups (see appendix), which can help evert the nipple when worn for 5 to 10 minutes prior to breastfeeding. The device uses gentle suction to slowly expand the nipple. It can be used during the last 3 weeks of pregnancy with birth attendant or OB approval.

» Avoid pacifiers and bottles. Start expressing your milk if the baby isn't latching and nursing.

» Nurse as soon after birth as possible.

» Avoid engorgement by frequent nursing or pumping.

» Sandwich the breast, holding behind the areola, and push back against your chest wall.

» If it hurts after the baby starts sucking, start over.

» Use a breast pump to pull the nipple out and start milk flow.

» With supervision, a nipple shield may help. It is a thin yet firmer plastic hat that fits over your nipple and areola (see nipple shield). Try to wean off as soon as possible. Once the baby learns that milk comes from the breast, he will try hard to figure out how to attach.

» Be aware that you can overcome this detour in your breast-feeding plan. Keep your milk flowing with regular expression and the baby will start nursing soon.

Dimpled Nipples

A dimpled nipple appears partially inverted but can be unfolded. Since babies do not nipple suck, this type of nipple is usually less problematic, unless the areola is very thick.

How to Overcome Dimpled Nipples

1. Position the baby so that he can plant his chin below the nipple. Unfold the nipple and tilt up.
2. Listen for sucks and swallows. If you feel pain or don't see active feeding, start again.
3. Pump after feeds if the baby doesn't soften the breast.
4. Be sure that the nipple is dry after nursing. Either hold it open or pat dry.

Double Nipples

Some women appear to have divided nipples, connected or separate from each other. Some are non-functioning while others have their own ductal system (Walker, 2014). A tiny newborn can have a hard time getting all the nipple tissue in his mouth. This can affect milk transfer and the mother's comfort with breastfeeding. Multiple nipples can also challenge pumping.

Feeding Plan for Double Nipples

» Using your thumb and forefinger, sandwich the breast just outside the areola, compressing as much as possible so that the baby can get the nipples and areola in his mouth.

» Protect your milk supply by pumping after breastfeeding until your baby is big enough to handle the amount of tissue needed to stimulate the breasts sufficiently.

» Work closely with a lactation consultant to select the correct pump flange kit that fits your unique anatomy so you can avoid causing trauma to the breast.

Long and Large Nipples

Nipples and babies are paired in many sizes and combinations. A small, sleepy baby will be more challenged with a long and large nipple than will a large, hungry, and awake baby. A small newborn nursing on a long nipple (more than an inch or 2.54 cm long) or a large nipple (larger than a quarter) might be challenged to pull the areola deep enough into his mouth to create a vacuum strong enough to draw milk. His superficial grasp will likely cause nipple soreness which, over time, may decrease the mother's milk supply. He could be getting enough to stay hydrated but not substantial nutrition to gain weight. Some babies lose weight.

You can detect this problem if you observe that while nursing the baby doesn't have the whole nipple and some areola in his mouth. You hear infrequent swallows. The baby looks sleepy but when you try to switch breasts or stop feeding, he wakes up and cries. At first, these infants act unsettled but after a few days, they can become passive and less demanding. Mothers with this anatomy are shocked when their baby is weighed, and they learn that he has not gained enough weight, even though they were breastfeeding frequently. To overcome, the baby will need to learn how to have a deeper hold of the nipple. Time is your friend. Most babies will nurse more efficiently as soon as their mouth size increases if their mother continues to breastfeed and pump as much as possible.

Feeding Plan Tips for Long or Large Nipples

» Make sure the baby is wide awake before attempting to nurse.

» Try using a football hold or side-lying position.

» Pull the breast away from the infant's chin to make sure the lower lip is curled down on the chin with some areola gathered in his mouth. Use the breastfeeding checklist on page 25 to assess the nursing position and milk transfer.

» If the baby nurses better on one breast over the other, nurse the preferred and pump the other.

» Check your breast before and after nursing. Did it soften? Is the baby content?

» Log your baby's stool and urine output and cross-check it with the diaper output chart on page 269.

» Pump after nursing and supplement with expressed breast-milk if a test weight on an accurate clinical scale shows inadequate weight gain.

» If the infant's weight gain is inadequate, consider supplementing the baby at your breast until breastfeeding improves (see supplementer-at-the-breast on page 240).

» Keeping your baby at the breast for frequent feeds will preserve breastfeeding as you give time a chance to fix the problem.

NURSING DIFFICULTIES DUE TO THE BABY

Some babies have a weak tongue that is more visible than usual or a very strong tongue that retracts. A retracted tongue does not come forward and covers the baby's lower gum while breastfeeding. You will know because it feels like he is biting down on your nipple. These are issues beyond the scope of this book. For any one of these conditions, you will need a plan of care from a skilled lactation consultant in conjunction with a pediatric occupational therapist, physical therapist, or speech pathologist that has Neurodevelopmental Training to work with infant sucking and swallowing skills.

Infant Anatomy or Nursing Style

There are times when the way the baby's body is injured or molded (shaped) at birth affects breastfeeding. You'll need to reflect on his experience thus far and make some observations. You might notice that his head is flat on one side or one part of his face is fuller than the other. Did he have a shoulder or clavicle injury at birth? Is his face severely bruised? When he nurses, does he easily lose the breast, or do you feel his gums bite after he latches? Were you told that he is a tongue sucker? If so, you will feel a very weak tug of your nipple when the baby nurses and see a dimple in his cheek. Does he have a tight neck that impacts his ability to turn his head to one side?

All of the above, plus many other newborn variations and injuries, can lead to suckling issues. With any of these or other muscular skeletal variations, the baby's milk intake and weight gain can be impacted because it takes a tremendous amount of muscles and nerves in the head, neck, and shoulders to nurse effectively. It also takes a copious milk supply, and a well and alert baby. Some mothers have so much milk that, early on, some of these sucking problems are missed. The following are a few suggestions for the more common sucking issues seen in practice. Always seek professional help if you suspect any of the previously mentioned issues.

Trouble on Left or Right Breast

A newborn may reject one breast if he was injured during labor and delivery, or if neck muscles are tight from the way he was positioned in the womb (Kroeger & Smith, 2004). If your baby has a strong preference for turning to the right or left, or trouble feeding on one side, have the infant examined for a possible broken clavicle or torticollis (tight neck). Other uncommon reasons for breast rejection are facial asymmetry or facial paralysis. With this condition, one side of the baby's cheeks and jaw appear fuller than the other. When there is an injured facial nerve, the baby's smile appears crooked and milk leaks out the side of the mouth. Milk let-down may be overwhelming for this baby.

Feeding Plan for Breast Rejection

» Have the infant examined by his healthcare provider. Point out that he can't take the breast into his mouth on one side.

» Maintain the milk supply in the affected breast by hand expression or an electric pump.

» See a lactation consultant to develop a feeding plan.

» If the baby nurses well on one side, keep his body positioned in the same direction on the more difficult side. This is when knowing the football hold is helpful.

» Request a referral to an occupational therapist or physical therapist trained to treat infants.

Most babies eventually take both breasts. Have peace of mind— babies can get enough nourishment from one breast. If this is a long-term issue, the body will likely compensate and fluctuate the supply to be greater in the breast that is used the most. Be aware that rejecting one breast is rarely a sign of a medical problem in that breast. If the problem persists, have your health professional thoroughly examine that breast to be sure.

Poor Suction at the Breast

A baby needs to have a strong hold of the nipple, so his jaw and tongue can work together to milk the breast without letting go. He must use this suction to pull the nipple and areola deep into his mouth and hold it there while he lifts and lowers his jaw. A baby that does not have a strong suction will easily let go of the breast, then cry. Often, he will choke and cough when his mother's milk lets-down because he isn't controlling the flow. He will most likely not adequately milk the breast, which could lead to slow or no weight gain. For the mother, it could potentially cause delayed onset of milk production and, overall, a decreased milk supply.

How to Examine Your Baby for Weak Suction

If you notice that your baby is very sleepy at the breast, coughs, and easily lets the nipple fall out of his mouth, do the following:

1. Check his mouth. Does his palate (roof) look deep instead of domed and shallow?

2. Let the baby suck on a clean finger. Does the finger easily come out of his mouth? Your finger should be pressed tightly against his upper mouth and feel surrounded by his tongue. When his tongue moves, your finger should stay in place. In most instances, a strong suction will require you to break suction to remove your finger, unless the baby has fallen asleep.

3. Does the infant easily slip off the breast? While nursing, gently press against your baby's forehead. If he comes right off, unless asleep, it is most likely due to weak suction.

Feeding Plan for Poor Suction

If you think a high-arched palate or weak suction is the problem, you will need to have skilled assistance. In the meantime, do the following:

1. Start expressing your breasts with a clinical-grade pump after nursing.
2. Have the baby examined and weighed. If the weight gain is insufficient, start feeding the baby extra milk (see supplementation for amounts). With tongue issues, a Dr. Brown bottle works well. If this is discovered before your milk comes in, small amounts of colostrum are best fed with a spoon (see spoon-feeding on page 248).
3. Keep track of the infant's stools and wet diapers.
4. Feeding in a football hold, laid-back position, or side-lying is usually most effective.
5. Support the breast or lean way back with the baby on top.

TONGUE- AND LIP-TIES

Today, tongue-ties (ankyloglossia) and lip-ties are commonly diagnosed. The rational for surgery for anything other than classic tongue-tie, described later, is based upon interpretation of dated ultrasound function of the tongue and lips, claiming that this procedure will correct breastfeeding challenges and prevent other potential problems of the teeth and oral cavity. The practitioners cite studies that have poor scientific validity to justify a surgical procedure (Douglas, 2013). Tongue-tie clinics have since sprung up all over the world.

Expensive alternative treatments, such as cranial sacral and chiropractic care, are being recommended to augment the surgery. In some instances, surgery is repeated as many as 3 to 5 times without fixing the breastfeeding problem. When the baby's wound heals closed instead of remaining an open-V-shape at the base (the practitioner's goal), the parents may be blamed for not following post-surgical instructions to use their fingers to lift and stretch the raw wound to prevent closure.

It is interesting to note that pediatric medicine has shifted from not recognizing a classic tongue-tie, which is known to impact tongue function, to identifying many of the normal variations of tongue and lip as a pathological deviation (Douglas, 2013). As Douglas says, it is wonderful that well-meaning practitioners have turned our attention to the many functions of the infant's tongue, but unfortunate that so many babies are being treated for conditions that are not proven scientifically based.

What Is a Frenulum?

During fetal development, the frenulum anchors the forming lips and tongue. As the fetus matures, the frenulum moves back and frees the tongue for movement. In some infants, this band is short, thick, and/or inelastic, restricting the tongue's movement, known as a tongue-tie. It is important to note that there are many variations of "normal" lip and tongue appearances—just look inside the mouths of those close to you.

How does the tongue move and why is it so important? Until recently, it was thought that a stripping movement of the tongue was essential to remove milk (Woolridge et al., 1986). The interpretation was that the tongue tip stayed forward and squeezed the milk out of milk sinuses, located behind the nipple, by lifting and gently waving. It was thought that the base of the tongue needed to be free to lift against the palate (upper mouth). It was also believed that a wide mouth or gap was important before bringing the baby to the breast.

A recent review demonstrated that when we use the baby's natural reflexes in conjunction with instinctive maternal holding, the baby doesn't open wide, but rather, when he feels the nipple and areola with his lips and chin, automatically, his mouth opens, and his tongue scoops the areola tissue into his mouth. With each suckle, the breast goes deeper in the baby's mouth and the lips act as a seal (Douglas & Geddes, 2018). The tongue moves in unison with the jaw, dropping to create a vacuum. Downward motion and the mother's let-down fills the baby's mouth with milk. It is the created vacuum, not the tongue action, that moves the milk. Then, the mid-tongue lifts to join the baby's palate to seal the upper mouth, and lifts against the breast with the lower jaw to seal off the flow while the baby swallows.

To optimize nursing, the baby's body needs to be fully supported while the mother holds the infant in a way that gives him freedom to move. Often, we swaddle babies, which restricts needed arm-movement. Sometimes the mother's fingers, which are supporting the breast, are in the baby's chin space. When the baby attempts to take the breast, he can't get a deep enough hold, resulting in frustration. Meanwhile, the baby gets tense, his mouth and entire body tighten, retracting or humping the tongue. He fusses, arches, or may even shut down.

Observing these infant behaviors in conjunction with maternal nipple pain have made professionals search for answers. Tests to evaluate infant mouth function during breastfeeding have been developed based on muscle action we thought was necessary for breastfeeding (Hazelbaker, 1993). A recent study found that tongue-tie is not a common source of breastfeeding problems. It emphasized the importance of holding the baby correctly. Researchers examined the tongues of 200 healthy babies during their first 3 days of life, using an infant tongue-tie identification tool, known as the Coryllos Tongue-Tie Classification System (Coryllos, 2004). Researchers were blinded to any breastfeeding problems. They found that 199 of the 200 babies were identified with one of the four types of tongue-tie. However, only 3.5% (7 babies) had breastfeeding problems related to tongue restriction (Haham et al., 2014). A tongue-tie revision solved the breastfeeding problem in only 5 of these 7 babies. Considering this new research, it seems that surgery is not the immediate solution. We need to go back to feeding on-cue in conjunction with finding ways to comfortably and effectively breastfeed, based on anatomy.

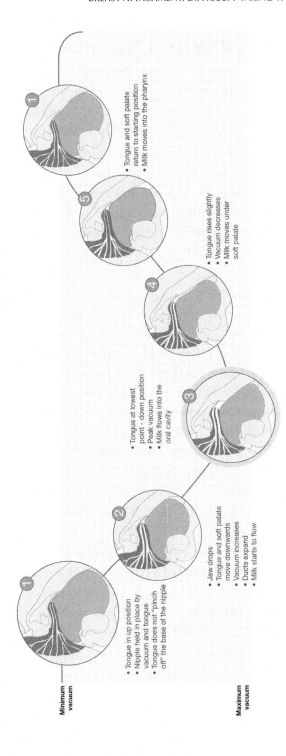

- Tongue in up position
- Nipple held in place by vacuum and tongue
- Tongue does not "pinch off" the base of the nipple

- Jaw drops
- Tongue and soft palate move downwards
- Vacuum increases
- Ducts expand
- Milk starts to flow

- Tongue at lowest point - down position
- Peak vacuum
- Milk flows into the oral cavity

- Tongue rises slightly
- Vacuum decreases
- Milk moves under soft palate

- Tongue and soft palate return to starting position
- Milk moves into the pharynx

Minimum vacuum

Maximum vacuum

ILLUSTRATION 14.3 - Anatomy & Physiology of Lactation & Milk Removal.
Source: ©Medela 2018. Used with Permission.

How Do I Know My Baby Has a Tongue-Tie?

The classic tongue-tie is fairly easy to see. The tongue tip will appear heart-shaped. You will see a small strip of skin in the middle of the tongue that anchors it to the floor of the mouth. When the baby cries, the tongue won't lift. He will not be able to stick his tongue out. This type of tongue-tie is a simple fix with scissors in the hand of a trained professional.

The type of tongue-tie that is questionable is the hidden-posterior tongue-tie. This type of tie is more often felt rather than seen. The examiner will lift the tongue and feel for a speedbump. This type of tie is deeper and needs more aggressive surgery with intensive aftercare.

There is much more to this assessment that can determine whether your baby's attachment issues are a result of a tongue-tie or perhaps another issue, like torticollis. Did you have a long, difficult delivery, resulting in a sleepy baby with a bruised head? Was the baby's shoulder stuck in the birth canal? Does he keep his head turned to one side or prefer one breast over the other? An affirmation to any of these questions is a possible cause to your baby's trouble and should be checked. This, combined with your own anatomy, will influence how well your baby nurses and whether you experience nipple pain or breastfeeding issues. For instance, a mother with poor stretch of her nipple skin will experience more pain. If your milk is delayed in coming in, your tense baby will suck harder and more often, trying to help get the milk going.

If your baby is diagnosed with more than a simple classic tongue-tie, give yourself and your baby time before allowing a deep surgical incision. After your milk comes in, the engorgement abates, and the baby recovers from birth, all may improve. Meanwhile, if you are in pain or your baby is not thriving, feed him your expressed milk (see supplementation).

Lip-Ties

Another oral area of concern is that of lip-ties. Treatment is being recommended with the objective of a more comfortable and effective breastfeeding experience. Parents are told that it may prevent tooth decay from trapped food, and the later need for braces. Surgically releasing a lip-tie in a young baby is based upon the belief that the lip needs to flange. In actuality, a flanged lip will decrease the mouth opening. Notice how you can't open your mouth wide when your lips are flanged. In infants, the upper-lip frenulum is more prominent and typically recedes as the baby grows. Good dental hygiene and preventative care with help deter future issues. It is only a problem if it is so rigid and thick that the lip has no mobility.

Blaming breastfeeding problems on the appearance of the baby's tongue or lips is a simple explanation for a complex process with potentially many consequences for the mother and baby (Douglas, 2013). How a baby's mouth fits on his mother's unique anatomy is a learning process. Usually, time and patience will get you to your breastfeeding goals.

NEWBORN BEHAVIORAL CONCERNS

Disinterest in Nursing

The First 24 Hours – A Baby Without Risk Factors

During the first day, some newborns are reluctant to nurse, appearing disinterested in breastfeeding. They are more curious about looking around and resting. If you have a totally healthy baby that is term and asymptomatic following a low-risk pregnancy and uncomplicated vaginal delivery, keep the baby skin-to-skin and look for feeding cues. Every time he nuzzles up to the breast, encourage him to feed but don't force him. In a hospital setting, where protocols must be met, staff may tend to push the baby to breastfeed. This can create a breast aversion—it's virtually taking a normal behavior and turning it into a dysfunction. Hand expressing a little colostrum to the tip of the nipple can offer a scent attraction to entice your newborn to the breast. Minimize distractions and promote private bonding by asking visitors to leave, and darkening and quieting the room. Typically, after a day, these babies "wake up" and breastfeed vigorously, and often, for the next 12 to 24 hours. Be prepared for the feeding frenzy. However, if your newborn is still disinterested after 24 hours, start the following protocol.

Plan for Disinterested Newborn with No Risk Factors after 24 Hours

1. Insist that the infant be evaluated by the baby's medical practitioner.

2. If you have any risk factors for low milk supply, hand express your colostrum as soon as possible after birth and every few hours around the clock until your baby starts nursing. Begin supplementation.

3. As the milk starts increasing in volume, start expressing your breasts regularly (8 to 10 times per 24 hours) with a multi-user (hospital-grade), double-electric breast pump.

The First 24 Hours - High-Risk Infant

A baby reluctant to nurse during the first day may have a problem when there are risk factors. Consider your medical history. Did you have a high-risk pregnancy? Did you have an infection during your pregnancy, such as beta strep, treated with antibiotics during your labor? Were you given a lot of pain medication during labor? Was your second stage of labor (pushing) longer than 4 hours? Did you have an instrument delivery with the use of a vacuum or forceps? Was the baby born before 40 weeks? Do you see any lumps, bruising, or bumps on your newborn's head or skeletal bones? If you can answer yes to any of the preceding questions, it may take your baby longer to begin nursing. Focus on the following action plan.

Immediate Plan for Disinterested Baby with High-Risk Factors

1. Be sure the infant gets a medical evaluation, particularly for any observed symptoms.

2. Keep your newborn skin-to-skin and hand express some colostrum to the nipple.

3. Start hand-expressing or pumping your milk right away (at least 8 to 10 times in 24 hours) to jumpstart your milk supply and preserve it.

4. Spoon or dropper-feed your baby to keep him nourished and hydrated (see supplementation).

5. Although you may feel disappointed, realize that your newborn is just not ready. Don't force the baby to breastfeed. Choose patience over giving up.

Breast Refusal after Day 2

If the baby was taking the breast and suddenly begins to refuse it after 2 to 4 days, check for engorgement. Infants often seem mystified by the change of texture in the breast. When the breast is too firm, the little mouth may have a hard time grasping it. The milk flow from a full breast can overwhelm the baby. Engorgement needs to be relieved. Laid-back nursing and reverse-pressure softening can help. If the baby continues to refuse the breast, seek professional help.

Eager but Struggling to Take the Breast

Some babies are eager to nurse but become frustrated in their attempts to take the breast. They typically try to attach, and either shut down or scream while arching and pushing away. It can feel like a wrestling match. Mothers say, they feel rejected by their baby, or think their newborn finds their nipple unappealing. Do the following assessments:

» Are your areolae still swollen? See reverse-pressure softening on page 299. Is your baby able to lift both arms? An injured shoulder or fractured clavicle can make the infant scream at the breast.

» Are you waiting too long to nurse, resulting in a tense, over-eager baby?

» Does the infant sound congested? If his nose is blocked, he will let go of the breast. Babies are nose-breathers and have trouble breathing through their mouth.

If the behavior continues following these interventions, see his medical practitioner for an assessment and seek lactation help.

The Good-Baby Syndrome

Because of our cultural expectations, there is a belief that a content, well-fed baby sleeps and cries when hungry. The "Good Baby" has subtle feeding cues. When hungry, instead of rooting and crying, he self-soothes by sucking on his tongue or hands. If not responded to and brought to the breast frequently, these babies are at risk for insufficient or low weight gain. Many a mother has been shocked to find that their "good baby" is still under birthweight when they bring the infant to their medical practitioner for a well-baby examination.

Tips to Overcome Underfeeding the Calm Baby

» Be sure to offer the breast on a regular basis.

» Baby watch so you don't miss the subtle early-feeding cues.

» Encourage the baby to nurse when your breasts signal you (feeling firmer or leaking).

Fussy Baby

An unhappy baby who wants to nurse all the time may not be getting enough to eat due to poor milk transfer or insufficient milk supply. This is usually seen after the first week. Fussiness is a problem if the baby has had excessive weight loss. Evaluate yourself for minimal engorgement, sore nipples, or even a lack of soreness. The potential cause could be a large nipple, hypotonic tongue, high-arched palate, or tight frenulum. If you have one or more risk factors for low milk supply, it would be appropriate to take this into consideration, although your body still needs to be given a chance to produce an adequate milk supply, which could take up to 10 weeks.

Brand new babies that consistently fuss every time they are put in the nursing position should be checked by a medical professional for any evidence of birth trauma, such as a broken clavicle, hematoma, torticollis, or shoulder dystocia. Make sure the baby is breathing well at the breast. To overcome these problems, first seek an assessment from your medical professional to eliminate medical causes, and in conjunction, work with a breastfeeding professional.

Difficult to Calm

Some babies have rapid state changes. They are instantly hungry without much warning. Calming enough to nurse may be a challenge. If your baby cries a lot, doesn't seem content overall, and you are experiencing very tender nipples, seek professional help and try the following.

Plan for the Difficult-to-Calm Baby

1. Reduce noise, visitors, and light. Ask for the baby to be examined again for any birth injuries. Try swaddling for the latch, and then loosen the swaddle once the baby is relaxed.

2. Offer the breast every few hours.

3. If the baby is stuck in a crying state, don't try to force him to the breast. Instead, first swaddle, go to a dark quiet room, and rock him. Once he is calm, very slowly and carefully turn the baby into the breast. Express a little milk to the tip of the nipple and see if he will latch on. Usually, this will work. If not, start over.

4. If this is happening frequently in a 24-hour period and you find that the baby isn't nursing at least seven times, start expressing your milk on a regular basis.

5. If this problem persists, seek skilled help and support to overcome it.

Sleepy Baby

As previously described, during the first 24 hours after birth, a healthy term baby will do one or two good feeds, then behave sleepily for the next 10 to 20 hours. On the second day, the baby should wake up and start being much more demanding and eager to nurse frequently. It is normal for newborns to need more help staying awake during a feed. The baby who wakes up, does short feeds, and quickly falls asleep, seeming to never finish a meal, needs to be assessed for a proper attachment at the breast. Check to make sure that the baby has a good hold of the areola, nipple, and breast, and you hear audible swallows. You'll know attachment is a factor if, shortly after falling asleep, the baby wakes right back up and acts like he never had a meal.

A sleepy baby is very hard to wake up, will nurse for a short time, and then quickly fall asleep. If your baby seems to sleep a lot and you have very tender nipples, seek professional help. He may not be eating enough. Swaddling in the first few days can keep a baby from waking up and eating as often as he should, so keep a sleepy baby un-swaddled. If you are on pain meds, try to time them with the feeds to reduce the level of medication that gets into your breastmilk. The pain medication is at its highest level in your body 2 hours after you take it. Ask your healthcare provider about substituting Ibuprofen. It won't make the baby sleepy.

It takes time (up to 15 to 20 minutes) and patience to wake a sleepy baby. Dr. Katherine Barnard describes several ways to help, called variety-to-awaken techniques. Babies are programed to seek your face and to hear your voice. Follow these steps slowly and watch for cues to make sure your efforts are not having the opposite effect (i.e., the baby pushes his hand toward your face, making a halt sign, or falls into a deeper sleep).

Variety-to-Awaken Techniques

1. Start slowly by taking off the baby's blanket. Then, undress the infant.

2. Put your face 7 to 8 inches away from your baby.

3. Talk to him and vary your voice, making it high or low.

4. Sit your baby up.

5. Gently brush his cheek (Barnard & Thomas, 2014).

Be aware that excess sleepiness could indicate a sign of illness. Call the baby's medical provider if he doesn't arouse for feedings or his breastfeeding patterns change.

The Baby Makes Clicking Sounds

Many babies make a loud clicking sound while nursing. If this behavior doesn't cause you pain and the infant is thriving, it is just an annoyance and may embarrass you a little when in public. Babies that click during milk let-down may be overwhelmed by the flow, so they use their tongue to push back and slow it. If this is the case, leaning way back will help decrease the clicking. If it causes nipple pain, examine your baby's mouth. Does he appear to have a tongue-tie or high palate? If you suspect this may be a cause, see a breastfeeding consultant for an evaluation. If the baby clicks and you see a dimple in the cheek, the baby is most likely tongue-sucking. To test for tongue-sucking, gently pull your breast away from the baby. A well-positioned baby won't let go. If the baby easily lets go, unless done feeding, it indicates inappropriate suction. Most often, the tongue-sucking baby will continue sucking his tongue when you take him off the breast. If you have nipple trauma from the baby clicking, and the following treatment plans do not help, see a skilled lactation consultant.

How to Overcome a Clicking Problem

» For too much milk, do laid-back or side-lying positioning.

» For the tongue-sucking baby, let him suck on your finger before the breast. Offer a clean finger with the pad up against the baby's palate. Once he begins sucking, gently press down on the tongue and stroke forward. If he gags, stop. Try slipping the baby on the breast after.

» Some babies click due to a sore and bruised head following a difficult and/or vacuum delivery, or from being stuck in the birth canal too long. A lot of molding or a cephalohematoma (soft swelling under the scalp, where blood is confined to one bone) can cause the tongue to not work correctly. This is something you'll need to seek skilled lactation support for.

NIPPLE SHIELD: APPROPRIATE USE OR MISUSE

A nipple shield is a thin, silicone, nipple-shaped cover that fits over the nipple. They come in various sizes and shapes. The shields are used for difficulty taking the breast, infant suckling issues, sore nipples, and transitioning from bottle-feeding to the breast. Years ago, shields were thicker and larger. Their usage often lowered infant weight gain and diminished many a mother's milk supply, endangering the babies' lives. Lactation consultants were proactive regarding this issue and able to impact retail sales, causing the shields to disappear from store shelves and maternity hospitals. More recently, a thinner shield was developed. It came in a larger selection of sizes. Infants were able to nurse more efficiently with these shields and several studies showed that the baby's weight gain was equal to those nursing without the shield (Chertok, 2009). Once again, nipple-shield use is increasing. History repeats itself and we are once more debating their overuse and safety. From clinical experience, shields are useful if chosen for appropriate reasons, combined with careful follow-up and weaning from their usage as soon as possible.

How to Use a Nipple Shield

Do try to avoid using one until your milk is in. Be aware that the artificial nipple shape and texture of the shield may impact the baby's sucking skill. Marsha Walker, RN, IBCLC, cautions that special cells in the infant's mucus membranes produce sensory cues, such as shape, texture, curvature, and edges to form a neural (brain) image in the infant's mouth (Walker, 2016). Babies adapt their sucking skills on this neural memory, so it can potentially change the baby's sucking pattern. See a skilled lactation profession to have the shield fitted correctly. There should be a gap between the end of your nipple and the end of the crown of the nipple shield.

How to Use a Nipple Shield

1. To apply the shield, do the following, or your baby's strong suction will pull your nipple into the holes and cause nipple injury.

   » Position any cut-outs where the baby's nose will touch the breast.

   » Sit the shield on the nipple. Have the brim turned up, facing away from the nipple. Press the nipple portion of the shield into your nipple, then while spreading your fingers around the diameter, snuggly pull the brim onto your breast. It should suction on.

   » Moistening the edges may help hold it in place. Use either hot water, coconut oil, or lanolin.

   » Express some milk into the nipple portion to entice the baby.

2. Understand that your baby drinking milk at your breast when using the shield is key to success. Look for the following:

   » The baby's mouth is open wide.

   » His chin is pressed into your breast.

   » The baby's lips are over the brim of the nipple shield, not just the nipple portion. The infant's lower lip is curled down on his chin and you see long draws of your milk. You should see the baby's smooth, round cheek against your breast. If you observe a deep indentation around the nipple portion of the shield and the brim pulls away from your breast, it usually indicates that the baby is not nursing correctly. If he is sleepy while nursing and you don't hear gulps, reposition the infant. If you still don't hear long draws of milk, supplement your baby.

» You see an active suck/pause rhythm and hear audible swallows.

» The baby is content after nursing. Your nipple is not sore and does not appear abraded.

» You should see milk in the shield when the baby comes off the breast.

3. Clean your hands, then wash the shield with hot, soapy water. Dry and store it in a clean container. Keep the shield out of reach of pets. Many a mother has needed to replace their shield after it was taken by their pet and became a chew toy.

4. Have the baby weighed at least twice a week to assess weight gain. Monitor his stool output. If the number of stools decreases, have the infant weighed again.

5. Remember, continuous use can result in a poor milk supply for yourself and inadequate weight gain in your baby. The shield is to be used as a temporary nursing aid and should be discontinued as soon as possible.

CHAPTER FIFTEEN

Cause for Concern: Overcoming Early Medical Problems

Chapter Goal: Protect your milk supply during stressful times.

MEDICAL HURDLES

After a safe delivery and a short go at breastfeeding, many parents are surprised by results of laboratory tests that show cause for concern. The required treatment may interrupt breastfeeding and possibly separate the mother and baby, requiring an alternate method to feed the infant. A mother may feel like the treatment, although medically necessary, is hampering their start with breastfeeding. Realize that these are usually slight detours. With the right care, your precious baby will be nuzzling up to nurse in no time. The following briefly details some of the most common medical problems that arise during the newborn's first week.

JAUNDICE

Normal Physiologic Jaundice

Almost all newborns have skin that appears slightly yellow on the second day of life, increasing in intensity by 36 to 48 hours (ABM, 2017). It is typically harmless and goes away during the first 2 weeks of life. This is not illness but the norm. Looking at these babies; you will see that they are active and eating well. Some researchers postulate that this yellow glow, known as jaundice, has an anti-inflammatory effect (Vitek & Ostrow, 2009).

Jaundice stems from special red blood cells the fetus needs to provide more oxygen for his developing body. The cells are constantly produced and broken down, then excreted through the placenta. After birth, the baby's lungs take over this function and these unnecessary fetal red blood cells are replaced by mature red blood cells. The extra fetal blood cells are then broken down and need to be eliminated. The byproduct of red cell break down is bilirubin. Our bodies constantly break down and eliminate red blood cells. The liver steadily processes the bilirubin and then we excrete it through urine and stools. A new baby's liver, however, is immature and, often, the bilirubin gets ahead of the system. The reddish-brown colored bilirubin gets stored in the baby's fat for later processing, giving the skin its yellow glow. Increasing levels of the excess bilirubin found in the blood are correlated with yellowing of the newborn's eyes, skin, urine, and stools. High levels can cause toxicity and illness.

The sooner the baby clears his intestines of meconium (the first stools), the less likely he will develop an exaggerated form of physiological jaundice. Colostrum has a laxative effect and can stimulate the passage of bilirubin-rich stools, preventing it from being reabsorbed by the baby's intestines (Mohrbacher, 2010). The trick is getting the colostrum into your newborn's stomach and ruling out other factors that cause high bilirubin, such as infant bruising, prematurity, mother-infant blood incompatibility, or illness. The most common cause of jaundice in healthy breastfeeding newborns is poor feeding. The baby is at the breast but not doing a good job. If a baby is becoming sleepy, not waking up to eat, has yellowing skin, and is not stooling, he is most likely not getting enough to eat.

Problematic Jaundice

When a baby is sleepy and not nursing well from the start, or the mother's milk is slow to come in, he may develop jaundice, caused by a lack of breastmilk, because he isn't eating enough to have bowel movements and thus, reabsorbs the excess bilirubin (ABM, 2017). The baby then develops hyperbilirubinemia, or levels of harmful bilirubin. The high levels make the newborn too sleepy to eat, which then results in less urine and stool output. The baby's body continues to reabsorb the bilirubin and it builds up in his blood.

Breastmilk Jaundice Syndrome

Some breastfed babies develop a safe form of jaundice, known as breastmilk jaundice syndrome (ABM, 2017). These infants show yellowing of the skin after the fourth day, which lasts up to 12 weeks (ABM, 2017). They are, otherwise, healthy and gaining weight. The cause of breastmilk jaundice is not totally understood but scientists believe that it's linked to an enzyme. With continued successful breastfeeding, it goes away naturally and varies from baby to baby. It is important to make sure breastfeeding is going well. Breastmilk jaundice should be monitored by the pediatrician to prevent toxicity caused by high bilirubin levels. Some doctors may suggest formula-feeding to prove this diagnosis or to speed up the treatment. If this occurs, express your breastmilk as frequently as the baby eats (at least 8 times daily). Typically, doctors will not interrupt breastfeeding if the diagnosis is breastmilk jaundice.

Hyperbilirubinemia: Breastfeeding During Treatment

Your medical provider will consider many factors before starting treatment to prevent or decrease harmful bilirubin levels. It will depend upon the baby's age in hours and how fast the blood bilirubin level is increasing. The baby's physical appearance and history are very important. Skilled medical professionals are aware of the health factors in both mother and baby that put babies at risk for this condition. A yellow appearance at birth is a sign of newborn illness and will alert your caregivers. Rarely, extremely elevated levels of bilirubin can cause brain damage. There are signs that warn us this condition is developing. The babies are very lethargic, difficult to arouse, and have poor feeding behavior.

Light therapy is the usual treatment for elevated bilirubin in conjunction with good feeding (hydration) and monitoring the blood levels of the bilirubin. Babies wear eyepatches to protect their eyes from the ultraviolet light. The Academy of Breastfeeding Medicine (ABM) recommends that babies be kept with their mothers and allowed to breastfeed without the light and eyepatches for 30-minute intervals. Breastfeeding should be evaluated to assure that the baby is feeding well. If he needs to be supplemented, it should first be his mother's own milk, next choice being human donor milk, and the last resort is formula (ABM, 2017).

In the United States, the American Academy of Pediatrics recommends that all babies have either a formal risk assessment for high levels of bilirubin or are tested for a bilirubin blood level before hospital discharge. Many hospitals follow the protocol set by the Joint Commission of Hospitals, requiring a screening bilirubin test at 36 hours of age. Of course, it is done sooner if any abnormal jaundice is noticed.

How to Reduce the Risk of Lack of Breastmilk Jaundice

Not all jaundice can be prevented but the risk of your baby developing starvation jaundice can be greatly reduced by following the ABM's protocol (ABM, 2017):

» Breastfeed within the first hour after birth.

» Feed frequently and respond to early hunger cues.

» Breastfeed exclusively and avoid giving your baby a pacifier.

» Be sure that your baby is nursing correctly and seek professional help to correct any issues.

Remember, the more food babies eat, the more they excrete. You can motivate your infant to eat more often by having skin-to-skin contact. Your warmth and smell will encourage feeding and arouse the newborn to nuzzle up to the breast and latch on, even in a sleepy state.

HYPOGLYCEMIA

Hypoglycemia means low levels of glucose (a type of sugar) in the blood. Research shows that nearly all newborns experience a safe level of low blood sugar following separation from the womb until they begin nursing with good milk transfer (Srinivasan et al., 1986). Healthy term newborns have a natural mechanism, called "counter-regulation," that produces its own form of energy to protect the brain and organs until the baby receives his mother's colostrum (Hawdon et al., 1992). This natural adaptation essentially provides a grace period during the first hours after birth until the newborn breastfeeds and glucose levels rise at about 24 hours postpartum (Hawdon et al., 1992). The Academy of Breastfeeding Medicine says that healthy term newborns without significant risk factors do not require blood glucose monitoring. In fact, the ABM, along with many other world authorities, believe that testing these babies would be disruptive to early breastfeeding. If you follow the subsequent ABM recommendations, you will help your baby's glucose levels return to normal and prevent complications.

How to Limit Abnormal Hypoglycemia (Wight et al., 2014)

1. Breastfeed by 30 to 60 minutes after birth.

2. Spend the first hour skin-to-skin to help your baby conserve his energy needed to stay warm.

3. Bring your baby to the breast on-cue before he begins to cry.

4. If he is willing, breastfeed 10 to 12 times per 24 hours for the first few days of life.

5. Breastfeed exclusively and avoid routine supplementation of water, glucose water, or formula to prevent interfering with the body's normal metabolic compensation.

Clinical Hypoglycemia

Babies with risk factors for a harmful form of hypoglycemia should be tested to prevent complications (Wight et al., 2014). Maternal risk factors include diabetes (gestational or type 1), a complicated and stressful labor and delivery, some drug treatments, and a medical problem identified during pregnancy. Infant risk factors for hypoglycemia include prematurity, low birthweight, a baby that is small or large for gestational age, and an infant who is stressed at birth and showing signs of low blood sugar. What specific levels and duration of low blood glucose can cause brain damage is still unknown (Wight et al., 2014). In a maternal/child hospital setting, medical staff is trained to assess your baby for signs of hypoglycemia.

If your newborn is diagnosed with clinical hypoglycemia but is not symptomatic, ideally, you would breastfeed with good milk transfer every 1 to 2 hours. If this is not happening, your baby would be given expressed breastmilk, donor pasteurized human milk, or formula. After a certain amount of time, the blood would be tested again. If the newborn's blood sugar level results are still low (below 20 to 25 mg/dL) and he is showing symptoms of hypoglycemia, then IV therapy will likely be started. The Academy of Breastfeeding Medicine recommends that the baby remain skin-to-skin while you continue breastfeeding with this treatment. The goal of any treatment is to reach an ideal blood glucose concentration between 40 and 50 mg/dL or higher that can be maintained, even if the baby sleeps for 4 hours (Wight et al., 2014). During this course, keep your infant as close as possible. If he can't feed well, ask the hospital to provide you with a double-electric breast pump so that you can express your milk and maintain production when feedings are missed, or the baby is supplemented with something other than your milk.

These conditions are frightening and may leave you feeling like your baby is ill and vulnerable for a long time. Make sure you talk about this with a professional and feel comfortable getting your questions about your baby's health answered. Parents who do not get this kind of emotional/informational support are at risk of becoming overly anxious about their baby's health (Chambers et al., 2011).

Communicating with Your Doctor

If your doctor tells you to do something, be sure to ask why and for how long. Then ask, "when do you want to see us again?" It's very important to be your baby's advocate in today's medical climate, where doctors have to see many patients a day to cover high overhead costs in the face of low insurance reimbursements. Request a copy of your reports and take a good look at them. If there is any confusion, go back and ask questions. Not that you shouldn't trust your doctor, but mistakes do happen with computerized charting. It's as simple as a wrong click or drop-down selection.

BABIES DISCHARGED BETWEEN 34 AND 38 WEEKS GESTATIONAL AGE

Babies born earlier than expected, then discharged after a few days, are still immature and should be monitored closely. Why include these babies in a book about term babies? For many years, it was thought that it was safe to induce labor or schedule C-sections earlier than 40 weeks. Several years ago, research and awareness began increasing about risks and complications that occur when treating early babies like term newborns. In the well area of the mother/baby hospital floor, routine care means less observation for complications and inappropriate preventative education. In 2013, the American Association of Obstetrics and Gynecology recommended new guidelines for the safe gestational age to induce or schedule a planned cesarean beginning at 39 weeks. This change reflects a growing body of research findings, showing that key developmental processes occur between 37 weeks and 39 weeks. The use of "term" previously indicated gestation between 37 weeks and 42 weeks. It has been replaced with these gestational age designations (Walker, 2017):

> » Late preterm: Babies born 34 to 36 weeks
> » Early-term: Babies born 37 weeks through 38 weeks and 6 days
> » Full-term: Babies born 39 weeks through 40 weeks and 6 days
> » Late-term: Babies born 41 weeks through 41 weeks and 6 days
> » Post-term: Babies born 42 weeks and beyond

Risks for Babies Born 34 to 38 weeks and 6 Days

Late preterm babies born 34 to 36 weeks are at risk of experiencing breathing problems, trouble maintaining their body temperature, low blood sugar, feeding challenges, jaundice, and rehospitalization. They are also more at risk for SIDS. After delivery, the early term baby born 37 to 38 weeks and 6 days may have breathing difficulties and require NICU admission. These babies often have longer hospital stays, usually due to jaundice and hypoglycemia. They are also more at risk for breastfeeding difficulties because their nursing reflexes are immature, muscles are weak, they tire before finishing a meal, and can't stay awake and alert as well as the term baby. In fact, waking these babies is very hard. As a mother, you may observe the following difficulties: poor state control (can't stay awake); poor breathing coordination while breastfeeding, noted by choking, sputtering, and a nursing pattern of "suck, suck, suck, suck," then "breathe, breathe, breathe"; poor milk intake; and needing more help to maintain their temperature, thus needing extra warmth in skin-to-skin bonding (Walker, 2017).

How to Overcome Breastfeeding Challenges with the Immature Newborn

If faced with an early delivery and your baby is in this gestational age group, there are things you can do to prevent the problems that we often see.

1. Right after delivery, keep your baby skin-to-skin, if possible, but do keep the baby covered or under a warmer (a special heating lamp positioned on top of you and the baby).

2. Make sure your baby is positioned correctly with support and has a deep, strong hold of the breast. Because the baby has weaker muscles, he must be positioned in a way that keeps the airway open. Laid-back nursing or a cross-cradle hold will often accommodate.

3. Once the infant starts sucking, test the strength of his suction by pulling him away from the breast. If he easily comes off, his hold is not strong enough. Babies need to create a strong vacuum in their mouth while lowering and raising their lower jaw to let the milk flow (Geddes et al., 2012).

4. One sign of poor milk flow will be a frustrated baby that easily and repeatedly loses the breast. In response, he will either cry or seem to be asleep again. A nipple shield may be helpful for this problem.

5. To prevent jaundice and hypoglycemia, start expressing your milk by hand expression after the baby eats, and if directed, start supplementing him with your expressed colostrum. This can be done by spoon or syringe.

6. Squeeze in extra feeds by bringing the baby to the breast when you see light sleep cues.

7. Look for early feeding cues: sucking movements, rapid eye movements, hand-to-mouth gestures, wiggling, and small sounds.

8. Feed hourly during the first 4 hours after birth and then every couple of hours after that.

9. Once your milk is in, it is highly recommended that you use a clinical-grade breast pump that can pump both breasts at the same time after every feed. We call this insurance pumping because a baby who is immature and weighs under 7 pounds usually won't relieve the engorged breast. This signals the breasts to make less milk. Meanwhile, a breast pump can help until the baby is more alert and awake enough to do a good job at the breast.

10. If triple feeding (nursing, expressing, then feeding the supplement to the baby) is becoming overwhelming, just pump and feed the baby the milk by your chosen method at night. Make sure to pump at least twice during the night. If there is adequate expressed breastmilk to feed the baby, most mothers find that they can skip a midnight pumping while a partner or relative feeds the baby at that time. This allows the mother to get some rest. Just don't skip the 3 am and 6 am expressions or allow your breasts to become too engorged.

11. If a lactation assessment reveals that the baby is not drinking milk when nursing, you will most likely have to start supplementing the infant with expressed milk.

12. Observe your baby's skin daily. Place the infant on a white sheet and check all over in a well-lit room. Call the baby's medical professional if you see that the yellow skin color is increasing in intensity and creeping down his body and into his extremities.

13. Seek medical attention if your baby is becoming too hard to wake up and/or his stool and urine output is less than normal (see diaper output on page 269).

We call these babies "little imposters" because they act alert when first born, but often begin to show that they really are immature when they develop problems. Good follow-up with your medical practitioner and a lactation consultant will help prevent potential complications. Support your milk supply by frequent nursing, followed by good milk expression, and feed the baby. If not at all at your breast, remember that your milk will keep him healthy. The goal is to get your baby to term and over 7 pounds, then things should get better.

DAIRY ALLERGY/SENSITIVITY

In a minority of infants who suffer from frequent irritability and excessive crying, a reaction to cow's milk or other food allergens may be the cause (Hiscock & Jordan, 2004). Symptoms of a food allergy include vomiting, blood or mucus mixed with diarrhea, poor weight gain, wheezing, and eczema (Hiscock & Jordan, 2004). Baby acne that is all over the face, appears very red and flaky, and spreads to the chest, back, and scalp may also be a sign of a food sensitivity. Stop all dairy for 24 to 72 hours. If dairy is the cause, you will see the baby's skin clear up. See your health professional before any treatment.

During the first 1 to 3 months of life, the incidence of cows' milk-protein intolerance is about 2 to 5% of babies, so it is relatively rare (Host et al., 1995). Parents should get a medical diagnosis before eliminating milk and dairy products from the mother's diet for more than a few days. If dairy is stopped, ask your medical professional about taking a calcium supplement.

GERD

When crying proves problematic, gastroesophageal reflux (GERD) may be the cause if the baby also vomits frequently, about five times a day (Hiscock & Jordan, 2004). You might also notice insufficient weight gain or weight loss, hiccupping, choking, gagging, and frequent irritability. When the milk mixed with stomach acids regularly comes up the baby's esophagus, causes irritation, and then goes back down without notable spit-up, this is known as silent GERD. A baby with GERD often seems happy after eating, then suddenly arches and screams once digestion sets in. Some babies bring milk up while nursing when the mother's milk is letting down. These babies pull off the breast, arch, swallow, then scream.

Nearly all babies spit-up sometimes or often after eating. Upwards of 50% of all 2-month-olds regurgitate at least twice a day (Brazelton & Sparrow, 2003). A ring of muscle, known as the lower esophageal sphincter, lies at the base of the esophagus, where it connects to the stomach. A mature sphincter opens when the healthy person swallows and remains closed at other times, preventing stomach contents from flowing backward. But since young infants have a pure liquid diet and an immature sphincter, contents from a full belly sometimes come back up when the baby is lying down, or the sphincter relaxes at the wrong times. Most babies spit-up and continue to smile and behave contentedly, making it more of a laundry problem than a medical one. Babies with GERD, however, have a lot more stomach fluid that builds up in the esophagus. The stomach acid, mixed with the milk, irritates, burns, and causes pain. It can be so severe that it causes damage to the esophagus.

GERD can affect sleep and nap patterns. Many babies peacefully drift off to sleep at the end of a feed. For the baby with GERD, however, reflux sets in about 10 to 15 minutes after the meal. The baby gets a rude awakening as milk comes up the esophagus, causing him to cry from the pain. You may need to find another way to help your baby fall asleep that does not include nursing, so reflux does not interrupt sleep. Try rocking, then nursing when he wakes up.

Over a period of days or weeks suffering from GERD, a baby may associate feeding with pain and become apathetic to breastfeeding. This negative association can lead to breast refusal. Changing how you manage breastfeeding can help. For example, try bringing the baby to the breast when he's in a drowsy state immediately after a nap/sleep, before he is totally alert and aware. This new timing of feeding after waking can also help prevent the problem of reflux waking your baby after being nursed to sleep.

If you observe GERD symptoms and behaviors, keep a log for several days, noting the timing of its occurrence (symptoms or behaviors) related to breastfeeding. Make an appointment with your medical practitioner and be sure to bring your log of evidence. You can even take a recording with your smartphone to illustrate the behavior for your healthcare provider. Request a thorough infant physical and assessment to rule out any other reasons for these symptoms. If your baby does, in fact, have GERD, the doctor will assess the severity to determine if medication to reduce the stomach acid will help treat symptoms and discomfort. If your baby is prescribed medication and does not respond to it, return to your medical practitioner for further assessment. Most babies with GERD grow out of it and no longer need medication after a few months because the muscle that prevents stomach contents from coming up matures. Trying management techniques to treat GERD before medication is recommended, such as:

» Holding the baby upright for about 45 minutes after a meal (a sling can help)

» Offering frequent, small breastfeeds

» Talking to your physician about a safe way to elevate the baby while sleeping

» Avoiding maternal intake of dairy and caffeine

» Trying the breastfeeding, sleep timing, and management tips discussed earlier

» Have a breastfeeding evaluation to see if you have overabundant milk

PYLORIC STENOSIS

Rarely, a fussy baby has a condition, genetic in nature, called pyloric stenosis (Quinn et al., 2011). It is usually seen in firstborn boys, showing up around 20 to 40 days of age (Quinn et al., 2011). The main symptom is vomiting that is forceful and slowly increases to every feed. The baby is hungry and wants to suckle constantly. As the condition worsens, he becomes more fretful and thinner. Urine and stool output greatly decrease. Doctors can feel an olive-shaped mass at the top of the stomach after the baby vomits. If your baby is vomiting after every meal for more than 4 to 8 hours, then seems hungry, call your practitioner immediately.

MATERNAL CONDITIONS AND ILLNESS

Mastitis

The sudden occurrence of flu-like symptoms in a breastfeeding woman, such as a fever of 101.3°F. or higher, aches, and chills may mean the onset of mastitis or inflammation of the breast. Women with mastitis typically think they have the flu before they notice a red triangular area on their breast that feels hot, swollen, and tender. Mastitis is usually caused by obstruction to milk flow or infection. Bacterial infection may or may not be present (Amir et al., 2014).

It is safe to continue breastfeeding, as there are no known risks to healthy infants (WHO, 2000).

Mastitis can occur anytime during lactation but is most common during the first 6 weeks postpartum (Amir et al., 2014) because of contributing factors during the establishment of breastfeeding, particularly milk build-up, sore nipples, and engorgement. Risk factors can increase a mother's likelihood of developing mastitis, including damaged nipples, not breastfeeding often enough, scheduled feedings, missed feedings, poor milk removal caused by incorrect attachment or suckling, a sick mother or baby, overabundant milk supply, rushed weaning, uneven pressure on the breast (i.e., caused by a bra or seatbelt), a blocked duct or nipple pore (bleb), maternal stress, and fatigue (Amir et al., 2014). Since mastitis is often a result of milk build-up, milk removal is the first and most effective way to manage it when symptoms have been present for less than 24 hours. The Academy of Breastfeeding Medicine (ABM) recommends the following (Amir et al., 2014):

Treatment Plan for Mastitis

1. Breastfeed more frequently, starting with the affected breast. If pain is preventing your milk from letting-down, start on the other breast. Once let-down occurs, switch to the affected breast. A heat pack or warm shower can help let-down.

2. You can expedite milk removal by pumping after breastfeeding.

3. A cold compress applied for 15 minutes after nursing can reduce pain and nipple edema.

4. Ask about taking Ibuprofen. It can also help reduce pain and inflammation, which can support the let-down reflex.

5. Drink lots of fluids and ask for support so you can get adequate rest.

6. If you do not see improvement within 12 to 24 hours, or start feeling worse, you may need a course of antibiotics.

7. If the mastitis is not resolved within several days, follow up with your clinician for further diagnosis and treatment. Most

doctors start with a standard antibiotic, but you may need a different medication. Take the medication for a full 10 to 14 days or as prescribed.

Abscess

Recurrent or unresolved mastitis can lead to a breast abscess, especially if you promptly cease to breastfeed or pump. Research shows that this happens in about 3% of mastitis cases (Amir et al., 2004). If you followed the treatment plan for mastitis, including antibiotics, and you still have a firm, raised, red area on your breast with or without pain, you should suspect that your infection hasn't healed. It may have progressed to an abscess. Seek professional medical treatment, immediately.

EMOTIONAL CONCERNS

Because breastfeeding concerns can make emotional changes worse, it is important to discuss normal and potential problematic family adjustments after birth. At some point, you might find yourself reflecting, "do I have the 'baby blues' or am I really having a problem?" Part of the baby blues are the changes happening in your brain. They are the new feelings when we, as women, become mothers. Your right brain is making remarkable connections to make you responsive to your baby. Baby blues may make you feel weepy and lonely. Some estimate that 50 to 80% of women in Western countries experience these feeling while their high levels of pregnancy hormones decrease (Beck, 2006). The symptoms are usually short-term and don't interrupt activities of normal living. Tears well up out of nowhere. Partners are shocked by these tearful outbursts. You begin to realize that the time your baby spends as a newborn is a minuscule part of his life and you don't want to miss a single moment. You may feel guilty looking away, not rushing to his cries, or tending to a household chore in lieu of holding your baby. The baby blues are real, but they are more than fluctuating hormones. It's when we, as mothers, are faced with conflicting thoughts and an ever-so-true reality that this beautiful part of our lives with this tiny miracle is short-lived.

In addition, you may not be accustomed to being home all the time. You may feel guilty when thoughts of resentment pop up. It can cause a stir-crazy sensation. You may feel lonely if you live away from close friends and relatives or are missing a lost loved one who you wish was by your side. So, don't discount the baby blues as hormones gone array. The feelings are real too. Sleep deprivation and the overwhelming reality of all the new responsibilities are also contributing to the heavy emotions.

POSTPARTUM DEPRESSION

Postpartum depression is a mood disorder related to childbirth, occurring in about 15 to 25% of births. It can occur anytime during the year after birth but commonly begins between a week and a month after delivery. It is possible to have symptoms as soon as you become pregnant. There are many causes of this condition. Chemical brain changes stimulated by the levels of hormones decreasing and other hormones increasing after childbirth trigger the mood swings. Some experiences can escalate the condition, such as loss of sleep, any birth trauma, including an unexpected cesarean delivery after a very long and painful labor, or subsequent pain. According to the National Institute of Mental Health, some of the more common symptoms a woman may experience include (NIMH, 2018):

» Loss of appetite or overeating

» Sleep disruption (either oversleeping or being unable to sleep, even when the baby is asleep)

» Feeling sad, hopeless, empty, or overwhelmed. Experiencing anger or rage

» Crying more often than usual or for no apparent reason

» Unusual worrying or acting overly anxious. Feeling moody, irritable, or restless

» Having trouble concentrating, remembering details, and making decisions

» Loss of interest in activities that are usually enjoyable

» Suffering from pain, such as physical aches, frequent headaches, and/or stomach problems

» Isolating yourself or avoiding friends and family

» Doubting your ability to care for the baby

» Thinking about harming yourself or the baby (get help immediately)

If you have any of these symptoms, call your healthcare provider right away. Postpartum depression usually requires treatment.

What Else Can You Do If You Think You Have Postpartum Depression?

» Call Postpartum Support International 1-800-944-4773, or www.postpartum.net, to find referrals for your geographical area. Your local hospital may also have a referral system or support group.

» Call 911 or go to the nearest ER if you feel that your life or the baby's safety is in danger.

» Call the toll-free 24-hour hotline of the National Suicide Prevention Lifeline at 1-800-273-TALK (1-800-273-8255); TTY: 1-800-799-4TTY (4889).

Postpartum depression is very different from baby blues. For one, the symptoms last longer. It is often misdiagnosed or ignored. Mothers may have difficulty getting others to hear their fears or complaints. Feelings of sadness and anxiety can become so extreme that it endangers the mother and infant, or affects her ability to care for her baby. A mother might blame herself when experiencing these symptoms, but it is not her fault. While there are risk factors, it can affect any woman, regardless of age, race, ethnicity, or economic status. Alert your medical professionals if you have or have had any of the following risk factors:

» Previous or family history of depression or mood disorder, such as anxiety or panic disorder

» History of depression with a previous pregnancy

» A recent stressful experience, such as domestic abuse, family catastrophic illness, job loss

» Mixed feelings about the pregnancy

» Isolation from close friends or family

» Traumatic birth or infant health issues

» Current or past addiction to alcohol or drugs

STRANGE EMOTIONAL FEELINGS WHEN NURSING

For a small number of women, feelings of anger, depression, or even panic may occur in reaction to their milk letting-down and lasts for several minutes. This phenomenon, called dysphoric milk-ejection reflex, is often a hidden but rare condition. It can be shocking and may make the mother consider weaning. Women may be ashamed to mention it because breastfeeding is supposed to be pleasurable. She will feel the dysphoria (sadness, irritability, anxiety, or anger) before her milk sprays. As the milk slows down, the feeling decreases. The symptoms vary from mother to mother and can be mild to severe. To reduce mild to moderate symptoms of the dysphoric milk-ejection reflex log and track the episodes, listing things that may be triggers (i.e., stress, dehydration, low blood sugar, and caffeine) and things that relieve symptoms (i.e. rest, hydration, protein, and exercise) (Heise & Wiessinger, 2011). Medication may be needed in the case of a severe let-down response. There is an excellent website that explains it further with additional resources, called D-Mer.org.

• • • • • • • • • • • • • • •

CHAPTER SIXTEEN

Breastfeeding Culprit #1: Perceived or Real Insufficient Milk Supply

Chapter Goal: Prevent sabotaging your success and avoid the premature weaning common during this difficult phase of infancy due to perceived insufficient milk supply.

MIXED MESSAGES

In a charming San Luis Obispo, California cottage gathers dozens of mothers with their new babies. The nurslings nuzzle up to their respective mother's breast in unison as Pediatric Nurse Practitioner/ Lactation Consultant Andrea Herron listens to their parents' many concerns: "My baby has become so gassy. Could she be allergic to my milk?" "My little guy hasn't pooped in days. Is he constipated?" "My breasts are not firm anymore. They don't leak like they used to. Am I losing my milk supply?" "My 6-week-old has been really fussy and wants to nurse all the time. I'm worried I don't have enough milk. Should I start her on a bottle?" These are the same concerns voiced at the Growing with Baby Breastfeeding Support Group held weekly for the last 30 years.

Changes in a baby's behavior frequently send mixed signals to the parents, leaving them distraught with worry. Some common normal behaviors that babies do as they develop can easily be mistaken for breastfeeding problems. Beware of mislabeling these normal behavioral changes. Have appropriate expectations so that you can stay on the right track with your baby and avoid some of the typical mistakes mothers make that potentially sabotage their breastfeeding goals.

THE CHANGING BABY, THE CHANGING BREAST

Normal changes in the dynamics of breastfeeding cause mothers to lose confidence in their breastfeeding. Once engorgement sets in during early milk production, women often use the feel of their breasts to detect adequate infant milk intake. They become accustomed to the fact that their firm breasts soften after the baby is done feeding. They listen to sucks and swallows while nursing and observe how long the baby is content after a feed. They count wet and dirty diapers. They log the time, aiming for the prescribed 20 minutes per breast. Suddenly, between 3 to 6 weeks postpartum, breasts that hardened when it was time to breastfeed the baby now feel soft, even at feeding times. Meanwhile, an infant who was signaling often to feed and taking 45 minutes or more to finish a meal may now be done in 10 minutes. The sleepy baby seems more demanding or hungrier than before. Stools that were associated with every feed slow down to every 1 to 6 days and look different. All of these changes are normal but not typically expected, so it tends to cause mothers to doubt the adequacy of their milk supply.

PERCEIVED INSUFFICIENT MILK SUPPLY

A common reason mothers cite for quitting breastfeeding within the first 10 weeks is not their free will and desire, but the belief that they do not make enough milk to meet their baby's demand (Kent et al., 2013; Li et al., 2008). In polls, they report that "my breastmilk alone did not satisfy my baby" (Li et al., 2008). This belief is so prevalent, that there is actually a lactation diagnosis known as Perceived Insufficient Milk Supply (PIMS), usually seen at 6 weeks but a concern throughout the breastfeeding experience. It is described in breastfeeding research "as a woman perceiving that her [milk] supply is inadequate either to satisfy her infant's hunger (based on the infant's behavior, including the frequency and duration of breastfeeding sessions) or to support adequate weight gain" (Kent et al., 2013). It essentially means that a mother feels like she doesn't make enough milk when she may, in fact, have plenty.

The trouble is that many mothers are coming to the erroneous conclusion that their milk supply is inadequate and, in response, make changes that eventually do undermine breastfeeding. They misunderstand their body's changes in combination with their baby's cues and conclude that they have inadequate breastmilk. An integrative review of research studies conducted by the University of Pennsylvania's Center for Health Disparities found that few "researchers, clinicians, and breastfeeding women" evaluate the actual milk supply and the baby's growth as true indications of a problem and merely rely on the mother's report (Gatti, 2008). Without proper diagnosis, it is difficult to discern who has enough milk and who really doesn't.

The assumption that the majority of women are not able to make the amount of milk their baby needs could not possibly be true. If it were a fair representation of genuine supply issues, the human race might not have progressed to a world population of more than 7 billion people. Mammals are designed to lactate to provide ample nourishment for their young infants. The failure rate must be much lower than 50%—think Darwinism and evolution.

Sure, there are times when certain factors delay the milk or interfere with early building of milk. However, apart from women with physical abnormalities and medical problems, it is not too little, too late; time is on her side. There are ways to demand more milk of the body and stimulate an increase in production, especially because the breasts continue to build the supply during the first few weeks (Kent et al., 2016), and for some women, through 2 1/2 months postpartum. Unfortunately, many women don't make it that long. They either quit or begin supplementing the baby's diet with formula as early as the second day in the hospital. This can prevent the mother from developing a normal supply if not done under the guidance of a skilled lactation professional who can guide her in a way that protects and builds the milk supply.

The changes that lead many mothers to suspect a milk quality or quantity problem begin at 3 weeks postpartum, when their snuggly newborn hits the first of several developmental milestones (see Chapter 17). The baby becomes more demanding while the mother's breasts start to soften. The less one understands these normal changes when they occur, the more confusing the infant's behaviors can be. Learn what changes to expect and you can avoid the trap that many parents fall into—the one that sabotages their own breastfeeding success. Soon, you will have the key to shelve Breastfeeding Pitfall #1 for good, right next to that free can of formula.

Remember, perceived insufficient milk supply is just a PERCEPTION. The following are signs of normal breast and baby changes occurring around 6 weeks after full-term birth (NOT an indication of low milk supply):

» Your baby seems fussier than before.

» You nurse more than the average 8 to 10 times a day.

» The baby used to stool every time he ate. Now, it's once every few days.

» Your breasts don't feel firm anymore.

» Your breasts no longer leak.

» You've pumped your breasts and yielded less milk than expected.

What may be an indication of a supply problem is described ahead. If, after reading and understanding this chapter, you continue to believe your milk supply is inadequate, seek a professional diagnosis before supplementing with bottles of infant formula because research shows it can lead to a cycle of ever-decreasing breastmilk production (Hill & Humenick, 1996; Kent et al., 2013). In the interim, stimulate your breasts frequently by pumping or hand-expressing your milk after breastfeeding.

ASSESSING MILK-SUPPLY CONCERNS

Typically, breastfeeding mothers rely on infant behavior and the way their breasts feel to determine the sufficiency of their milk. While this is good practice to determine when to nurse and the effectiveness of an individual feed, it has proven to be an unreliable indicator of a mother's milk production (Meier et al., 1994). Comparing your breastfeeding experience to that of your sister, your peers, or by-the-book averages is also not a good indication of how your milk supply measures up. Bottle-fed babies are often overfed because they tend to drink beyond satiety to satisfy their non-nutritive suckling needs. While bottle-feeding, parents can easily miss the cues that the baby is full because it takes more time to digest formula compared to breastmilk. The baby appears full for longer. It is thought that bottle-feeders become more passive eaters; feeding is something that is done to them. Breastfed babies learn to be active participants. While this is natural and correct (and preventative against obesity), it can conflict with parenting norms and lead to misperceptions. If a mother doesn't understand these normal baby behaviors and then thinks it has to do with her breastmilk, she might be tempted to wean.

Common Misperceptions

Often, a mother will begin to question her milk when she uses a breast pump for the first time and pumps less than expected. Beware about using a breast pump to measure your breastmilk capacity. Pumping is a learned art and supply varies, depending on the timing interval and 24-hour cycle. Also, the way your body responds to a cold, mechanical pump is different than how it responds to your warm bundle of love. An alert, healthy baby that is capable of taking the breast correctly nurses efficiently, triggers more let-downs (milk flow), and is better at building your supply. Also note that the volume and nutritional breakdown of milk contained in your breasts varies throughout the day. Most women are fuller in the morning. Your baby's increasing physical growth is the best determinant of whether you have a sufficient milk supply.

Do not allow averages or comparisons to chip away at your confidence, or comments like "didn't you just feed the baby?" There are very wide variations of what is considered normal breastfeeding frequencies, suckling times, and amounts of breastfeeding between mother-baby couplets (Kent et al., 2012), and sometimes the patterns change day-to-day. For example, one day, you might breastfeed six times while another, you might exceed 12 sessions. One baby might be satisfied after nursing on one breast for 15 minutes, while another suckles for more than an hour with a short break in between breasts. Not every minute is spent taking in milk or gulping through a let-down. Babies often come to the breast for comfort or thirst alone.

Normal Milk Supply

Normal maternal milk production of an exclusively breastfed infant between 1 and 6 months old is considered 750 to 800 ml/day (25 to 26.5 ounces) but a range of 440 to 1220 ml/day (14 to 40 ounces) can also be perfectly healthy if the baby is thriving and growing (Kent et al., 2006). As your baby gets bigger, his energy requirement decreases. Naturally, one would assume that a larger baby needs more milk, so this fact is very much counterintuitive. Henceforth, by 1 month postpartum, if all goes well, your daily milk production will remain constant if you are exclusively breastfeeding (Butte, 2005).

Diagnosis

There are ways of detecting a milk-supply problem and methods for giving it a boost, which will be covered ahead. Several parameters should be used to evaluate concerns before doubting your milk supply or offering bottles of milk. First, see your baby's medical professional for an evaluation. Once that's done, get an assessment from a skilled lactation consultant, which needs to include the following:

» A complete feeding history for you and the baby
» A physical examination of the baby, including an observation of the infant's skin color, alertness, hydration, and muscle tone
» A physical examination of your breasts

» Tracking of the infant's weight gain and growth to analyze consistency. The baby's weight and height should be plotted on the WHO Growth Charts developed for infants 0 to 2 years found at www.cdc.gov/growthcharts. If the baby was born earlier than 40 weeks, the growth should be adjusted for the baby's true gestational age in weeks.

» Accurate test weights (with a digital scale accurate to 2 grams), which requires weighing the dressed baby before and after a breastfeed without changing his clothes or the diaper before each test weight. The difference will tell you how much he drank in that feed.

» Observation of a complete nursing session

» A record of your baby's 24-hour urine and stool output

» A feeding plan that includes adequate calories for your baby's growth and stimulation to develop your milk supply

Signs of Real Insufficient Milk Supply

We've discussed at length many of the behaviors and changes that confuse parents and make a mother worry about her milk supply. So, what are the signs of true insufficient milk supply?

» The baby is not starting to gain weight after your milk comes in day 2 to 4 postpartum (note that this can be an infant-sucking issue).

» The baby is not back to birthweight after a normal 5 to 7% loss by day 7 to 10 after birth.

» The baby is gaining less than 5 to 7 ounces each week.

» Inadequate infant output—stools and wet diapers (see Diaper Output).

» The baby is unhappy after nursing or too sleepy to nurse at least 6 to 9 times in 24 hours.

» The infant falls asleep quickly when put to the breast, then cries when put down.

» The baby shuts his eyes when feeding and does intermittent sucks and audible swallows with frequent, long pauses. Very few audible swallows are heard.

» The baby pulls off the breast frequently and cries, or tugs on the breast while nursing.

» You never felt hard, full breasts. (This can be normal for some women if the baby is content and thriving.)

» The breasts don't feel full before nursing followed by a softening after the baby finishes.

» Your nipples are more than slightly tender at the beginning of a feed. They hurt throughout the nursing session and into the next time the baby wants to feed.

» Instinctively, you feel worried.

Realize that the milk supply has the potential to build as milk cells activate during the first several weeks after childbirth. Ways to boost the milk supply will be covered ahead.

GREAT GROWTH EXPECTATIONS

Parents really mean it when they tell you, "Enjoy, because they grow so fast." Who has not heard that? One might think, "yes, how obvious." However, when you discover that the changes are happening before your eyes, you might reflect on that popular comment, and perhaps even be the next person to utter it to a mom-to-be. For the parents of the baby who is not thriving, however, it can be the heart of all concern. Breastfeeding mothers can be consumed with worry over their infant's growth. The last thing a mother wants is to realize she is affecting her child's growth by her body's inability to produce enough milk. A first-and-foremost question mothers have is, "how many ounces is the baby taking?" For a bottle-feeding parent, that answer is simple but for the nursing mother, she must follow the baby's cues, listen to her intuition, and reflect on her own response. By now, you have read about your baby's potential cues for hunger and satiation during the first 10 weeks. You know how to tell when the baby is nursing correctly and is gulping at the breast. You feel your breasts get fuller between feeds and soften after the baby nurses.

When analyzing your baby's growth, monitor changes week to week rather than day to day. Growth rates fluctuate. There are also variables, such as bowel movements, mood, and appetite, which can account for daily differences in milk intake and weight. During the first 10 weeks, the average female gains 34 grams (a little more than an ounce) per day, males average 40 grams (about 1.3 ounces) per day, while the minimum expected weight gain if the baby is content is 20 grams (3/4 of an ounce) per day (Walker, 2017). After 6 weeks of age, growth should follow a standard curve on the WHO Growth Chart. Some babies gain 3 ounces a day, but this fast weight gain may be accompanied by fussiness and gassiness because the infant is dealing with too much milk intake (see overabundant milk supply on page 286).

After 3 to 4 months, the baby's rate of growth slows down. An infant who was gaining at least an ounce per day now gains 16 ounces per month. If the baby is gaining 1/2 an ounce or less per day during the first 3 months, this could be a sign of either a faltering milk supply or an infant-intake issue (Mohrbacher, 2010). Growing and mothering a breastfed baby well requires intuition and cognitive judgments. As the provider of nurturance, sometimes it means sorting through a maze of concerns. It's why this text is coaching you on how to follow your intuition, by reading cues and evaluating your own response.

"Is my baby getting enough to eat?"

For the young infant, the daily energy needs are the highest during the first month. After that, most breastfed babies take in the same amount of milk (between 19 to 30 oz or 570 to 900 ml daily) until age 6 months (Kent et al., 1999). Once you know your baby is gaining weight steadily, feed on cue. Some days, it will seem that your baby can't get enough and there will be other days when he just does not seem that hungry. The problem is that breasts are not always comfortable under that pattern. So, always pay attention to your body. If you feel you need relief, use your pump or hand express enough milk to feel comfortable.

One of the most unsettling parts of early breastfeeding for new mothers is the fact that you can't see how many ounces your baby is drinking at the breast, unless you do a test weight before and after he eats. In contrast, when bottle-feeding, every ounce can be quantified. If only our breasts came with a gauge. You will know your baby is getting enough to eat when:

» Hunger cues are followed by signs of satiation. When the baby first latches on the breast, the suction is strong, and his fists are tight. The moment your milk lets down, you will see the baby's eyes widen and you will hear gulping. After a while of rhythmic sucking and swallowing, the baby's hands become relaxed and he loosens hold of the breast, or passively, intermittently suckles and swallows. He may fall asleep, full and satisfied.

» Your nursling softens the breast by the end of the feeding.

» He is content for at least 90 minutes after he eats during the day. Do not be confused by evening cluster feeds.

» He has at least 3 to 4 ample yellow, loose, seedy stools a day (after day 5). Note that during the first few weeks of life, many babies stool each time they eat. This changes during the second month.

» He has a wet diaper before his next meal.

» He is growing out of his newborn or zero to 3-month-old clothes.

» The newborn or size one diapers are getting tight or too small.

» He has returned to or surpassed his birthweight by 7 to 12 days of age.

If your detective work gives you reason to believe your baby is not thriving, have him weighed—a sure method for tracking growth. Note: Not all scales are calibrated the same, so be aware about making determinations based on measurements from two different scales. If there are growth concerns, see a medical professional skilled in lactation. The consultant can do a test weight to determine the baby's milk intake. The baby should be weighed naked. Then, be dressed and weighed again once before breastfeeding and then again after in the same diaper and clothes. The difference in the two weights will tell you how many ounces your baby took during the feed. It is important that an accurate scale, developed for this purpose, is used. Keep in mind that this is one weight—only one piece of the puzzle.

REAL CAUSES OF MILK-SUPPLY PROBLEMS

Successful lactation typically occurs when a mother has developed adequate mammary tissue, supported by intact nerves and ducts in a body that is releasing appropriate levels of various hormones, plus a healthy baby who nurses vigorously. There are multiple causes of milk-supply issues. Some start with inherent physical issues of the mother's breast development, past surgeries, or medical issues. Others start with the infant. Most milk-supply problems stem from medical causes or mismanagement of breastfeeding. If you are worried, it is important to obtain a professional medical diagnosis to assess your milk supply. Formula is not an end-all solution. Not just for the sake of breastfeeding but because sometimes, true insufficient milk supply masks an underlying medical problem that needs attention.

Risk Factors for Delayed or Insufficient Milk Supply

Check all that apply and inform your practitioner.

[_] I have had breast surgery.

[_] I have been diagnosed with obesity, metabolic syndrome, and/or type 1 or type 2 diabetes.

[_] I have a history of infertility or other hormonal conditions, such as hypothyroidism or polycystic ovary syndrome.

[_] I have a chronic medical or mental illness.

[_] I have been told I have hypoplastic breasts, breasts that did not develop adequate glandular tissue.

[_] My nipples are bigger than a half-dollar coin (large nipples).

[_] My nipples are short and don't stretch (short/inelastic nipples).

[_] My nipples do not evert (inverted nipples).

[_] I had a long, stressful, and/or difficult labor and delivery.

[_] I had a traumatic labor and delivery, which led to a cesarean delivery.

[_] I had postpartum hemorrhage or retained placenta.

[_] I have pain so bad that it impairs my ability to move.

[_] I have been experiencing unrelieved engorgement.

[_] I'm not sure if I'm positioning the baby correctly at the breast.

[_] My baby is feeding less than six times a day so that I can maintain a feeding schedule.

[_] My baby was delivered prematurely.

[_] I am taking medication daily that may impact my milk supply (check with your doctor or IBCLC).

Maternal Reasons

The physical characteristics of the breasts that interfere with milk transfer include, but are not limited to, inverted nipples, nipples that might be flat or too large, or short, inelastic nipples (Mohrbacher, 2010; Riordan & Wambach, 2016), and underdeveloped milk glands (a very small percentage), known as hypoplasia (Neifert, 2001). Any surgical incisions or changes to the breast, especially near the areola, may sever ductal and neurological pathways, and interfere with the normal production process (Kent et al., 2012). Even something as simple as nipple piercings are potentially disrupting (Neifert, 2001).

Research shows that women with hormone issues may have their milk production impacted (Foong et al., 2015). Such problems include body mass index >30 (Nommsen-Rivers et al., 2012), diabetes (Riddle & Nommsen-Rivers, 2016), thyroid disease, polycystic ovarian syndrome (Vanky et al., 2012), and history of infertility (Foong et al., 2015). Medical conditions that interfere include severe illness, postpartum hemorrhage (Thompson et al., 2010), infection, hypertension, or retained placental fragments (Neifert, 1981). Postpartum mothers must be careful to prevent engorgement with unrelieved emptying because it signals the breasts to make less milk. The pressure makes the milk cells shrink and decrease in number (Neifert, 2001).

Mothers who face severe sore nipples, chronic pain, mastitis, abscesses, fatigue, exhaustion, PTSD from a history of sexual abuse or other trauma, or depression can also struggle to maintain a sufficient milk supply through insufficient emptying. Parents report that returning to work can be a detriment to their milk supply and ability to exclusively breastfeed. Due to the job responsibilities, finding a time to relax and express their milk is challenging. The first sign of pregnancy may also lead to a decrease or abrupt end to a mother's milk supply.

Hypoplastic Breasts

A small percentage of women fail to develop enough milk cells (sufficient glandular tissue) to produce adequate breastmilk. Red flags that you have this condition are the following: failure to increase at least one cup size during pregnancy, not seeing an increased appearance of blood vessels, areolar darkening, or leaking colostrum (note that some women don't get bigger or leak colostrum), and never feeling engorgement. When looking at your breasts, you may see a marked difference between their size; the breasts might be spaced further than 1.5 inches apart. One or both breasts will appear tubular shaped and the areola may be large and appear to be bulging. Some describe a hypoplastic breast as appearing long and narrow. Most of the breast feels smooth and firm, with very little bumpy glandular tissue found.

Starting Birth Control and Other Medicines

At the 6-week check-up with their obstetrician, women typically begin a birth control method. Birth control medications that contain hormones may affect the milk supply. Clinically, lactation consultants have reported seeing mothers who faced loss of milk immediately after the introduction of hormone-based prescriptions. Before you start a birth control (pill, device, injection) or have an IUD inserted, have the baby weighed. Then, follow up with another weight check after 1 week of the medication. If everything is on track (4 to 7 ounces of weight gain per week) but you see the baby's behavior change, have the weight checked again the next week. The following birth control methods are not recommended while breastfeeding because they can potentially inhibit a normal milk supply: combined-hormone birth control before 6 months postpartum; progesterone-only birth control pills; Depo-Provera shot; and hormonal IUD before 6 weeks postpartum. Be cautious any time you start a hormone when lactating. Even cream suppositories with hormones can impact supply. Avoid decongestants (Berens et al., 2015).

INFANT ISSUES

Milk supply may be impacted when an infant is premature or late preterm, born with a neurologic problem, has cephalohematomas (large spongy bumps on the head) or oral anatomic problems (tongue-tie or cleft palate) (Geddes et al., 2008), any metabolic issues, heart problems, illness, or experienced a long, difficult birth. A common reason is a sleepy baby—particularly one with jaundice (Walker, 2017). In these cases, a faltering milk supply is caused by poor feeding, which leaves the breast engorged or under stimulated.

What if You Can't Breastfeed?

Know that you can still be a good mother, even if you don't reach your breastfeeding goals. If you feel that pain and/or prolonged difficulties are keeping you from bonding with your baby, seek the advice of a caring professional who can help you assess whether to continue. Close and continuous physical contact in an attachment relationship is necessary for children to thrive emotionally (Bowlby, 1970). What matters most is that you can smile, interact, and love. Know that there are many ways to bond with your baby and form attachment. Since humans are adaptable, attachment can still happen later after birth (Klaus & Kennell, 2000).

Any duration of breastfeeding is beneficial for your baby—the more, the better. Even a single day of colostrum is more valuable than no breastmilk at all. It is so meaningful that in Neonatal Intensive Care Units, doctors cherish any amount the infant's mother can give. With just drops of colostrum, NICU specialists coat the inside of the premature baby's mouth, kick-starting the digestive and immune systems. Every drop is a priceless gift and if you have managed to give that you have already succeeded.

We understand that coping with severe breastfeeding difficulties can be lonely and burdensome. What's important is that you develop your place as a mother, regardless of whether you are breastfeeding, so you can be the best parent you can be. Wipe away the tears and shed the guilt. You'll have more opportunities to create a lifetime of health benefits through the formation of a diet rich in natural whole foods.

BREASTFEEDING MANAGEMENT

Mismanagement of breastfeeding, such as limiting or scheduling feeds, impacts milk supply. When lactating breasts are not stimulated and emptied sufficiently, it often leads to a decrease in milk supply (Hill & Aldag, 2005). Practices that contradict responsive parenting and on-cue feeding are frequently spawned by cultural norms, not biological feeding norms.

Scheduled Breastfeeds

Many women are told to get their newborn baby on a schedule so the mother can maintain control. There are numerous reasons that have been discussed throughout the book, explaining why schedules are not conducive to breastfeeding. Not allowing unlimited access of the baby to the breast due to maternal misunderstanding of normal infant-feeding patterns is a risk factor for milk-supply problems (Riordan & Wambach, 2016; Walker, 2017). Shortening feeds for whatever reason, rather than allowing the baby to breastfeed until satiated, calibrates a smaller demand than what he needs for his individual growth. In addition, for many women, offering one breast per feed lengthens intervals of breast stimulation between feeds and impacts the milk supply. In the beginning, most newborn babies need to nurse from both breasts to complete a feed and build adequate milk. Some babies almost always need to nurse from both breasts until solids are introduced in order to thrive.

Supplementing

Babies who cry at night, or after nursing during the evening hours, often lead the mother to believe, based on the infant's behavior, that her milk supply is insufficient (Sachdev & Mehrotra, 1995). The women report that their breasts feel empty and they have no more to give. They test their baby's hunger after nursing by offering a bottle. Note that newborn babies have a strong sucking drive and will eagerly suck on a bottle, even after nursing. This practice often reinforces the belief that she does not have enough milk. Studies show that while breastfeeding has become more and more popular, babies are often fed bottles of formula to supplement breastfeeding, usually without medical necessity, within days after birth (Cloherty et al., 2004). As mentioned before, supplementation can lead to premature weaning.

Devices

A temporary tool that solves one problem may create another if not used moderately or discontinued at the right time. Early on, giving babies bottles, artificial nipples, or pacifiers replace time stimulating the breasts and activating milk producing cells. Extended use of nipple shields has also been found to slow milk production (Walker, 2017). Sucking on a pacifier may diminish the infant's interest in suckling at the breast. Delaying feeds or shortening nursing sessions by using a pacifier satisfies his normal suckling needs and may leave you with less milk. You may soon notice a slow weight gain in the baby.

Be aware that many babies are ready to take the second breast within 30 minutes of finishing at the first. This completes a full breast-feed. Some parents who don't understand this rhythm, especially because it contradicts bottle-feeding culture, will offer a pacifier after the first breast. Over time, it can impact the mother's milk supply through insufficient breast stimulation. Unless directed by a skilled breastfeeding professional, wait on pacifiers until your milk supply is fully established.

BOOSTING MILK PRODUCTION

When you have reason to believe your milk supply is not enough, you'll want to see a medical professional skilled in lactation to evaluate you and the baby. Ideally, you would be given a feeding plan based on the diagnosis of the problem, including how much additional milk the baby needs to drink for adequate growth. It may be as simple as you are not feeding the baby enough times in 24 hours. Maybe someone told you not to wake a sleeping baby. Perhaps you were offering only one breast because you hear about foremilk and hindmilk but for your anatomy and milk storage capacity, your baby needs two breasts. Your baby may have tight muscles or a bruised head from delivery, which affects his efficiency in removing milk from your breasts. You may need to use a breast pump in addition to breastfeeding while your baby recovers. Without risk factors for insufficient milk, supply largely relies on emptying the breasts (Mohrbacher, 2010). For many mothers, though, they just need a little help understanding normal baby feeding behaviors to boost their confidence. If the assessment reveals more complicated reasons for insufficient milk, the plan may include some of the following recommendations.

ACTION PLAN

Tips for Making More Milk
Get an Assessment
Try Correcting the Latch
Drain the Breasts with a Pump
Reduce Stress = Release More Milk
Get Blood Work
Use a Supplementer
Try an Herbal Remedy

Correcting the Latch

Many breastfeeding clinicians believe that in conjunction with a normal mother and baby, how the infant takes the breast in his mouth is critical. When the baby is not positioned and holding the breast correctly, his intake is less, often leaving the breast engorged. Over time, this can lead to a dwindling supply. Correcting how the baby is held and making sure he takes the breast deeply into his mouth will allow the infant to milk the breast more efficiently, get more milk, and activate milk producing cells to further develop the milk supply (see breast attachment on page 293).

Promoting Let-Down

You could have plenty of milk, and the problem could quite simply rely on the release of it, especially if you are worried about your milk supply. Stress can inhibit milk ejection and lead to insufficient milk supply (Geddes, 2007). Without the milk ejection, the baby is not able to extract much milk to create the chain reaction of supply and demand (Hartmann, 1991).

Focus on ways to reduce any anxiety, which is surely amplified by a lack of sleep and learning to breastfeed. Try skin-to-skin contact with your baby before breastfeeding. Lay down on your side in your bedroom to nurse in private instead of sitting upright in the living room among the excitement of the household. A horizontal posture for even a few minutes throughout the day can offer respite. Quietly play your favorite music. Nibble on some comfort food, your favorite snack, hot tea with honey, an organic broth, or even a lollipop.

Take 5-minute breaks outside throughout the day while you take big breaths and allow the sun to beat down on your face. Short walks can reduce stress significantly. Ask your partner to rub your feet or massage your shoulders. These are just a few ideas. Of course, sleep is healing for the mind and the body, if it's possible. Try to put yourself first every so often and think, "what can I do for myself in this moment?" If you don't stop and think about it, those times will be few and far between.

Focusing on Thorough Drainage

The more a breast is drained, the faster the milk is made (Daly et al., 1993). You can take control and increase your milk production by optimizing drainage. For starters, make sure you've verified that you understand correct breastfeeding techniques. Holding the baby correctly will allow him to efficiently and comfortably milk the breast. Consider nursing more often. Taking the time for skin-to-skin contact may stimulate your baby's natural feeding and searching behaviors. It might allow you to squeeze in a few extra feeds. If the baby does not soften the breasts or show interest in the second after his normal pause, express remaining milk in each breast. Research shows that pumping for a few minutes beyond milk flow can boost production (Slusher et al., 2003).

Another way to drain the breasts adequately to increase milk output is a technique called power pumping. It mimics a baby's vigorous feeding pattern during a cluster feed or unsettled growth behaviors. It tells your body to release more prolactin, which triggers the breasts to make more milk. Substitute one regular pumping session a day with the following method: (1) Pump for 20 minutes; (2) Rest for 10 minutes; (3) Pump for another 10 minutes; (4) Rest for 10 minutes; (5) Pump a third time for 10 minutes.

Another way to stimulate more milk in an hour of pumping with breaks is to watch a TV program at the same time. Turn off the pump during commercials. Start it again when the break is over. Enjoy the show while your pump does its job. Or, set your pump up somewhere convenient and try to get an extra 5 to 10 minutes of pumping in as many times that fit your busy life. No need to wash your plastic parts each time if you start with a clean kit. Wash your hands prior to each usage. When finished, place it in the refrigerator or a cooler.

Keeping the Baby Interested

If the baby's weight gain is slightly low (1/2 oz per day) and the mother is healthy, with normal-appearing breasts, we sometimes recommend switch nursing to keep the baby interested. Listen for sucks and swallows. Switch sides as soon as the baby shuts his eyes and swallows become intermittent (i.e., suck, suck, suck, swallow instead of a rhythmic suck, swallow, breathe with that wonderful "ka" sound). Switch breasts over and over each time his sucking and swallowing slows down. If there is a worry about your baby's weight gain, don't spend more than 30 to 40 minutes on this technique.

Alternate Breast Compression

Several years ago, Dr. Jack Newman introduced the lactation world to the technique of alternate breast compression. It is a helpful way to expedite breast drainage and it keeps the baby interested (Newman, 2017). This technique requires your Baby-Watching skills.

1. Hold the breast, cupping it from underneath with the thumb on one side, fingers on the other.

2. Watch the baby's swallowing. The milk flows more rapidly when the infant is drinking with an open, pause, close-type of suck. Open, pause, close is one suck; the pause is a swallow.

3. When the baby stops swallowing and goes into an irregular pattern or quicker suckle, gently squeeze and hold the breast. You will see vigorous swallows again if the baby is drinking.

4. Hold the pressure until he stops the suck-pause pattern. Then, shift your hand to another area of the breast. Switch breasts when this no longer keeps the baby actively swallowing.

5. Do lean back because the compressions will more forcefully release the milk. This technique keeps the baby more vigorously sucking and releases more fat. It is also very helpful when using an electric breast pump. If you have breast implants, be careful not to press directly over the implants to avoid rupturing the sac.

If the assessment suggests more complicated reasons for insufficient milk, the plan may include some of the following recommendations.

Blood Work for Chronic Low Milk Supply

If you have persistent low milk supply, your healthcare provider may order blood tests to ascertain underlying issues. If you were anemic during pregnancy or had more than normal bleeding during labor and delivery, ask to have a blood test for anemia. Your thyroid function is very important for a good milk supply, so a thyroid level test should be included in the blood work. Gestational theca lutein cyst has been identified as a possible cause for delayed lactogenesis II (milk coming in). To test for this condition, a blood test to check testosterone levels is needed. Prolactin should be drawn before and after a feed, waiting at least 45 minutes, then measuring the increase (West & Marasco, 2009). Type 1 and 2 diabetes is correlated with low milk supply.

A blood test will review your general health, such as a metabolic or chemistry panel to look at your blood sugar level, kidney, and liver functions.

Some issues, such as retained placenta and gestational ovarian theca lutein cysts, may resolve during the first several weeks after birth. Others, such as hypothyroidism, require treatment. Both treatment and spontaneous resolution can lead to a quick increase in a mother's milk supply. Testing for polycystic-ovary syndrome (PCOS)-related milk supply problems is less clear. PCOS has received special attention during recent years as a major and often over-looked factor in true low milk supply (Marasco, 2014). However, symptoms and hormonal imbalances present differently among women, making this condition difficult to diagnose.

Use a Supplementer

Whether you are building your milk supply, or you have been diagnosed with low milk, one of the best ways to protect breast-feeding while maintaining or continuing to build your milk supply is to feed your baby extra milk right at your breast. Ask your lactation consultant to set you up with a tube system that can attach to your nipple and provide extra milk to your baby while you nurse, such as a Medela Supplementary Nutritional System (SNS), a Supply Line, or a 1 oz syringe or bottle connected to an infant-feeding tube. Although, this is not what you dreamed of when you imagined breastfeeding your baby, if you can think of this new reality as a means to maintaining a breastfeeding relationship with your baby, you can still be successful, and your baby will not be able to tell the difference (see supplementer-at-the-breast on page 241).

Experiment with an Herbal Remedy

After all of the above tactics have been exhausted and proven to be ineffective at increasing the milk supply, continue to try these measures in combination with an herbal treatment. Herbal galactagogues are substances known to promote lactation in humans by increasing the body's prolactin levels. There is limited scientific evidence of their safety and effectiveness (Mortel & Mehta, 2013). Nonetheless, mothers have reported a noticeable increase in their milk supply while taking fenugreek or blessed thistle. Traditionally, fennel hops and anise are also used as galactogalogues. There are many others, including herbal combinations. A lactation consultant or naturopathic doctor can help you choose an appropriate herb. The book, *The Breastfeeding Mother's Guide to Making More Milk* by Diana West and Lisa Marasco, is an excellent resource on appropriate selection of both medication and herbal solutions known to enhance milk supply. Always consult your health practitioner before taking a medication or herbal supplement, especially if your baby is sick or premature.

Lastly, be sure to consume a diet rich in protein, grains, fruits, and vegetables. Stay hydrated but don't overdrink. If your urine is dark and concentrated, you are drinking too little. Urinating every hour in large, clear, amounts means overhydration. Overhydration can decrease your milk supply (Walker, 2017).

. . . .

CHAPTER SEVENTEEN

Learning Curves and Growing "Pains": Breastfeeding the Unsettled Baby

Chapter Goal: Learn how growth spurts and developmental changes affect how you might feel about your breastfeeding progress.

"I CAN'T GET NO SATISFACTION"

For Jessica, it's week 2 postpartum. She's starting to recover from childbirth and beginning to feel more settled with her newborn daughter, Bella. Jessica yearns for sleep but is hopeful that her body will soon acclimate. Breastfeeding appears to be going well. Around week three, things start to change. Her sleepy newborn is more alert and fussier. It seems that the baby has found her voice. Bella nurses much more than before, yet she seems less satisfied. The mother begins to lose confidence and questions whether she has enough milk. By week 6, the fussiness continues and appears to get worse by the day. Each night, Jessica feels exhausted from Bella's hours of crying and cluster feedings. Her confidence is officially compromised. She begins to question whether she has enough breastmilk.

Jessica's mother-in-law arrives from overseas to meet Bella. She suggests, "You should eat raw onions. It's good for your milk." "What the [expletive]?" Jessica thinks. Grandma warns the new mother not to hold the baby too much. Hours later, Jessica's husband arrives home from work and finds his wife frustrated to the point of tears. He says, "Why don't you just give her a bottle? Wouldn't it be easier?" He knows how hard Jessica has been trying to make breastfeeding work and how important it is for their baby. She takes out the free formula sample sitting in her pantry—thus setting in motion the beginning of the end of breastfeeding for this family.

This story is all too familiar. Many new moms turn to formula within the first few weeks of their newborn's life. In fact, four out of five mothers who birthed in U.S. hospitals started breastfeeding in 2013, according to the U.S. Centers for Disease Control & Prevention's 2016 Breastfeeding Report Card (CDC, 2016). By their baby's 3-month mark, many mothers were already offering formula as a means of supplementation or exclusively bottle-feeding. At 3 months post-partum, the number of mothers who were exclusively breastfeeding dropped from the initial 81% to about 44%, the report shows. That's nearly half that couldn't keep it up.

Around 6 weeks postpartum, research shows that many mothers begin to believe that they don't have enough milk to nourish their baby because of increased infant fussiness and crying, particularly in the evenings (Hill, 1991). This, associated with other simultaneous changes described in Chapter 16, like the softening of the breasts, which occurs when the milk supply reaches its full development, and changing infant stool patterns, fuels the misperception. They begin supplementing with formula or abandon nursing altogether. This may reduce the milk supply, thus making the previously mentioned perceived insufficient milk supply a reality.

Often, the fussiness and overall dissatisfaction in a growing baby during the first 2 months of life is completely normal and due to a phase of growth and neurological development. Wonderful research out of the Netherlands explains exactly what's driving your baby's behavior. "A number of indications in babies of approximately 4 to 5 weeks show that they are undergoing enormous changes that affect their senses, metabolism, and internal organs," writes Doctors Hetty van de Rijt and Frans Plooij in The Wonder Weeks.

Specifically, the researchers explain, at about 3 to 4 weeks of age, there are big brain changes, including glucose metabolism and a sizable increase in the infant's head circumference (van de Rijt & Plooij, 2013). These internal changes, which most people are not aware of, manifest dramatic external behaviors. Babies become particularly clingy, want to nurse more often than usual, may need motion or the breast to fall asleep, and once asleep, may awake the moment they are put down to bed. Notably, the infant's maturity appears to have regressed.

Unfortunately, these internal developments make things harder on you before they get easier. Simple, everyday tasks that you finally worked into a rhythm are disrupted. Finding time to eat and sleep well might be out of the question. You might find yourself asking, "what is wrong with my baby?" or "what is wrong with my milk?" It might even warrant a visit to the pediatrician. (Please don't ever fear overreacting when it comes to seeking a medical assessment. It's your job to be a strong advocate for your baby.)

The Netherlands' research explains that all infants undergo fussy periods around the same age, as determined by the date of conception. During the first year of life, there are eight major phases when they behave all out-of-sorts, according to Doctors van de Rijt and Plooij. During each phase, more organization takes place in the central nervous system, which builds the foundation of behavioral development. After each difficult period, the scientists subsequently observed a leap in mental development, and then a settled phase, according to *Wonder Weeks*.

Even after we learn about Baby Watching, we must infuse ourselves with knowledge about normal breast changes during lactation, and developmental milestones that affect infant behaviors because, combined, they do alter the dynamics of the breastfeeding experience. This chapter summarizes how you can expect your breastfed baby to behave during the first 10 weeks of life as he goes through some major developmental phases, including the first of many growth spurts to come.

NEWBORN DEVELOPMENT: STAGES AND PHASES

The first 10 weeks of an infant's life are a whirlwind as they cycle through the first phase of being disorganized and unsettled to more organized and settled. It's this overall unsettledness that defines dissatisfaction in babies and leads mothers to believe that their milk is not enough or is causing difficult behaviors in their baby. The following summarizes the common experience during each phase of the first 10 weeks.

Birth to 10 Days: The Transitional Period

If feeding is going well during the first 10 days, the average neuro-logically mature newborn appears very sleepy and quiet. People think that they have the easiest baby. You basically have to undress them to get them awake enough to eat. These babies can habituate (shut down) to block stimuli, so they appear to be sleeping much of the time when they are not eating.

10 Days to 9 Weeks: The Unsettled Baby

At 10 days to 3 weeks, babies typically wake up. By now, the medications and effects of childbirth have worn off. Several things start happening. They begin to cry a lot because they are more affected by stimulation in their environment. They also have a diminishing capability to habituate because they are more aware. So, they spend the day being subjected to new sights and sounds that they try to process. When it's too much, they shut down, and by the evening, they begin to fuss and give their parents a series of mixed messages and confusing cues. They act hungry but may just be overtired. Regardless, they really may not settle down until they have had about 3 to 4 hours of cluster feedings. What follows may be a nice, long sleep.

Overall, babies are more awake, irritable, and gassy, particularly in the evening. As the weeks go on, this fussiness accelerates, peaking around 6-weeks-old. Parents become so concerned that they typically blame the mother's diet. She takes out that list of potential foods that can irritate the baby (possibly given to her in a breastfeeding class) and starts eliminating major food groups, unnecessarily depleting her nutrition. Other changes (i.e., softer breasts and less frequent dirty diapers. See perceived insufficient milk) lead her to think that he is not getting enough to eat. At around 8 weeks, there is a small growth spurt, so the baby is still unsettled but not as fussy as at 6 weeks. The changes that begin at 3 weeks get mothers thinking and by 6 weeks, there seems to be enough *proof* to confirm a milk-supply problem or an allergy. Women who do not have good support or proper information often begin supplementing formula at this time or stop breastfeeding all together.

Week 10: The Settled Baby

If you have been paying attention to your infant's need cues with responsive care, things will naturally begin to improve after this stage of infancy reaches its climax. Those that weaned from nursing to feed formula will have the perception that their milk was the issue, noted by the improved baby behavior, thus reinforcing this common belief. Then, at 10 weeks, it is as though a major hurdle has been crossed. The baby can happily stay awake longer and is more rested. A 10-week-old is not as bothered by stimulation in his environment. By simply looking away, he can shut out disturbances without shutting down. He can comfort himself by sucking on his hands. A larger stomach and more mature digestive system makes him capable of taking in more food so he's not constantly hungry. He is alert, social, and smiley. Best of all, he can interact more and sleep longer.

Some moms worry when their baby begins to nurse less. Know that infants become more efficient as they grow older. They can self-comfort by sucking on their hands. Meet the settled baby. The question is, how can you help teach your baby to be more organized so that you can enjoy a settled baby rather than one that is overwhelmed by the world around him? The answer lies in your response to your baby's communication. If you have been a good Baby Watcher, it means you have been paying attention.

If you have identified his cues, responded the best you could, and accommodated his sensitivities, then you have helped him reach this settled state.

GROWTH SPURTS

When people talk about growth, we tend to think about weight gain and other physical changes that we can see. We believe that the baby needs more food for growth. The developments that are happening inside the baby's body, however, are even more remarkable and occur not only from nutrition but time and responsive parenting (attachment).

The brain and nervous system grow tremendously during the first 10 weeks of life. Newborn babies start with only about one third the size of an adult brain (Jackson, 2002). Scientific evidence shows that, immediately after birth, the brain is tasked with turning billions of existing cells into functioning neurons. These connections are the basis of your child's future social and emotional intelligence. Growth is not linear. Children have times when they are more settled when their system is in equilibrium, and they have times when they are out-of-sorts, called disequilibrium. These periods are short within the first year.

"Neurological studies have shown that there are times when major, dramatic changes take place in the brains of children younger than 20 months. Shortly after each of them, there is a parallel leap forward in mental development," according to *The Wonder Weeks* (p. 2). "Babies all undergo these fussy phases at around the same ages. During the first 20 months of a baby's life, there are ten developmental leaps with their corresponding fussy periods on onset. The fussy periods come at 5, 8, 12, 15, 23, 34, 42, 51, 60, and 71 weeks" (van de Rijt & Plooij, 2013, p. 13). These dates are for full-term babies and may vary by a week or two. The fussy periods can last as little as a few days, although it feels like longer. As the baby gets older, the changes in the brain are more advanced and it may take longer to adjust. The fussiness may go on for a week or as long as 6 weeks (van de Rijt & Plooij, 2013).

During growth spurts, babies need their mother to hold them a lot and allow them to nurse more often. They don't necessarily take in more milk, but rather, need extra comfort while they feel out-of-sorts. The experience during a growth spurt is taxing on parents, as babies customarily exhibit fussiness, difficulty getting settled, a desire to nurse frequently, clingy behavior, frequent night waking, and difficulty napping. If breastfeeding is going well, don't be afraid to use a pacifier after nursing to help settle the baby.

Because the behaviors are so confusing and exhausting, it may not be clear that the baby is undergoing a spurt until the period of the increased growth has passed. But when it is over, the parents can expect a reward for their extra hard work in the form of something new from their baby, whether it's a purposeful smile, he can reach a little further, or accomplish one of the many developmental milestones of infancy. When you suspect your baby appears to be in a growth spurt, have his weight checked to make sure he is gaining on track. Also, rule out any signs of illness, such as fever and/or congestion, because infants do similar behaviors when they are fighting illness. If there are no signs of sickness, your baby has been gaining weight steadily, and you have a normal milk supply, the fussy phase is likely developmental. If you have been struggling and you know your baby is not happy, make sure you have him weighed.

The First Growth Spurt

"Between 4 and 5 weeks old, your baby goes through a whole set of changes that affect his senses—the way he feels, even the way he digests his food," explains doctors van de Rijt and Plooij in *The Wonder Weeks* (p. 46). "His whole world feels, looks, smells, and sounds different."

Imagine waking up to discover that things have changed. You were just beginning to feel safe and brave in this strange new world and now everything that you perceived to be true is different. Your feelings of contentment would surely be replaced with anxiety in this atmosphere of changing sensations. A newborn can't communicate his fears. Instead, he cries. And he can't ask questions. He must cling to what he knows is safe. Sometimes, babies lose every bit of control and work themselves up into a screaming fit—one that lasts for hours. Subsequently, the parents' next Google search is "colic."

Soon after the baby adjusts to this "new world," you may observe a developmental leap. A 6-week-old baby of a responsive mother can calm himself down when put on her lap as she prepares to nurse. He can settle a bit when he knows food is coming (the beginning of patience). During these first 10 weeks, one milestone quickly follows the next. Around 8 weeks, a big change in the brain enables the baby to perceive simple patterns for the first time (van de Rijt & Plooij, 2013). Waking to a world full of patterns will have your baby behaving like he woke up on the wrong side of the bed. The discovery of patterns means his perception of his environment is changing once again. The baby's new awareness may make him desperate for Mom.

Behaviors to Expect

While not all developmental changes are noticeable as physical growth, a growth spurt can be identified by the following behaviors, which are commonly confused for breastfeeding problems:

> » The baby fusses more often, especially during the evening.
> » He refuses to be put to sleep in his crib. He cries desperately when put down.
> » At times, he cries inconsolably and appears to have a stomachache. He pulls his legs up and arches his body.
> » There are periods when he roots constantly and never seems to get enough of the breast.
> » He requires the breast or motion to fall asleep.
> » He shows a desire to be carried around a lot, and calms when you do so.

Be able to identify these behaviors so that you can distinguish them separately from what you already know are need cues. Because these phases of difficult behavioral changes are a major source of frustration for parents, it is pertinent that you are aware of them to avoid the utter confusion that might lead you to make a choice that would undermine your breastfeeding success (i.e., unnecessary supplementation). During these unsettled periods, babies are very labor intensive. If you had developed a nursing pattern by this point, it could officially be derailed. Abandon the idea of a schedule and continue to nurse on-cue.

CHECK-LIST

If you are confused by your baby's unexpected behaviors, look for the following signs of a normal developmental spurt, not to be confused with a breastfeeding problem:

[_] The baby fusses more often, especially during the evening.

[_] He refuses to be put to sleep in his crib.

[_] At times, he cries inconsolably and appears to have a tummy ache.

[_] Sometimes, he roots constantly and never seems to get enough.

[_] My baby requires the breast or motion to fall asleep.

[_] He needs me to carry him around a lot but calms when I do.

[_] I thought breastfeeding was going well.

[_] My baby is gaining weight as expected, 4 to 7 ounces per week.

[_] There are no symptoms of illness, such as fever, skin rash, or congestion.

THE SETTLED BABY

Caring for a newborn can be overwhelming. Parents are tired and anxious about their new responsibilities. Keep in mind that this is a learning period and that your baby is healthy and resilient. Hold him and love him. Keep him warm, fed, and clean, and you will do well. As your baby nears 10-weeks-old, you may begin to feel like you are turning a corner. Evenings are no longer hysterical, breastfeeding feels more comfortable, and the confidence-seeds sprout.

Breastfeeding Patterns Change

You might also notice a welcome change in your baby's breastfeeding pattern. Feeds will have progressed from very long—a period when you spent most of your time nursing—to progressively shorter. You will also likely see a change in the frequency of feeds and intervals between them. Research shows that between the first and third months, babies who exclusively breastfeed nurse less often but take in more milk at each session, while the daily milk intake remains the same (Kent et al., 2013). Essentially, breastfeeding becomes more efficient. The exception is the baby who started out with a low feeding frequency. In this case, you might not see a decrease in feeding duration. Instead, it would likely remain stable for as long as you exclusively breastfeed or about 6 months (Kent et al., 2013). These normal pattern changes arrive once your milk supply is established, the baby's stomach can stretch to hold more volume, and he becomes more alert and proficient at eating. Anticipate this development because it is commonly confused as an indication of insufficient milk supply (Kent et al., 2013). It's not a sign of a breastfeeding problem, but rather, breastfeeding success—an outcome of a healthy, normal nursing relationship (Kent et al., 2013). After 3 months of lactation, breastfeeding patterns for frequency of feeding, duration, and milk intake stay relatively stable for the remainder of exclusive breastfeeding or about 6 months (Kent et al., 2013). Overall, babies spend less time eating than they did during the first 3 months but have the same daily intake.

Making Milestones

During his first 10 weeks, your baby makes leaps and bounds, overcoming the first major developmental period. Rest assured that he is developing normally if you see these behaviors:

» His neck appears stronger, having more control over the weight of the head.

» Your baby makes good eye contact at close distances.

» He focuses on things.

» He interacts with his caregivers.

» He shows interest in objects with contrasting colors.

» He turns his head to a shaken rattle.

» He shows excitement by kicking his feet.

» He can bring both hands up to his mouth equally.

» He uses all four limbs symmetrically.

» He is starting to have distinct cries, which are different for hunger and pain.

CHECK-LIST

Look for the following signs that your baby is developing normally:

[_] The neck appears stronger, having more control over the weight of the head.

[_] He is starting to have distinct cries, which are different for hunger and pain.

[_] He makes good eye contact at close distances.

[_] He focuses on things.

[_] He interacts with his caregivers.

[_] He shows interest in objects with contrasting colors.

[_] He turns his head to a shaken rattle.

[_] He shows excitement by kicking his feet.

[_] He can bring both hands up to his mouth equally.

[_] He uses all four limbs symmetrically.

When week 10 approaches, celebrate because you established breastfeeding and made it past the first major hurdles. Be proud of the remarkable mother (parents) you are for the sacrifices you made to give your baby the best nutrition and emotional start possible. Your reward should begin to set in. Now, he should be entering a settled phase, which will afford you temporary relief and changes, which this time, are more predictable. Look for the following signs that indicate that your baby is entering a settled phase:

» He can stay awake longer than before.

» He seems to have a longer visual acuity, focusing at greater distances.

» He shows an interest in his surroundings.

» He sometimes reacts to things around him.

» He smiles on purpose.

» He is less fragile—not startling as often.

» He can handle let-down easier, seen by choking less.

» He seems more efficient at the breast, nursing faster.

» His digestion is more under control, observed by less spitting up and burping.

» When he cries, real tears come out.

Notice that some reflexes are beginning to fade away. They were controlled by primitive centers in the lower brain and vanish to make way for developments in the higher levels (van de Rijt & Plooij, 2013). The new levels of organization that have taken place over the last several weeks open a world of new possibilities for your baby. You know his cues. You know his nursing pattern. You understand the signs when he is growing. Now you know how to discover the traits of his individual temperament and emerging personality, which will begin to blossom into the third month.

CHECK-LIST

Look for the following signs that your baby is past the first developmental milestone and now entering a settled phase around 10 weeks:

[_] My baby is able to stay awake longer than before.

[_] He seems to have a longer visual acuity, focusing at greater distances.

[_] He shows an interest in his surroundings.

[_] He sometimes reacts to things around him.

[_] He smiles on purpose.

[_] He is less fragile—not startling as often.

[_] He can handle let-down easier, seen by choking less.

[_] He seems more efficient at the breast, completing a breastfeed faster.

[_] His digestion is more under control (vomiting and burping less).

[_] When he cries, real tears come out.

COPING WITH THE ADJUSTMENT TO PARENTHOOD

Adjusting to parenting is a time of great upheaval. The baby is developing and so are the parents. You are learning a new job while exhausted and undergoing emotional and biological surges. Both parents are physically and mentally adapting, and usually feeling out-of-sorts—a rollercoaster of ups and downs. For the mother, the hormones of pregnancy and the growth and development the body undergoes starts to prepare her. Fathers also evolve as they respond to their partner's new behaviors, different body shape, and attitudes. Parents have expectations of this mystery child. There may be preconceived ideas in response to the way the baby kicks and moves. Pregnant Mary stated, "I know this one will be active. She never lets me rest."

Reality sets in soon after birth, beginning with the appearance of the baby, the fatigue, and the emotional ride of parenthood with the young infant. Who is that woman who cries at the blink of an eye? She thrusts the baby at her partner, who just walked in the door. Left with a screaming infant makes him feel resentful and helpless. The coparent often feels slighted, and in response, may seem either distant or angry—too ashamed to admit to feeling jealous of this helpless baby. Throwing in another sibling intensifies sentiments of lost time together. A parent may also grieve the loss of their old body shape, active sex drive, and previous identity. All this and much more compounds this period of disorganization.

A new birth changes the household dynamics, which stresses the family system. Breastfeeding challenges compound the difficulties. Before the baby was born, everybody in the family knew their roles, when they would have time and energy to finish all the household tasks, and when they could relax, work on hobbies, and have fun. Now, the needs of the helpless infant take up much of that time. Everybody will feel frustrated if roles fail to shift. Often, women take on most of the household work. If you were employed outside the home before the baby was born, you might feel obligated to do all the household tasks in addition to caring for the baby because your partner has taken over the financial burden. Some fathers are expected to do more of the household and baby care, but maybe he is having difficulty taking on the new tasks. How your own father role-modeled parenting often influences your expectations of your mate. Unless couples communicate and negotiate how to accomplish household tasks in a manner that feels good for both parties, their relationship may be strained. A mother cannot do everything without feeling resentment, extreme fatigue, and stress. Some days, especially if the baby is ill or fussy, completing a single household task can be frustrating and seemingly impossible. By figuring out what needs to be done and reallocating the household jobs, everyone will feel better. The following stress reduction techniques may help:

>> Learn to set limits. You cannot possibly do everything you did before the baby was born. If you are accustomed to having to "wait" on certain friends or relatives when they come, you may have to delay their visit until you have adjusted and recovered. Say "no" to social pressure unless promised help, or the friends and family make you feel supported.

>> Reduce your standards on things that aren't top priority and accept imperfection.

>> Sleep-in with your newborn, staying in bed together until you receive enough cumulative night-sleep. Nap when the baby naps and nurse lying in bed throughout the day.

>> Take a bath. Put the baby nearby in an infant chair with toys hanging.

>> Take care of your physical self, including hygiene, exercise, and a balanced diet, rich with whole, unprocessed foods. Take walks daily and get some sun for a needed vitamin D boost.

>> Simplify dinner, hire help if you can afford it, or accept help from others.

>> Realize that this is a short time in your life, a transition. Soon, you will have new rhythms.

>> Give yourself time to learn and strengthen your relationships.

» Find a trusted source for advice, such as a pediatric nurse, wise aunt, or parent educator.

» Communicate with your partner using "I" statements: "I feel overwhelmed," instead of, "you aren't helping me!"

» Show empathy, not jealousy, for the other parent. Put yourself in your partner's shoes.

New babies, while such a joy, at the same time, put a tremendous strain on relationships. Families are learning new jobs and developing new roles while healing from childbirth and often feeling grumpy from sleep deprivation and hormone surges. If you feel the strain is too much, seek the help of a therapist. Usually, your obstetrician or midwife can make recommendations for an appropriate mental health professional. Try not to take your partner's grumpiness or lack of energy and enthusiasm too personally. Instead, strive to develop better communication abilities. These are the moments in relationships that build the foundations of a lifetime.

Nursing On:
A Heartfelt Message
from the Authors

To Nursing Mothers

This is just the beginning. You may go on to breast-feed for a year or even more, as long as you find it beneficial to you and your baby. We hope that in having a basic understanding of early infant development and breastfeeding, you will have the confidence and the knowledge to rely on your intuition because mother knows best. Best wishes for a healthy and safe start.

To World Leaders

We ask you to develop policy that supports mothers in their first 6 months postpartum, so that they CAN exclusively breastfeed their babies. First and foremost, work to prevent separation of mothers and newborns. Recognize the power of breastfeeding as one of the most cost effective, protective, and lifesaving preventive healthcare measures. Strengthen each and every nation by putting families first.

APPENDIX

REFERENCES

AAP (American Academy of Pediatrics) Task Force on Sudden Infant Death Syndrome. 2016. Policy Statement.

AAP (American Academy of Pediatrics) Task Force on Sudden Infant Death Syndrome. 2005. The Changing Concept of Sudden Infant Death Syndrome: Diagnostic Coding Shifts, Controversies Regarding the Sleeping Environment, and New Variables to Consider in Reducing Risk. *Pediatrics* 116:1245-1255.

AAP (American Academy of Pediatrics). 2012. Breastfeeding and the Use of Human Milk: Section on Breastfeeding. *Pediatrics* 129(3):e827-e841.

AAP (American Academy of Pediatrics). 2016. Task Force on Sudden Infant Death Syndrome. SIDS and Other Sleep-Related Infant Deaths: Updated 2016 Recommendations for a Safe Infant Sleeping Environment. *Pediatrics* 138(5):e20162938.

ABM (Academy of Breastfeeding Medicine Protocol Committee). 2008. ABM Clinical Protocol #6: Guidelines on Co-Sleeping and Breastfeeding. *Breastfeeding Medicine* 3(1):38-43.

ABM (Academy of Breastfeeding Medicine Protocol Committee). 2009. ABM Clinical Protocol #3: Hospital Guidelines for the Use of Supplementary Feedings in the Healthy Term Breastfed Neonate, Revised 2009. *Breastfeeding Medicine* 4(3):175-182.

ABM (Academy of Breastfeeding Medicine Protocol Committee). 2010. ABM Clinical Protocol #7: Model Breastfeeding Policy (Revision 2010). *Breastfeeding Medicine* 5(4):173-177.

ABM (Academy of Breastfeeding Medicine Protocol Committee). 2017. ABM Clinical Protocol #22: Guidelines for Management of Jaundice in the Breastfeeding Infant Equal to or Greater Than 35 Weeks' Gestation. *Breastfeeding Medicine* 12(5):250-257.

Alekseev, N. P., E. V. Omel'inuk, and N. E. Talalaeva. 2000. Dynamics of milk ejection reflex during continuous rhythmic stimulation of areola-nipple complex of the mammary gland. *Rossiiskii Fiziologicheskii Zhurnal Imeni I. M. Sechenova* 86(6):711-719.

Aljazaf, K., T. W. Hale, K. F. Ilett, P. E. Hartmann, L. R. Mitoulas, J. H. Kristensen, and L. P. Hackett. 2003. Pseudoephedrine: effects on milk production in women and estimation of infant exposure via breastmilk. *British Journal of Pharmacology* 56(1):18-24.

Allen, J. C., R. P. Keller, P. Archer, and M. C. Neville. 1991. Studies in Human Lactation: milk composition and daily secretion rates of macronutrients in the first year of lactation. *The American Journal of Clinical Nutrition* 54(1):69-80.

Amir, L. H., and the Academy of Breastfeeding Medicine Protocol Committee. 2014. ABM Clinical Protocol #4: Mastitis, Revised March 2014. *Breastfeeding Medicine* 9(5):239-243.

Amir, L. H., D. Forester, H. McLachlan, et al. 2004. Incidence of breast abscess in lactating women: Report from an Australian cohort. *BJOG* 111(12):1378-1381.

Anderson, J. E., N. Held, and K. Wright. 2004. Raynaud's Phenomenon of the Nipple: A Treatable Cause of Painful Breastfeeding. *Pediatrics* 113(4):e276-e282.

Armstrong, K. L., A. R. Van Haeringen, M. R. Dadds, and R. Cash. 1998. Sleep deprivation or postnatal depression in later infancy: separating the chicken from the egg. *Journal of Paediatrics and Child Health* 34:260-262.

Armstrong, K. L., R. A. Quinn, and M. R. Dadds. 1994. The sleep patterns of normal children. *Medical Journal of Australia* 161(3):202-6.

Asnes, R. and R. L. Mones. 1982. Infantile Colic: A Review. *Journal of Developmental & Behavioral Pediatrics* 4:1.

Baby-Friendly USA. Jan. 2016. The Ten Steps to Successful Breastfeeding.

Baddock, S. A., B. C. Galland, B. J. Taylor, and D. P. G. Bolton. 2007. Sleep Arrangements and Behavior of Bed-Sharing Families in the Home Setting *Pediatrics* 119;e200.

Ball, H. 2014. Sleep Ecology and Development in Early Infancy. Parent-Infant Sleep Lab, Anthropology, Durham University. Gold Learning Webinar.

Ball, H. L. 2003. Breastfeeding, bed sharing, and infant sleep. *Birth* 30:181-188.

Ball, H. L. 2014. Reframing what we tell parents about normal infant sleep and how we support them. *Breastfeeding Review* 22(3):11-12.

Barnard, K., and K. A. Thomas. 2014. *Beginning Rhythms: The Emerging Process of Sleep Wake Behavior and Self-Regulation, 2nd edition.* NCAST Programs: Seattle, Washington.

Barr, R. G. 2001. "Colic" is Something Infants Do, Rather than a Condition They "Have": A Developmental Approach to Crying Phenomena, Patterns, Pacification and (Patho)genesis in *New Evidence on Unexplained Early Infant Crying: Its Origins, Nature and Management.* Johnson & Johnson Pediatric Institute Division of Johnson & Johnson Consumer Companies, Inc. P. 87-104.

Barr, R. G., M. Konner, R. Bakeman, and L. Adamson. 1991. Crying in !Kung San infants: a test of the cultural specificity hypothesis. *Developmental Medicine and Child Neurology* 33:601-610.

Barr, R., M. S. Kramer, B. I. Pless, C. Boisjoly, and D. Leduc. 1989. Feeding and Temperament as Determinants of Early Infant Crying/Fussing Behavior. *Pediatrics* 84(3):514-21.

Beck, C. T. 2006. Postpartum depression: it isn't just the blues. *American Journal of Nursing* 106(5):40-50.

Benckert, J., N. Schmolka, C. Kreschel, M. J. Zoller, A. Sturm, B. Wiedenmann, and H. Wardemann. 2011. The majority of intestinal IgA+ and IgG+ plasmablasts in the human gut are antigen-specific. *Journal of Clinical Investigation* 121(5):1946–1955.

Berens, P., M. Labbok, and The Academy of Breastfeeding Medicine. 2015. ABM Clinical Protocol #13: Contraception During Breastfeeding, Revised 2015. *Breastfeeding Medicine* 10(1):1-9.

Bergman, N. 2007. Perinatal Neuroscience and Skin-to-Skin Contact. goldlearning.com

Bergman, N. 2007. Restoring the Original Paradigm for Infant Care. goldlearning.com

Binns, C. W., and J. A. Scott. 2002. Breastfeeding: Reasons for starting, reasons for stopping and problems along the way. *Breastfeeding Review* 10(2):13-19.

Blair, P. S., P. Sidebotham, A. Pease, and P. J. Fleming. 2014. Bed-Sharing in the Absence of Hazardous Circumstances: Is There a Risk of Sudden Infant Death Syndrome? An Analysis from Two Case-Control Studies Conducted in the UK. *PLOS ONE* 9(9):e107799.

Blass, E. M., and C. A. Camp. 2003. Biological bases of face preference in 6-week-old infants. *Developmental Science* 6(5):524-536.

Blyton, D. M., C. E. Sullivan, and N. Edwards. 2002. Lactation is associated with an increase in slow-wave sleep in women. *Journal of Sleep Research* 11:297-303.

Boere-Boonekamp, M. M., L. L. van der Linden-Kuipper. 2001. Positional preference: prevalence in infants and follow-up after two years. *Pediatrics* 107:339-343.

Bowlby, J. 1970. *Child Care and the Growth of Love (2nd ed.).* Baltimore: Penguin.

Brazelton, T. B. 1962. Crying in infancy. *Pediatrics* 29:579-588.

Brazelton, T. B., and B. G. Cramer. 1990. *The Earliest Relationship: Parents, Infants, and the Drama of Early Attachment.* A Merloyd Lawrence Book: Addison-Wesley Publishing Company, Inc.

Brazelton, T. B. and J. Sparrow. 2003. *Calming Your Fussy Baby The Brazelton Way.* Perseus Publishing Da Campo Press.

Brazelton, T. B., and J. D. Sparrow. 2006. *Touchpoints.* Boston, MA: Da Capo Press.

Brazelton, T. B. and Nugent, J.K. 2011. *The Neonatal Behavioral Assessment Scale. 4th edition.* Blackwell Press.

Britton, J. R. 2011. Infant Temperament and Maternal Anxiety and Depressed Mood in the Early Postpartum Period. *Women & Health* 51:55-71.

Brown, E. W., and A. W. Bosworth. 1922. Studies of infant feeding XVI. A bacteriological study of the feces and the food of normal babies receiving breastmilk. *The American Journal of Diseases of Children* 23:243-258.

Buckley, S. J. 2014. Epidurals: Risks and Concerns for Mother and Baby. Gentle Birth: The Science and the Wisdom.

Bullen, C., P. Tearle, and M. Stewart. 1977. The effect of "humanized" milks and supplemented breast feeding on the faecal flora of infants. *Journal of Medical Microbiology* 10:403-413.

Butte, N. F. 2005. Energy Requirements of infants. *Public Health Nutrition* 8(7A):9-67.

Butte, N., and A. Stuebe. 2015. Patient information: Maternal health and nutrition during breastfeeding (Beyond the Basics). *UpToDate*. Available at www.uptodate.com/contents/maternal-health-and-nutrition-during-breastfeeding-beyond-the-basics?source=online_link&view=text&anchor=H3#H3. Accessed October 20, 2015.

Caffeine Informer. 2016. Caffeine Content of Drinks. Available at www.caffeineinformer.com. Accessed March 3, 2016.

Carlson, S. E. 2009. Docosahexaenoic acid supplementation in pregnancy and lactation. *American Journal of Clinical Nutrition* 89(2):678S-684S.

Carskadon, M.A., and W. C. Dement. 2011. Monitoring and staging human sleep. In M.H. Kryger, T. Roth, & W.C. Dement (Eds.), *Principles and practice of sleep medicine, 5th edition*, (pp 16-26). St. Louis: Elsevier Saunders.

CDC (Centers for Disease Control and Prevention). 2016. CDC Breastfeeding Report Card 2016. Accessed via: https://www.cdc.gov/breastfeeding/pdf/2016breastfeedingreportcard.pdf

CDC (Centers for Disease Control and Prevention). Dec. 30 2011. Media Statement - FDA and CDC Update: Investigation of Cronobacter bacteria illness in infants. Atlanta, GA: Centers for Disease Control and Prevention. www.cdc.gov/media/releases/2011/s1230_Cronobacter.html

Cernoch, J. M., and R. H. Porter. 1985. Recognition of maternal auxiliary odors by infants. *Child Development* 56:1593-1598.

Chambers, P. L., E. M. Mahabee-Gittens, and A. C. Leonard. 2011. Vulnerable child syndrome, parental perception of child vulnerability, and emergency department usage. *Pediatric Emergency Care* 27(11):1009-1013.

Chantry, C. J., L. A. Nommsen-Rivers, J. M. Peerson, R. J. Cohen, and K. G. Dewey. 2011. Excess weight loss in first-born breastfed newborns relates to maternal intrapartum fluid balance. *Pediatrics* 127:171-179.

Chertok, I. 2009. Reexamination of ultra-thin nipple shield use, infant growth and maternal satisfaction. *Journal of Clinical Nursing* 18: 2949-2955.

Cloherty, M., J. Alexander, I. Holloway. 2004. Supplementing breast-fed babies in the UK to protect their mother from tiredness or distress. *Midwifery* 20(2):194-204.

Colson, S. D., J. H. Meek, and J. M. Hawdon. 2008. Optimal positions triggering primitive neonatal reflexes stimulating breastfeeding. *Early Human Development* 84(7):441–49.

Coryllos, E., C. W. Genna, and A. C. Salloum. 2004. Congenital tongue-tie and its impact on breastfeeding. Breastfeeding: Best for Baby and Mother. *American Academy of Pediatrics Summer 2004:* 1-12.

Cubero, J., V. Valero, J. Sanchez, M. Rivero, H. Parvez, A. B. Rodriguez, and C. Barriga. 2005. The circadian rhythm of tryptophan in breast milk affects the rhythms of 6-sulfatoxymelatonin and sleep in newborn. *Neuroendocrinology Letters* 26(6):657-661.

Daly, S. E. J., R. A. Owens, P. E. Hartmann. 1993. The short-term synthesis and infant-regulated removal of milk in lactating women. *Experimental Physiology* 78:209-220.

Daly, S. E., A. Di Rosso, R. A. Owens, and P. E. Hartmann. 1993. Degree of breast emptying explains fat content, but not fatty acid composition, of human milk. *Experimental Physiology* 78: 741-755.

Davis, K.F., K. P. Parker, and G. L. Montgomery. 2004. Sleep in infants and young children: Part one: Normal sleep. *Journal of Pediatric Health Care* 18(2):65-71.

de Lauzon-Guillain, B. D., K. Wijndaele, M. Clark, C. L. Acerini, I. A. Hughes, D. B. Dunger, J. C. Wells, and K. K. Ong. 2012. Breastfeeding and Infant Temperament at Age Three Months. PLOS ONE 7.1.

DeCasper A. J., and W. P. Fifer. 1980. Of human bonding: newborns prefer their mothers' voices. *Science.* 208(4448):1174-1176.

Declercq, E. R., C. Sakala, M. P. Corry, S. Applebaum, and A. Herrlich. 2013. Listening to Mothers III: Pregnancy and Birth. New York: Childbirth Connection.

Dennis C. L., K. Jackson, and J. Watson. 2014. Interventions for treating painful nipples among breastfeeding women. *Cochrane Database of Systematic Reviews* 12:CD007366.

Dennis, C. L. 2002. Breastfeeding Initiation and Duration: A 1990-2000 Literature Review. *JOGNN* (in Review) 31(1):12-32.

Dewar, G. 2008-2014. The Infant Feeding Schedule: Why--breast or bottle-- babies benefit from being fed "on demand" http://www.parentingscience. com/infant-feeding-schedule.html#sthash.13Uil9jc.dpuf.

Dewey, K. G., L. A. Nommsen-Rivers, M. J. Heinig, and R. J. Cohen. 2003. Risk Factors for Suboptimal Infant Breastfeeding Behavior, Delayed Onset of Lactation, and Excess Neonatal Weight Loss. *Pediatrics* 112:607-619.

Di Mauro, A., J. Neu, G. Riezzo, and F. Indrio. 2013. Gastrointestinal function development and microbiota. *Italian Journal of Pediatrics* 39(1):15.

Doan, T., A. Gardiner, C. L. Gay, and K. A. Lee. 2007. Breast-feeding Increases Sleep Duration of New Parents. *Journal of Perinatal & Neonatal Nursing* 21(3):200-206.

Douglas, P. M., and D. Geddes. 2018. Practice-based interpretation of ultrasound studies leads the way to more effective clinical support and less pharmaceutical and surgical intervention for breastfeeding infants. *Midwifery* 58:145-155.

Douglas, P., and P. S Hill. 2013. Behavioral sleep interventions in 1st 6 months of life. *Journal of Developmental & Behavioral Pediatrics* 34:497-507.

Douglas, P., and R. Keogh. 2017. Gestalt Breastfeeding: Helping Mothers and Infants Optimize Positional Stability and Intraoral Breast Tissue Volume for Effective, Pain-Free Milk Transfer. *Journal of Human Lactation* 33(3):089033441770795.

Douglas, S. 2013. Rethinking Posterior Tongue-Tie. *Breastfeeding Medicine* 8(6):503-506.

Dupierrix, E., A. Hillairet de Boisferon, D. Méary, K. Lee, P. C. Quinn, E. Di Giorgio, F. Simion, M. Tomonaga, and O. Pascalis. 2014. Preference for human eyes in human infants. *Journal of Experimental Child Psychology* 123:138-146.

Eglash, A. L. Simon, and The Academy of Breastfeeding Medicine. 2017. ABM Clinical Protocol #8: Human Milk Storage Information for Home Use for Full-Term Infants. *Breastfeeding Medicine* 12(7):390-395.

Embleton, N., J. Katz, E. E. Ziegler. 2015. *Low-Birthweight Baby: Born Too Soon or Too Small.* Basel, Switzerland: Karger.

Erikson, E. H. 1950. *Childhood and Society.* New York: W.W. Norton & Company, Inc.

Eshach, A. O., M. Berant, and R. Shamir. 2004. New supplements to infant formulas. *Pediatric Endocrinology Review* 2:216-224.

Evans, A., K. A. Marinelli, J. S. Taylor, and The Academy of Breastfeeding Medicine. 2014. ABM Clinical Protocol #2: Guidelines for Hospital Discharge of the Breastfeeding Term Newborn and Mother: "The Going Home Protocol." 9(1):3-6.

FDA. 2017. FDA Confirms elevated levels of belladonna in certain homeopathic teething products. News Release.

Feldman-Winter, L. J., P. Goldsmith, and Committee on Fetus and Newborn, Task Force on Sudden Infant Death Syndrome. 2016. Safe Sleep and Skin-to-Skin Care in the Neonatal Period for Healthy Term Newborns. *Pediatrics 138*(3).

Ferrante, A., R Silvestri, and C. Montinaro. 2006. The importance of choosing the right feeding aids to maintain breastfeeding after interruption. *International Journal of Orofacial Myology* 32:58-67.

Field, T. M. 1981. Infant gaze aversion and heart rate during face-to-face interactions. *Infant Behavior and Development.* 4:307–315.

Field, T., M. A. Diego, M. Hernandez-Reif, O. Deeds, and B. Figuereido. 2006. Moderate versus light pressure massage therapy leads to greater weight gain in preterm infants. *Infant Behavior and Development.* 29(4):574-578.

Foong, S. C., M. L. Tan, L. A. Marasco, J. J. Ho, and W. C. Foong. 2015. Oral galactagogues for increasing breast-milk production in mothers of non-hospitalised term infants (Protocol). *Cochrane Database of Systematic Review* 4:CD011505. DOI:10.1002/14651858.

Francis-Morrill, J., M. J. Heinig, D. Pappagianis, and K. G. Dewey. 2004. Diagnostic value of signs and symptoms of mammary candidosis among lactating women. *Journal of Human Lactation* 20(3):288-295; 296-299.

Gable, S., and R. A. Isabella. 1992. Maternal contributions to infant regulation of arousal. *Infant Behavior and Development.* 15:95-107.

Gagnon, A. J., G. Leduc, K. Waghorn, H. Yang, and R. Platt. 2005. In-hospital formula supplementation of healthy breastfeeding newborns. *Journal of Human Lactation* 21:397-405.

Galbally, M., A. J. Lewis, K. McEgan, K. Scalzo, and F. A. Islam. 2013. Breastfeeding and infant sleep patterns: An Australian population study. *Journal of Paediatrics and Child Health* 49(2):E147-152.

Garcia-Lara, N. R., D. Escuder-Vieco, O. Garcia-Algar, J. De la Cruz, D. Lora, and C. Pallas-Alonso. 2012. Effect of freezing time on macronutrients and energy content of breastmilk. *Breastfeeding Medicine* 7:295-301.

Gartner, L. M., J. Morton, R. A. Lawrence, A. J. Naylor, D. O'Hare, R. J. Schlander, and A. I. Eidelman. 2005. Breastfeeding and the Use of Human Milk. *Pediatrics* 115(2):496-506.

Gatti, L. 2008. Maternal Perceptions of Insufficient Milk Supply in Breastfeeding. *Journal of Nursing Scholarship* 40(4):355-363.

Geddes, D. 2007. Inside the Lactating Breast: The Latest Anatomy Research. *Journal of Midwifery Women's Health* 52:556-563(6).

Geddes, D. T., D. B. Langton, I. Gollow, L. A. Jacobs, P. E. Hartmann, and K. Simmer. 2008. Frenulotomy for breastfeeding infants with ankylglossia: Effect on milk removal and sucking mechanism as imaged by ultrasound. *Pediatrics* 122(1):e188-1194.

Geddes, D. T., V. S. Sakalidis, A. R. Hepworth, H. L. McClellan, J. C. Kent, C. T. Lai, and P. E. Hartmann. 2012. Tongue movement and intra-oral vacuum of term infants during breastfeeding and feeding from an experimental teat that released milk under vacuum only. *Early Human Development* 88:443-449.

Genna, C. W. 2009. *Selecting and Using Breastfeeding Tools: improving care and outcomes.* Amarillo, TX: Hale Publishing.

Gerard, C. M., Harris, K. A., and B. T. Thach. 2002. Spontaneous Arousals in Supine Infants While Swaddled and Unswaddled During Rapid Eye Movement and Quiet Sleep. *Pediatrics* 110: e70.

Gerber, R. J., T. Wilkes, and C. Erdie-Lalena. 2010. Developmental Milestones: Motor Development. *Pediatrics in Review* 31:267-277.

Gert, K., N. Bergman, and F. M. Hann. 2001. Kangaroo Mother Care in the nursery. *Pediatric Clinics of North America.* 48(2):443-452.

Gessner, B. D., G. C. Ives, and K. A. Perham-Hester. 2001. Association between sudden infant death syndrome and prone sleeping position, bed sharing, and sleeping outside an infant crib in Alaska. *Pediatrics* 108:923-927.

Gidrewicz, D. A., and T. R. Fenton. 2014. Systematic review and meta-analysis of the nutrient content of preterm and term breast milk. *BMC Pediatrics* 14:216.

Glynn, L. M., E. P. Davis, C. D. Schetter, A. Chicz-DeMet, C. J. Hobel, and C. A. Sandman. 2007. Postnatal maternal cortisol levels predict temperament in healthy breastfed infants. *Early Human Development* 83:675-681.

Goldfield, E., M. Richardson, K. Lee, and S. Margetts. 2006. Coordination of sucking, swallowing, and breathing and oxygen saturation during early infant breast-feeding and bottle-feeding. *Pediatric Research* 60:450-455.

Gooding, J., J. Finlay, J. A. Shipley, M. Halliwell, and F. A. Duck. 2010. Three-Dimensional Ultrasound Imaging of Mammary Ducts in Lactating Women a Feasibility Study. *Journal of Ultrasound Medicine* 29(1):95-103.

Goodlin-Jones, B. L., M. M Burnham, E. E. Gaylor, and T. F. Anders. 2001. Night waking, sleep-wake organization, and self-soothing in the first year of life. *Journal of Developmental & Behavioral Pediatrics* 22(4):226-33.

Goodman, S. 1992. Presumed Innocents: Newborns: What Do They Know and When Do They Know It? *Modern Maturity* 26-27.

Graven, S. N. 2006. Sleep and Brain Development. *Clinical Perinatology* 33:696-702.

Graven, S. N., and J. V. Browne. 2008. Sleep and Brain Development: The Critical Role of Sleep in Fetal and Early Neonatal Brain Development. *Newborn & Infant Nursing Reviews* 8(4):173-179.

Greenberg, J. A., S. J. Bell, and W. Van Ausdal. 2008. Omega-3 Fatty Acid Supplementation During Pregnancy. *Reviews in Obstetrics & Gynecology* 1(4):162-169.

Greenspan, S. I. with N. B. Lewis. 1999. *Building Healthy Minds: The Six Experiences That Create Intelligence and Emotional Growth in Babies and Young Children.* New York, NY: Da Capo Press.

Greenspan, S. I., and N. T. Greenspan. 1985. *First Feelings: Milestones in the Emotional Development of Your Baby and Child.* New York, N.Y: Viking Penguin Inc.

Haham, A., R. Marom, L. Mangel, E. Botzer, and S. Dollberg. 2014. Prevalence of Breastfeeding Difficulties in Newborns with a Lingual Frenulum: A Prospective Cohort Series. *Breastfeeding Medicine* 9(9):438-441.

Hamosh, M., L. A. Ellis, D. R. Pollock, T. R. Henderson, and P. Hamosh. 1996. Breastfeeding and the working mother: Effect of time and temperature of short-term storage on proteolysis, lipolysis, and bacterial growth in milk. *Pediatrics* 97:492-498.

Handa, D., A. F. Ahrabi, C. N. Codipilly, S. Shah, S. Ruff, D. Potak, J. E. Williams, M. A. McGuire, and R. J. Schanler. 2014. Do thawing and warming affect the integrity of human milk? *Journal of Perinatology* 34:863-866.

Harrison, Y. 2004. The relationship between daytime exposure to light and night-time sleep in 6-12-week-old infants. *Journal of Sleep Research* 13(4):345-52.

Hartmann, P. E. 1991. The breast and breast feeding. In E. Philipp, M. Setchell, and J. G. Ginsberg (Eds.), Scientific Foundations of Obstetrics and Gynecology. Butterworth-Heinemann.

Hawdon, J. M., M. P. Ward Platt, and A. Aynsley-Green. 1992. Patterns of metabolic adaptation for preterm and term infants in the first neonatal week. *Archives of Disease in Childhood* 67(4):357-365.

Hazelbaker, A. K. 1993. The assessment Tool for lingual frenulum function (ATLFF) Use in a Private Lactation Consultant Practice (thesis). Pasadena, CA:Pacific Oats College.

Heise, A. M., and D. Wiessinger. 2011. Dysphoric milk ejection reflex: A case report. *International Breastfeeding Journal* 6:6.

Henderson, J. M., K. G. France, J. L. Owens, and N. M. Blampied. 2010. Sleeping through the night: the consolidation of self-regulated sleep across the 1st year of life. *Pediatrics* 12: e1081-1087.

Henderson, J. M., K. G. France, J. L. Owens, and N. M. Blampied. 2011. The consolidation of infants' nocturnal sleep across the first year of life. *Sleep Medicine Reviews* 15(4):211-220.

Herron, A., E. Weber. 1998. *Only the Best for My Baby: Learning to Breastfeed.* San Luis Obispo, CA: Growing with Baby.

Hill, P. D. 1991. The enigma of insufficient milk supply. *The American Journal of Maternal Child Nursing.* 16:31-36.

Hill, P. D., and J. C. Aldag. 2005. Milk volume on day 4 and income predictive of lactation adequacy at 6 weeks of mother of nonnursing preterm infants. *Journal of Perinatal Neonatal Nursing* 19(3):273-282.

Hill, P. D., J. C. Aldag, and R. T. Chatterton. 1999. Effects of pumping style on milk production in mothers of non-nursing preterm infants. *Journal of Human Lactation* 15(3)209-216.

Hillman, N, S. G. Kallapur, and A. Jobe. 2012. Physiology of Transition from Intrauterine to Extrauterine Life. *Clinics in Perinatology* 39(4):769-783.

Hiscock, H., and B. Jordan. 2004. Problem Crying in Infancy. *MJA Practice Essentials Paediatrics* 181:507-12.

Holmberg, H., J. Wahlberg, O. Vaarala, and J. Ludvigsson. 2007. Short duration of breastfeeding a risk factor for B-cell autoantibodies in 5-year-old children from the general population. *British Journal of Nutrition* 97:111-116.

Hopkinson, J. M., R. J. Schanler, and C. Garza. 1988. Milk production by mothers of preterm infants. *Pediatrics* 81(6)815-820.

Host, A., H. P. Jacobsen, S. Halken, and D. Holmenlund. 1995. The natural history of cow's milk protein allergy/intolerance. *European Journal of Clinical Nutrition* 49(1):S13-S18.

Howard, C. R., F. M. Howard, B. P. Lanphear, S. Eberly, E. A. De Blieck, D. Oakes, and Ruth A. Lawrence. 2003. Randomized Clinical Trial of Pacifier Use and Bottle-Feeding or Cupfeeding and Their Effect on Breastfeeding. *Pediatrics* 111:511-518.

Hunziker, U. A., and R. G. Barr. 1986. Increased carrying reduces infant crying: A randomized controlled trial. *Pediatrics* 77:641-648.

Iacovou, M. and A. Sevilla. 2013. Infant feeding: the effects of scheduled vs. on-demand feeding on mother's wellbeing and children's cognitive development. *The European Journal of Public Health* 23(1):13-19.

Institute of Medicine (US) Committee on Sleep Medicine and Research; Colten, H. R., B. M. Altevogt, editors. 2006. *Sleep Disorders and Sleep Deprivation: An Unmet Public Health Problem*. Washington (DC): National Academies Press (US).

Ip, S., M. Chung, G. Raman, P. Chew, N. Magula, D. DeVine, T. Trikalinos, and J. Lau. 2007. Tufts-New England Medical Center Evidence-based Practice Center. Breastfeeding and maternal and infant health outcomes in developed countries. *Evidence Report/Technology Assessment* (Full Rep) 153(153):1-186.

Jackson, B. 2002. *The Role of Experience on the Developing Brain*. Munroe-Meyer Institute. Omaha, NE.

Jenni, O. G., and M. A. Carskadon 2009. Life cycles: Infants to adolescents. In C. Amlaner and P. M. Fuler (Eds.), *SRS basics of sleep guide* (pp. 33-41). Westchester, IL: Sleep Research Society.

Jenness, R. 1974. Biosynthesis and composition of milk. *Journal of Investigative Dermatology*. 63:109-118.

Jones, F., and M. R. Tully. 2006. *Best Practice for Expressing, Storing and Handling Human Milk in Hospitals, Homes and Child Care Settings 2nd Edition*. Raleigh, NC: Human Milk Banking Association of North America, Inc.

Jones, S. 1992. *Crying Baby Sleepless Nights: Why Your Baby is Crying and What You Can Do About It*. Boston. MA: The Harvard Common Press. p.1-2, 5, 14-16.

Joseph, D., N. W. Chong, M. E. Shanks, E. Rosato, N. A. Taub, S. A. Petersen, M. E. Symonds, W. P. Whitehouse, and M. Wailoo. 2015. Getting rhythm: how do babies do it? *Archives of Disease in Childhood Fetal Neonatal Edition* 100:F50-F54.

Kalra, R., and M. L. Walker. 2012. Posterior plagiocephaly. *Child's Nervous System* 28:1389-1393.

Karp, Harvey. 2002. *The Happiest Baby on the Block: The New Way to Calm Crying and Help Your Newborn Baby Sleep Longer*. New York, NY: Bantam Dell.

Kearney, M., L. Cronenwett, and R. Reinhardt. 1990. Cesarean delivery and breastfeeding outcomes. *Birth* 17: 97-103.

Kellams, A., C. Harrel, S. Omage, C. Gregory, C. Rosen-Carole, and the Academy of Breastfeeding Medicine. 2017. ABM Clinical Protocol #3: Supplementary Feedings in the Healthy Term Breastfed Neonate, Revised 2017. *Breastfeeding Medicine* 12(3):1-10.

Kendall-Tackett, K. 2007. A new paradigm for depression in new mothers: the central role of inflammation and how breastfeeding and anti-inflammatory treatments protect maternal mental health. *International Breastfeeding Journal* 2:6.

Kent, J. 2007. How Breastfeeding Works. *Journal of Midwifery & Women's Health* 52:564-570.

Kent, J. C., H. Gardner, and D. T. Geddes. 2016. Breastmilk production in the First 4 Weeks after Birth of Term Infants. *Nutrients* 8(12):756.

Kent, J. C., L. Mitoulas, D. B. Cox, R. A. Owens, and P. E. Hartmann. 1999. Breast volume and milk production during extended lactation in women. *Experimental Physiology* 84(2):435-47.

Kent, J. C., L. R. Mitoulas, M. Cregan, D. T. Ramsay, D. A. Doherty, and P. E. Hartmann. 2006. Volume and Frequency of Breastfeedings and Fat Content of Breast Milk Throughout the Day. *Pediatrics* 117(3).

Kent, J. C., A. R. Hepworth, J. L. Sheriff, D. B. Cox, L. R. Mitoulas, and P. E. Hartmann. 2013. Longitudinal Changes in Breastfeeding Patterns from 1 to 6 Months of Lactation. *Breastfeeding Medicine* 8(4):401-407.

Kent, J. C., D. K. Prime, and C. R. Garbin. 2012. Principles for Maintaining or Increasing Breast Milk Production. *Journal of Obstetric, Gynecologic and Neonatal Nursing* 41(1):114-121.

Kent, J. C., L. R. Mitoulas, M. D. Cregan, D. T. Geddes, M. Larsson, D. A. Doherty, and P. Hartmann. 2008. Importance of vacuum for breastmilk expression. *Breastfeeding Medicine* 3(1):11-19.

Klaus, M., and P. Klaus. 2000. *Your Amazing Newborn*. Boston, MA: Da Capo Press.

Kroeger M., and L. J. Smith. 2004. *Impact of birthing practices on breastfeeding: Protecting the mother and baby continuum*. Sudbury, MA: Jones & Bartlett Publishers.

Kurcinka, M. S. 1991. *Raising Your Spirited Child: A Guide for Parents Whose Child Is More Intense, Sensitive, Perceptive, Persistent, and Energetic*. New York, NY: William Morrow.

LactMed. 2016. Available at http://toxnet.nlm.nih.gov/cgi-bin/sis/htmlgen?LACT. Accessed March 2, 2016.

Latz, S., A. W. Wolf, and B. Lozoff. 1999. Cosleeping in context: Sleep practices and problems in young children in Japan and the United Sates. *Archives of Pediatrics and Adolescent Medicine* 153:339-346.

Lawrence, R. A., and R. M. Lawrence. 2011. *Breastfeeding: A Guide for the Medical Professional Seventh Edition*. Maryland Heights, MO: Mosby/Elsevier.

Leach, P. 2010. *The Essential First Year*. New York, N.Y: Dorling Kindersley Limited. p. 78, 112.

Leach, P. 2010. *Your Baby & Child: From Birth to Age Five*. Knopf. p. 78.

Lee, K. A. 2003. Impaired sleep. In: *Pathological Phenomena in Nursing. 3rd ed*. St Louis, Mo: Saunders; 363-385.

Li, R., S. B. Fein, J. Chen, and L. M. Grummer-Strawn. 2008. Why mothers stop breastfeeding: mothers' self-reported reasons for stopping during the first year. *Pediatrics* 122(Suppl 2):S69–S76.

Livingstone, V. H., C. E. Willis, and J. Berkowitz. 1996. Staphylococcus aureus and sore nipples. *Canadian Family Physician* 42:654-659.

Lucassen, P. L., W. J. Assendelft, J. T. van Eijk, J. W. Gubbels, A. C. Douwess, and W. J. van Geldrop. 2001. Systemic review of the occurrence of infantile colic in the community. *Archives of Disease in Childhood* 84:398-403.

Lundström, J. N., A. Mathe, B. Schaal, J. Frasnelli, K. Nitzsche, J. Gerber, and T. Hummel. 2013. Maternal status regulates cortical responses to the body odor of newborns. *Frontiers in Psychology* 4:597.

MacDonald, P., S. Ross, L. Grant, and D. Young. 2003. Neonatal weight loss in breast and formula fed infants. *Archives of Disease in Childhood Fetal Neonatal Edition* 88(6):F472-F476.

Macknin, M.L., S. V. Medendorp, and M. C. Maier. 1989. Infant sleep and bedtime cereal. *American Journal of Diseases of Children* 143(9):1066-8.

Manganaro, R., C. Mami, T. Marrone, L. Marseglia, and M. Gemelli. 2001. Incidence of dehydration and hypernatremia in exclusively breast-fed infants. *Journal of Pediatrics* 139:673-675.

Mannel, R., P. Martens, and M. Walker. 2012. "Biochemistry of Human Milk by Linda J. Smith" *Core Curriculum for Lactation Consultant Practice Third Edition* Burlington, MA: Jones & Bartlett Learning.

Mao, A., M. M. Burnham, B. L. Goodlin-Jones, E. E. Gaylor, and T. F. Anders. 2004. A comparison of the sleep-wake patterns of co-sleeping and solitary-sleeping infants. *Child Psychiatry and Human Development* 35:95-105.

Marasco, L.A. 2014. Unsolved Mysteries of the Human Mammary Gland: Defining and Redefining the Critical Questions from the Lactation Consultant's Perspective. *Journal of Mammary Gland Biology and Neoplasia* 19(3-4):271-288.

March of Dimes. 2003. Understanding the Behavior of Term Infants. *Perinatal Nursing Education* 1-14.

Marinelli, K. A., G. S. Burke, and V. L. Dodd. 2001. A comparison of the safety of cupfeedings and bottlefeedings in premature infants whose mothers intend to breastfeed. *Journal of Perinatology* 21:350-355.

Matthiesen, A. S., A. B. Ransjö-Arvidson, E. Nissen, and K. Uvnäs-Moberg. 2001. Postpartum maternal oxytocin release by newborns: effects of infant hand massage and sucking. *Birth* 28(1):13-9.

Mawji, A., A. Robinson Vollman, J. Hatfield, D. McNeil, and R. Sauve. 2013. The Incidence of Positional Plagiocephaly: A Cohort Study. *Pediatrics* 132(2):298-304.

McClellan, H. L., J. C. Kent, A. R. Hepworth, P. E. Hartmann, and D. T. Geddes. 2015. Persistent Nipple Pain in Breastfeeding Mothers Associated with Abnormal Infant Tongue Movement. *International Journal of Environmental Research and Public Health* 12(9):10833-10845.

McCoy, R. C., C. E. Hunt, S. M. Lesko, R. Vezina, M. Corwin, M. Willinger, H. Hoffman, and A. Mitchell. 2004. Frequency of bed sharing and its relationship to breastfeeding. *Journal of Developmental & Behavioral Pediatrics* 25(3):141-149.

McKenna, J. 1994. Experimental studies of infant-parent co-sleeping: mutual physiological and behavioral influences and their relevance to SIDS. *Early Human Development* 38(3):187-201.

McKenna, J. J., S. S. Mosko, and C. A. Richard. 1997. Bedsharing promotes breastfeeding. *Pediatrics* 100:214-219

McKenna, J., and T. McDade. 2005. Why babies should never sleep alone: A review of the co-sleeping controversy in relation to SIDS, bedsharing and breast feeding. *Pediatric Respiratory Reviews* 6:134-152.

Medela. 2015. *Human Milk Magazine* Issue 1. McHenry, IL: Medela.

Meier, P. P., A. L. Patel, R. Hoban, and J. L. Engstrom. 2016. Which breast pump for which mother: an evidence-based approach to individualizing breast pump technology. *Journal of Perinatology* 1-7.

Meier, P. P., J. L. Engstrom, C. L. Crichton, D. R. Clark, M. M. Williams, and H. H. Mangurten. 1994. A new scale for in-home test-weighing for mother of preterm and high-risk infants. *Journal of Human Lactation* 10(3):163-168.

Meltzer, L. J. and H. E. Montgomery-Downs. 2011. Sleep in the family. *Pediatric Clinics of North America* 58(3) 765-774.

Mennella, J. A., L. M. Yourshaw, and L. K. Morgan. 2007. Breastfeeding and Smoking: Short-term Effects on Infant Feeding and Sleep. *Pediatrics* 120(3)497-502.

Michelsson, K., K. Christensson, H. Rothganger, and J. Winberg. 1996. Crying in separated and non-separated newborns: sound spectrographic analysis. *Acta Paediatrica* 85(4):471-75.

Middlemiss, W., D. Granger, W. Goldberg, and L. Nathans. 2011. Asynchrony of mother-infant hypothalamic-pituitary-adrenal axis activity following extinction of infant responses induced during the transition to sleep. *Early Human Development* 88(4):227-232.

Mindell, J. A, E. S. Leichman, J. Composto, C. Lee, B. Bhullar, and R. M. Walters. 2016. Development of infant and toddler sleep patterns: real-world data from a mobile application. *Journal of Sleep Research.* 25(5):508-516.

Mohrbacher, N. 2010. *Breastfeeding Answers Made Simple: A Guide for Helping Mothers.* Amarillo, TX: Hale Publishing, L.P., 58, 388.

Mohrbacher, N. 2010. *Breastfeeding Solutions.* Oakland, CA: New Harbinger Publications.

Mohrbacher, N. 2016. Pumping for Babies in the NICU. Powerpoint lecture.

Mohrbacher, N., and K. Kendall-Tackett. 2010. *Breastfeeding Made Simple: Seven Natural Laws for Nursing Mothers, Second Edition.* Oakland: New Harbinger Publications.

Moore, E. R., G. C. Anderson, and N. Bergman. 2007. Early skin-to-skin contact for mothers and their healthy newborn infants. *Cochrane Database System Review* July 18(3):CD003519.

Moore, T., and L. E. Ucko. 1957. Night Waking in early infancy: part I. *Archives of Disease in Childhood* 32(164):333-342.

Morrison, B. 2006. Care for Fullterm Infants: State of the Science Conference: Biennial Conference and Workshop of the International Network of Kangaroo Mother Care. Cleveland, Ohio.

Mortel, M., and S. D. Mehta. 2013. Systematic review of the efficacy of herbal galactogogues. *Journal of Human Lactation* 29(2):154-162.

Morton, J. 2016. Video Clip: Early Hand Expression Increases Later Milk Production. Stanford School of Medicine (Produced by Breastmilk Solutions) newborns.stanford.edu. Accessed online July 10, 2016.

Morton, J., J. V. Hall, R. J. Wong, L. Thairu, W. E. Benitez, and W. D. Rhine. 2009. Combining hand techniques with electric pumping increases milk production in mothers of preterm infants. *Journal of Perinatology* 29: 757-764.

Mosko, S., C. Richard, J. McKenna, and S. Drummond. 1996. Infant sleep architecture during bedsharing and possible implications for SIDS. *Sleep* 19(9):677-684.

Mosko, S., C. Richard, J. McKenna. 1997. Infant arousals during mother-infant bed sharing: implications for infant sleep and sudden infant death syndrome research. *Pediatrics* 100: 841-849.

Mozingo, J. N., M. W. Davis, P. G. Droppleman, and A. Merideth. 2000. "It Wasn't Working": Women's Experiences with Short-Term Breastfeeding. *MCN The American Journal of Maternal/Child Nursing* 25(3):120–126.

Munoz, L. M., B. Lonnerdal, C. L. Keen, and K. G. Dewey. 1988. Coffee consumption as a factor in iron deficiency anemia among pregnant women and their infants in Costa Rica. *American Journal of Clinical Nutrition.* 48:645-51.

Murray, L., C. Stanley, R. Hooper, F. King, and A. Fiori-Cowley. 1996. The role of infant factors in postnatal depression and mother-infant interactions. *Developmental Medicine and Child Neurology* 38:109-119.

Muscat, T., P. Obst, W. Cockshaw, and K. Thorpe. 2014. Beliefs About Infant Regulation, Early Infant Behaviors and Maternal Postnatal Depressive Symptoms *Birth* 41:2.

National Sleep Foundation. 2017. Sleepiness & New Parenthood: Tips To Improve Your Nighttime Routine. National Sleep Foundation sleepfoundation.org.

Naumburg, E. G., and R. G. Meny. 1988. Breast Milk Opioids and Neonatal Apnea. *The Pediatric Forum* 142:11-12.

NCAST Programs. 2018. Parent-Child Relationship Programs at the Barnard Center. Seattle, WA: University of Washington.

NCAST-AvenUW. 2003. *Baby Cues: A Child's First Language.* Seattle, WA: University of Washington.

National Institute of Mental Health (NIMH). Postpartum Depression Facts. U.S. Department of Health and Human Services. NIH Publication No. 13-8000. retrieved online July 2018.

Neifert, M. R., 2001. Prevention of breastfeeding tragedies. *Pediatric Clinics of North America* 48(2):273-297.

Neifert, M. R., S. L. McDonough, and M. C. Neville. 1981. Failure of lactogenesis associated with placental retention. *American Journal of Obstetrics and Gynecology* 140:477-478.

Nevo, N., L. Rubin, A. Tamir, A. Levine, and R. Shaoul. 2007. Infant Feeding Patterns in the First 6 Months: An Assessment in Full-Term Infants. *Journal of Pediatric Gastroenterology and Nutrition* 45(2):234-239.

Newman, J. 2017. Breast Compression Information Sheet. International Breastfeeding Centre. Ibconline.ca

Niegel, S., E. Ystrom, K. A. Hagtvet, and M. E. Vollrath. 2008. Difficult Temperament, Breastfeeding, and Their Mutual Prospective Effects: The Norwegian Mother and Child Cohort Study. *Journal of Development & Behavioral Pediatrics* 29:458-462.

Noble, R. and A. Bovey. 2016. When the Back of the Baby's Head is Held to Attach the Baby to the Breast. Health e-Learning. Retrieved online July 10, 2016.

Noel-Weiss, J., A. K. Woodend, W. E. Peterson, W. Gibb, and D. L. Groll. 2011. An observational study of associations among maternal fluids during parturition, neonatal output, and breastfed newborn weight loss. *International Breastfeeding Journal* 6:9.

Nommsen-Rivers, L. A., C. J. Chantry, J. M. Peerson, R. J. Cohen, and K. G. Dewey. 2010. Delayed onset of lactogenesis among first-time mother is related to maternal obesity and factors associated with ineffective breastfeeding. *The American Journal of Clinical Nutrition* 92(3):574-584.

Nommsen-Rivers, L.A., L. M. Dolan, and B. Haung. 2012. Timing of stage to the lactogenesis is predicted by antenatal metabolic health in a cohort of primiparas. *Breastfeeding Medicine* 7:43-49.

Nugent, J. K., C. H. Keefer, S. Minear, L. C. Johnson, and Y. Blanchard. 2007. *Understanding Newborn Behavior Early Relationships: The Newborn Behavioral Observation (NBO) System Handbook.* Baltimore, MD: Paul H. Brookes Publishing Co.

Ockwell-Smith, S., J. Hoffman, D. Narvaez., W. Middlemiss, H. Stevens, J. McKenna, K. Kendall-Tackett, and T. Cassels. 2013. Simple Ways to Calm a Crying Baby And Have a More Peaceful Night's Sleep. *Clinical Lactation* 4-2:79-82.

Office of the Surgeon General (US); Centers for Disease Control and Prevention (US); Office on Women's Health (US). 2011. The Surgeon General's Call to Action to Support Breastfeeding. Rockville (MD): Office of the Surgeon General (US). Barriers to Breastfeeding in the United States.

Ohgi, S., M. Fukada, H. Moriuchi, T. Kusumoto, T. Akiyama, J. K. Nugent, et al. 2002. Comparison of kangaroo care: Behavioral organization, development, and temperament in healthy low-birth weight infants through 1 year. *Journal of Perinatology* 22:374-379.

398 SUCKLE, SLEEP, THRIVE

Oo, C. Y., D. E. Burgio, R. C. Kuhn, N. Desai, and P. J. McNamara. 1995. Pharmacokinetics of caffeine and its demethylated metabolites in lactation: predictions of milk to serum concentration ratios. *Pharmaceutical Research* 12:313-6.

Owen, C. G., R. M. Martin, P. H. Whincup, G. D. Smith, and D. G. Cook. 2005. Effect of infant feeding on the risk of obesity across the life course: a quantitative review of published evidence. *Pediatrics* 115(5):1367-1377.

Palmér, L., G. Carlsson, M. Mollberg, and M. Nyström. 2012. Severe Breastfeeding Difficulties: Existential Lostness as a Mother—Women's Lived Experiences of Initiating Breastfeeding under Severe Difficulties. *International Journal of Qualitative Studies on Health and Well-Being* 7.0.

Paredes, M. F., D. James, S. Gil-Perotin, H. Kim, J. A. Cotter, C. Ng, K. Sandoval, D. H. Rowitch, D. Xu, P. S. McQuillen, J. M. Garcia-Verdugo, E. J. Huang, and A. Alvarez-Buylla. 2016. Extensive migration of young neurons into the infant human frontal lobe. *Science* 354(6308).

Parker, L. A., S. Sullivan, C. Krueger, T. Kelechi, and M. Mueller. 2012. Effect of early breast milk expression on milk volume and timing of lactogenesis stage II among mothers of very low birth weight infants: a pilot study. *Journal of Perinatology* 32:205-209.

Pascalis, O., S. de Schonen, J. Morton, C. Deruelle, and M. Fabre-Grenet. 1995. Mother's face recognition by neonates: A replication and an extension. *Infant Behavior and Development* 18:79-85.

Perez-Escamilla, R., S. Segura-Perez, and M. Lott. 2017. Feeding Guidelines for Infants and Young Toddlers: A Responsive Parenting Approach. Durham, NC: Healthy Eating Research.

Perrine, C. G., K. S. Scanlon, R. Li, E. Odom, and L. M. Grummer-Strawn. 2012. Baby-Friendly Hospital Practices and Meeting Exclusive Breastfeeding Intention. *Pediatrics.* 130(1):54-60.

Perry, B. D. 1997. Incubated in terror: Neurodevelopmental factors in the 'cycle of violence.' In Joy Osofsky (ed.), *Children, Youth, and Violence: The Search for Solutions.* New York: Guilford Press.

Pittard, W. B., K. M. Geddes, S. Brown, and T. C. Mintz. 1991. Bacterial contamination of human milk: Container type and method of expression. *American Journal Perinatology* 8(1):25-27

Powers, N. G., and W. Slusser. 1997. Breastfeeding update. 2: Clinical lactation management. *Pediatrics in Review* 18:147-161.

Puapornpong, P., K. Raungrongmorakot, P. Paritakul, S. Ketsuwan, and S. Wongin. 2013. Nipple length and its relation to success in breastfeeding. *Journal Medical Association Thai* 96(1):S1-S4.

Quinn, N., A. Walls, I. Milliken, and M. McCullagh. 2011. Pyloric Stenosis - Do Males and Females Present Differently? *The Ulster Medical Journal* 80(3):145-147

Rahm, V. A., A. Hallgren, H. Högberg, I. Hurtig, and V. Odlind. 2002. Plasma Oxytocin Levels in Women During Labor With or Without Epidural Analgesia: A Prospective Study. *Acta Obstetricia et Gynecologica Scandinavica* 80(11):1033-1039.

Ramsay, D. T., J. C. Kent, R. A. Hartmann, and P. E. Hartman. 2005. Anatomy of the lactating human breast redefined with ultrasound imaging. *Journal of Anatomy* 206(6):525-534.

Rand, K., and A. Lahav. 2014. Maternal sounds elicit lower heart rate in preterm newborns in the first month of life. *Early Human Development* 90:679-683.

Rapley, G., and T. Murkett. 2012. *Baby-Led Breastfeeding: Follow Your Baby's Instincts for Relaxed and Easy Nursing*. New York: NY: The Experiment. P. 104-105.

Righard, L., and M. O. Alade. 1990. Effect of delivery room routines on success of first breast-feed. *Lancet* 336(8723):1105-7.

Riordan, J. and K. Wambach. 2016. *Breastfeeding and Human Lactation*. Burlington, MA: Jones and Bartlett Learning.

Saarinen, K. M., K. Juntunen-Backman, A. Jarvenpaa, P. Kuitunen, L. Lope, M. Renlund, M. Siivola, and E. Savilahti. 1999. Supplementary feedings in maternity hospitals and the risk of cow's allergy: A prospective study of 6209 infants. *Journal of Allergy and Clinical Immunology* 104:457-461.

Sachdev, H. P., and S. Mehrotra. 1995. Predictors of exclusive breastfeeding in early infancy: operational implications. *Indian Pediatrics* 32:1287-1296.

Sadeh, A., L. Tikotzky, and A. Scher. 2010. Parenting and Infant Sleep. *Sleep Medicine Review* 14(2):89-96.

Sadler, S. 1994. Sleep: what is normal at six months? *Professional Care of Mother and Child* 4(6):166-7.

Savilahti, E., J. Tuomilehto, T. T. Saukkonen, E. T. Virtala, J. Tuomilehto, H. K Åkerblom, and The Childhood Diabetes in Finland Study Group. 1993. Increased levels of cow's milk and blactoglobulin antibodies in young children with newly diagnosed IDDM. *Diabetes Care* 16:984-989.

Savino, F. 2007. Focus on infantile colic. *Foundation Acta Pediatrica* 1259-1264.

Savino, F., S. Ceratto, A. De Marco, and L. Cordero di Montezemolo. 2014. Looking for new treatments of Infantile Colic. *Italian Journal of Pediatrics* 40:53.

Scher, A. 1991. A longitudinal study of night waking in the first year. *Child: Care, Health and Development* 17(5):295-302.

Schore, A. N. 1996. The experience-dependent maturation of a regulatory system in the orbital prefrontal cortex and the origin of developmental psychopathology. *Development and Psychopathology* 8:59-87.

Schore, A. N. 2001. Effects of a secure attachment relationship on right brain development, affect regulation, and infant mental health. *Infant Mental Health Journal* 22(1-2):7-66.

Schwarz, E. B., R. M. Ray, A. M. Stuebe, et al. 2009. Duration of lactation and risk factors for maternal cardiovascular disease. *Obstetrics Gynecology* 113(5):974-982.

Seehagen, S., C. Konrad, J. S. Herbert, and S. Schneider. 2014. Timely sleep facilitates declarative memory consolidation in infants. *PNAS* Early Edition 10.1073.

Sexton, S., and R. Natale. 2009. Risks and Benefits of Pacifiers. *American Family Physician* 79(8):681-685.

Shah, A., C. Hayes, B. C. Martin. 2017. Characteristics of Initial Prescription Episodes and Likelihood of Long-Term Opioid Use -- United States, 2006-2015. *Centers for Disease Control and Prevention* MMWR 66(10):265-269.

Shipster, C., D. Hearst, A. Somerville, J. Stackhouse, R. Hayward, and A. Wade. 2003. Speech, language, and cognitive development in children with isolated sagittal synostosis. *Developmental Medicine and Child Neurology* 45:34-43.

Simkin, P. 2015. Maternity Care and the Microbiome: How Birth Practices Dictate Future Health. Presentation.

Simkin, P. 2015. Scorecard: Practices that Disrupt the Infant Microbiome. Scorecard of Disruptive Events.

Slusher, T. R. Hampton, F. Bode-Thomas, S. Pam, F. Akor, and P. Meier. 2003. Promoting the exclusive feeding of own mother's milk through the use of hindmilk and increased maternal milk volume for hospitalized, low birth weight infants (<1800 grams) in Nigeria: a feasibility study. *Journal of Human Lactation* 19(2):191-198.

Smith, L. J. 2007. Impact of Birthing Practices on the Breastfeeding Dyad. *Journal of Midwifery & Women's Health* 52:621-630.

Spitzer, J., K. Klos, and A. Buettner. 2013. Monitoring aroma changes during human milk storage at +4 degrees C by sensory and quantification experiments. *Clinical Nutrition* 32:1036-1042.

Srinivasan, G., R. S. Pildes, G. Cattamanchi, S. Voora, and L.D. Lilien. 1986. Plasma glucose values in normal neonates: a new look. *Journal of Pediatrics* 109:114-117.

St. James-Roberts, I. 1993. Explanations of persistent infant crying in *Infant Crying, Feeding, and Sleeping: Development, Problems, and Treatments*. New York: Harvester Wheatsheaf. p. 26-46.

St. James-Roberts, I. 2001. Infant Crying and Its Impact on Parents in *New Evidence on Unexplained Early Infant Crying: Its Origins, Nature and Management*. Johnson & Johnson Pediatric Institute Division of Johnson & Johnson Consumer Companies, Inc. 5-24.

St. James-Roberts, I., S. Conroy, and K. Wilsher. 1995. Clinical, developmental and social aspects of infant crying and colic. *Early Development and Parenting* 4:177-189.

Stavchansky, S., A. Combs, R. Sagraves, M. Delgado, and A. Joshi. 1988. Pharmacokinetics of caffeine in breast milk and plasma after single oral administration of caffeine to lactating mothers. *Biopharmaceutics & Drug Disposition* 9:285-99.

Stifter, C. A., and T. L. Spinrad. 2002. The effect of excessive crying on the development of emotion regulation. *Infancy* 3:133-152.

Stocche, R. M., J. G. Klamt, J. Antunes-Rodrigues, L.V. Garcia, and A.C. Moreira. 2001. Effects of Intrathecal Sufentanil on Plasma Oxytocin and Cortisol Concentrations in Women During the First Stage of Labor. *Regional Anesthesia and Pain Medicine* 26(6):545-550.

Stratton, P. 1982. *Rhythmic Functions in the Newborn.* In P. Stratton (Ed.), Physchobiology of the human newborn. New York: Wiley.

Tait, P. 2000. Nipple pain in breastfeeding women: Causes, treatment, and prevention strategies. *Journal of Midwifery & Women's Health* 45(3):212-215.

Takikawa, D., and C. Contey. 2010. *What Babies Want: Five Simple Steps to Calming and Communicating with your Baby.* New York, NY: LTM Books.

Thatrimontrichai, A., W. Janjindamai, and M. Puwanant. 2012. Fat loss in thawed breastmilk: Comparison between refrigerator and warm water. *Indian Pediatrics* 49:877-880.

Thoman, E. B. 1975. How a Rejecting Baby Affects Mother-Infant Synchrony. *Parent-Infant Interaction* Ciba Foundation Symposium 33:177-200.

Thomas, A. and S. Chess. 1977. *Temperament and Development.* New York, NY: Bruner/Mazel.

Thomas, A., S. Chess, and H. G. Birch. 1968. *Temperament and Behavior Disorders in Children.* New York, NY: University Press.

Thompson, J. F., L. J. Heal, C. L. Roberts, and D. A. Ellwood. 2010. Women's breastfeeding experiences following a significant primary postpartum haemorrhage: A multicentre cohert study. *International Breast Feeding Journal* 5(5):11-12.

Thompson, R., S. Kruske, L. Barclay, K. Linden, Y. Gao, and S. Kildea. 2016. Potential predictors of nipple trauma from an in-home breastfeeding programme: A cross-sectional study. *Women and Birth* 29(4):336-344.

Thorley, V. 2015. Latch problems arising from mothers' fear response to anticipated pain. Gold Lactation 2015 Webinar.

Tilden, C. D., and O. T. Oftedal. 1997. Milk composition reflects pattern of maternal care in prosimian primates. *American Journal of Primatology* 41:195-211.

UC Davis Human Lactation Center. 2011. Secrets of Baby Behavior. Slideshow presented by Annmarie Golioto. The Regents of the University of California

van de Rijt, H. and F, Plooij. 2013. *The Wonder Weeks: How to stimulate the most important developmental weeks in your baby's first 20 months and turn these 10 predictable, great, fussy phases into magical leaps forward.* The Netherlands: Kiddy World Publishing.

Vanky, E., J. J. Nordskar, H. Leithe , A. K. Hjorth-Hansen, M. Martinussen, and S. M. Carlsen. 2012. Breast size increment during pregnancy and breast-feeding and mothers with polycystic ovary syndrome: a follow-up study of a randomized controlled trial on metformin versus placebo. *British Journal of Obstetrics and Gynecology* 11:1403-1409

Varendi, H., R. H. Porter, and J. Winberg. 2002. The Effect of labor on olfactory exposure learning within the first postnatal hour. *Behavioral Neuroscience* 116:206-11.

Vitek, L., and J. D. Ostrow. 2009. Bilirubin chemistry and metabolism: harmful and protective aspects. *Current Pharmaceutical Design* 15(25) 2869-2883.

Vorster, D. S. 1980. Crying and Non-Crying Babies. *British Medical Journal* 281(6232)58-59.

Walker, M. 2010. *The Nipple and Areola in Breastfeeding and Lactation: Anatomy, Physiology, Problems, and Solutions.* Amarillo, TX: Hale Publishing.

Walker, M. 2014. *Breastfeeding Management for the Clinician: Using the Evidence Third Edition.* Burlington, MA: Jones & Bartlett Learning. P. 211.

Walker, M. 2014. Nipple nuances: From pain to peppermint and what the textbooks don't cover. Powerpoint.

Walker, M. 2014. Supplementation of the Breastfed Baby "Just One Bottle Won't Hurt"--or Will It?

Walker, M. 2016. Nipple shields: what we know, what we wish we knew, and how best to use them, *Clinical lactation* 7(3):100-107.

Walker, M. 2017. *Breastfeeding Management for the Clinician: Using the Evidence, fourth edition.* Burlington, MA: Jones & Bartlett Learning.

Wall, R., R. P. Ross, C. A. Ryan, S. Hussey, B. Murphy, G. F. Fitzgerald, and C. Stanton. 2009. Role of Gut Microbiota in Early Infant Development. *Clinical Medicine: Pediatrics* 3:45-54.

Wambach, K., and J. Riordan. 2016. *Breastfeeding and Human Lactation Enhanced Fifth Edition.* Burlington, MA: Jones & Bartlett Learning.

Wells, J. C. 2003. Parent-offspring conflict theory, signaling of need, and weight gain in early life. *The Quarterly Review of Biology* 78:179-202.

West, D., and L. Marasco. 2009. *The Breastfeeding Mother's Guide to Making More Milk.* New York: Mc Graw Hill.

WHO (World Health Organization). 2000. *Mastitis: Causes and Management.* Publication number WHO/FCH/CAH/00.13. Geneva: World Health Organization.

WHO (World Health Organization). 2016. The World Health Organization's Infant Feeding Recommendation. http://www.who.int/nutrition/topics/infantfeeding_recommendation/en/. Accessed January 20, 2016.

Widström, A. M., G. Lilja, P. Aaltomaa-Michalias, A. Dahllöf, M. Lintula, E. Nissen. 2011. Newborn behaviour to locate the breast when skin-to-skin: a possible method for enabling early self-regulation. *Acta Paediatrica* 100(1):79-85.

Wight, N., K. A. Marinelli, and The Academy of Breastfeeding Medicine (ABM). 2014. ABM Clinical Protocol #1: Guidelines for Blood Glucose Monitoring and Treatment of Hypoglycemia in Term and Late-Preterm Neonates, Revised 2014. *Breastfeeding Medicine* 9(4):173-179.

Wilson-Clay, B. Hoover, K. 2017. *The Breastfeeding Atlas Sixth Edition.* Manchaca, Texas: Lact News Press, P. 63.

Wilson-Clay, B., and K. Hoover. 2008. *The Breastfeeding Atlas.* (4th ed). Manchaca, TX: BWC/KH Joint Venture.

Wood, R., G. Chibbaroo, and M. McGrory. 2013. Plagiocephaly, torticollis, lambdoid craniosynostosis: A spectrum of disease. A review of 9,683 patients with posterior plagiocephaly. Abstract presented at the International Society of Craniofacial Surgery, Sept. 10-14.

Wooding, A. R., J. Boyd, and D. C. Geddis. 1990. Sleep patterns of New Zealand infants during the first 12 months of life. *Journal of Paediatrics and Child Health* 26(2):85-8.

Woolridge, M. W. 1986. The Anatomy of infant sucking. *Midwifery* 2:164-171.

Woolridge, M. W. and C. Fisher. 1988. Colic, "Overfeeding," and Symptoms of Lactose Malabsorption in the Breast-Fed Baby: A Possible Artifact of Feed Management? *Lancet 2* 8607:382-384.

Woolridge, M. W., J. C. Ingram, and J. D. Baum. 1990. Do changes in pattern of breast usage alter the baby's nutrient intake? *Science Direct* 336(8712):395-397.

Zanardo, V., S. Nicolussi, G. Carlo, F. Marzari, D. Faggian, F. Favaro, and M. Plebani. 2001. Beta endorphin concentrations in human milk. *Journal of Pediatric Gastroenterology and Nutrition* 33:160-4.

Zangen, S., C. DiLorenzo, T. Zangen, H. Mertz, L. Schwankovsky, and P. Hyman. 2001. Rapid maturation of gastric relaxation in newborn infants. *Pediatric Research* 50:629-632.

Resources for Additional Support

The following are some resources to find additional reliable information, peer support, and professional assistance.

BUILDING A SUPPORT SYSTEM

» **La Leche League International:** For support groups, accurate information, finding a local leader. www.llli.org

» **Special Supplemental Nutritional Program for Women, Infants, and Children (WIC):** Breastfeeding assistance, education, and support for eligible low-income women. www.fns.usda.gov/wic/women-infants-and-children-wic

» **Nursing Mother's Council:** Get free breastfeeding help by phone, email, or in-person. www.nursingmothers.org

» **The National Breastfeeding Helpline:** Reach peer counselors who are available to answer common breastfeeding questions. 1(800) 994-9662

» **Breastfeeding Coalition:** Search online for your local breastfeeding coalition.

» **Baby-Friendly Medical Centers:** Locate a Baby-Friendly medical center near you. www.babyfriendlyusa.org

» **DONA International:** Find a birth or postpartum doula. www.dona.org/what-is-a-doula/find-a-doula/

FINDING A LACTATION CONSULTANT

» **International Lactation Consultant Association (ILCA):** Search for an internationally board-certified lactation consultant (IBCLC) near you. http://uslca.org/resources/find-a-lactation-consultant

» **Your Local Hospital:** Call your local hospital to seek a referral for breastfeeding assistance.

SAFETY OF MEDICATIONS

» **LACTMED:** Find information about drugs and their effect on lactation. LACTMED is associated with the United States National Library of

Medicine and its Toxicology Data Network.
www.toxnet.nlm.nih.gov/newtoxnet/lactmed.htm

» **Infant Risk Center:** A nonprofit helpline for breastfeeding and pregnant women, regarding drug ingestion and their effect on the fetus and baby. www.infantrisk.com (806) 352-2519

HOSPITAL-GRADE BREAST PUMPS AND SELECT SUPPLIES

» **Ameda Breastfeeding Products:** For breast pumps, information, and accessories. www.ameda.com

» **Medela:** Find breast pumps, nursing bras, and supplementation supplies. www.medela.com

» **Supple Cups:** To find supple cups, a product that helps with inverted nipples. www.supplecups.com/about.html

RELIABLE INFORMATION ONLINE

» **Academy of Breastfeeding Medicine:** For detailed protocols on various breastfeeding topics. www.bfmed.org

» **Kelly Mom:** For evidence-based breastfeeding articles written by IBCLCs. www.kellymom.com

» **BFAR:** An informative website for women who breastfeed after a breast or nipple surgeries, such as augmentation or reduction. www.bfar.org/index.shtml

» **Biological Nurturing:** British researcher Suzanne Colson on laid-back breastfeeding. www.biologicalnurturing.com

» **Breastfeeding.com:** Breastfeeding information, videos, and stories from breastfeeding moms.

» **Breastfeeding Inc.:** Excellent videos and breastfeeding education. www.breastfeedinginc.ca

» **Nancy Mohrbacher:** Wonderful up-to-date information on everyday issues, milk supply, adoptive nursing, and breastfeeding challenges. www.nancymohrbacher.com

SLEEP WEBSITES

» **Co-sleeping:** For guidelines from Dr. James McKenna, an expert on infant sleep safety. https://cosleeping.nd.edu/

» **Parenting Science:** Find child development articles based on evidence found in research in the following fields: psychology, anthropology, evolution, and cognitive neuroscience. www.parentingscience.com

KNOWING YOUR RIGHTS

» **National Conference of State Legislatures (NCSL):** Find state laws that protect breastfeeding in public and in the workplace. http://www.ncsl.org/research/health/breastfeeding-state-laws.aspx

» **The Office on Women's Heath (OWH):** For information on breastfeeding in public and going back to work. www.womenshealth.gov/breastfeeding; www.workandpump.com

ADDITIONAL RESOURCES AND TOOLS MENTIONED IN TEXT

» **Safe Baby Wearing:** Advisory showing safe and improper use of carrier slings. www.cpsc.gov/content/cpsc-educates-new-parents-on-safe-babywearing-infant-suffocation-deaths-in-slings-prompt

» **Infant Toddler Temperament Tool (IT3):** To assess "goodness of fit" and temperament traits. www.ecmhc.org/temperament/

» **Online Cranial Assessment:** An at-home assessment for head flattening. www.cranialtech.com/online-assessment/

» **Hand Expression Video:** To watch how to hand express your milk. http://med.stanford.edu/newborns/professional-education/breastfeeding/hand-expressing-milk.html

» **Newborn Weight-Loss Assessment Tool (Newt):** For weight loss and gain concerns, compare your newborn's weight with a large sample of babies the same age. www.newbornweight.org

Breastfeeding Challenges Symptom Checker

If you are experiencing pain or unusual symptoms use this chart to find the corresponding topic. The index will direct you to the page numbers in the book.

ASSESS PAIN & APPEARANCE	SEE CHAPTER TOPICS
Minor discomfort with no visible skin changes	Mild Nipple Pain
Redness, bruising, bleeding, cracked or flaky skin	Attachment; Cracked and Bleeding Nipples; Yeast Infection
Cracks with discharge	Cracked and Bleeding Nipples
White blister at the tip of the nipple	Blebs or a Milk Blister; Plugged Milk Ducts
Nipple pain persists through feed; latch correct	Strong Vacuum: Another Cause of Sore Nipples
Soreness at the top of the nipple	Lip-Tie; Positioning
Abraded nipple tip	Pressing to make an airway
Soreness on the bottom side of the nipple	Ineffective Hand Positioning; Tongue-Tie
Blister on any part of the nipple	Attachment: Difficulty Taking the Breast
Burning pain and blanched nipple with nursing or cold exposure	Vasospasm of the Nipples: Raynaud's
Itching, throbbing, burning pain; swollen red nipple and areola; pealing skin	Yeast Infection
Normal-shaped nipples during pregnancy have become flat	Areolar Engorgement/Edema
Hot, hard, tender breasts; stretched, shiny skin; throbbing; lumpiness	Engorged Breasts
Firm, red, tender part of the breast; flu-like symptoms: fever higher than 101 F., aches, chills	Mastitis
Tender and painful lump in the breast; may have a white dot at end of nipple	Plugged Milk Ducts

Acknowledgments

Andrea Herron

This book is dedicated to three very special people in my life. First, my role model and mentor, Ruth Wester, RN, PNP, co-founder of Well Start International. It is because of Ruth that I am a Pediatric Nurse Practitioner, followed her path in preventive healthcare, and became a lactation consultant. She mentored me through my early days of practice, motherhood, and writing this breastfeeding book. Second, my best friend and partner, Larry Herron. He never doubted me—said I could do anything. When I had to commute 4 hours to accomplish a graduate degree, he was unfazed. When I wanted to quit my job to start a breastfeeding practice, he said, "Let's do it." Throughout the many hours writing this book, he picked up the slack and assisted in every way he could. Last, to my amazing son Dan, the pride and joy of my life.

Lisa Rizzo

To my boys, Joe and Gianmarco, whom through breastfeeding, showed me the greatest love I have ever known. Special thanks to my husband Saro, and parents, Carolyn Jamieson and Joe Giancola, for their uncompromising support; Francesca Cappelletti and Courtney Anderson for the "life support"; sisters Leslie, Lori, and Lianna; and brother Joey, who gave me the determination I needed to complete this project.

Special Thanks

To our publisher, Praeclarus Press, and the wonderful team, including editor Kathleen Kendall-Tackett, production manager Ken Tackett, copy editor Chris Tackett, and designer Nelly Murariu. Thank you, photographer Lisa Maksoudian, for capturing our vision; Ruth Wester, Carolyn Jamieson, Dr. Larry Herron, and Rose Kast for your thorough review and edits; Phyllis Klaus, for your endorsement and thoughtful foreword; Amy Collins and Medela, for anatomy illustrations; Cal Poly State University interns Joella Oddi, Colette Long, and Oriana Bardinelli, for your research and transcriptions; and mother/baby models Erica and Sky, Sharlene and Zosa, Emily, twins Georgia and Grace, Belle, Maggi Jo, and Jordyn. Many thanks to Trisha Garrison and all the Breastfeeding Support Groups and mothers who shared their stories and questions.

Index

A

abnormal developmental outcomes 195
abscess(es) 337, 353
Academy of Breastfeeding Medicine
(ABM) 198, 230, 237, 238, 239,
258, 268, 326-328, 336, 406
active awake 91, 92, 123
activity level 49
adoptive nursing 406
alcohol 46, 52, 53
blood alcohol levels 52
alert state(s) 6, 91, 98-104, 121, 122, 138,
158
alertness 82, 83, 97, 107, 346
allergies xxi, 35, 48, 208, 238
milk allergy 69
alternate breast compressions 268
American Academy of Pediatrics (AAP)
xviii, 4, 33, 189, 265, 326
American Association of Obstetrics and
Gynecology (AAOG) 329
Anatomy of Lactating Breasts 41
areola 39-42, 49, 68
areolar edema/engorgement 20, 298-300
artificial nipple 45, 49
asthma 37, 53
atopic dermatitis 37
attachment xxiv, xxv, 7, 15, 19, 32, 39, 68,
74, 78, 86, 112, 117, 130, 138, 141,
142, 151, 156, 172, 186, 230, 242,
274, 282, 286, 290-293, 299, 312,
318, 336, 355, 358, 370
mother-infant bonding 7, 112
auditory response 104

B

Babinski reflex 99
baby acne 333
baby blues 189, 337-339
Baby-Friendly 230, 405
baby-led breastfeeding 12
Baby Watching iii-xxiii, 73, 76-84, 88, 93,
113, 115, 121, 142, 151, 159, 177-
181, 290, 360, 367
baby with a congenital anomaly 234

Ball, Helen 197
Barnard, Katherine 318
bedsharing 173, 193, 196-198
co-sleeping 163, 172-174, 184, 196-198,
407
Belladonna 70
beta strep 314
Biologic Breastfeeding 159
biologic nursing 15
birth control 51, 281, 354
birth experience 3, 6, 264
birth trauma 35, 317, 338
bisphenol A (BPA) 258
bleb(s) 285, 286, 336
milk blister 285
block-feeding 288
blood work for chronic low milk
supply 361
bottles xxi, 48, 245, 257, 258, 278, 302,
344, 346, 356, 357
bottle-feeding xix, xxii, 30, 117, 143, 167,
197, 228, 244, 245, 246, 248, 260,
320, 345, 348, 350, 357, 366
bottle-use 49
pace bottle-feeding 246
brain development 51, 140, 168
Brazelton Neonatal Behavioral
Assessment Scale 88
break suction 23, 274, 275, 307
breast attachment 151, 274, 293, 299,
358
breastfeeding challenges xv, 264, 266,
308, 406
breastfeeding consultation 265
breastfeeding management 355
breastfeeding patterns 319, 374
Breastfeeding Report Card xviii, 366
breastfeeding (typical pattern)
breastfeeding duration xxiii
breastfeeding frequency 270
typical breastfeed 48, 56
breast implants 283, 361
breast massage(s) 15, 257